Child Behavior Therapy

CHILD BEHAVIOR THERAPY
Principles, Procedures, and Empirical Basis

Alan O. Ross

State University of New York at Stony Brook

John Wiley & Sons
New York • Chichester • Brisbane • Toronto

Library of Congress Cataloging in Publication Data:

Ross, Alan O
   Child behavior therapy.

   Bibliography: p.

   Includes indexes.
   1. Behavior therapy.   2. Child psychotherapy.
I. Title.
RJ505.B4R67   618.92'89142   80-24109
ISBN 0-471-02981-5

Printed in the United States of America

10 9 8 7 6 5 4 3 2 1

To Ilse
—and 30 years of harmony

Preface

Child behavior therapy has undergone remarkable growth in recent years. The principles of psychology on which child behavior therapy is based are finding an ever wider range of applications in the treatment of the various psychological disorders and behavior problems of children and adolescents. Concomitantly, there is an increasing demand for individuals who are competent to offer this form of treatment. Many vacant positions exist for well-trained child behavior therapists in such facilities as clinics, schools, hospitals, correctional institutions, specialized treatment settings, and community organizations. To meet this need for trained personnel, colleges, universities, and professional schools are offering courses, seminars, workshops, and institutes in child behavior therapy not only for those preparing to enter the field but also for established professional people who seek to increase and update their skills through continuing professional education.

From the point of view of providing the rapidly expanding application of child behavior therapy with a sound empirical basis it is fortunate that research on its principles and practices has kept pace with this development. This is reflected in a constantly growing literature that, having outgrown existing publications, led to the appearance of edited compendia of contributed chapters and occasioned the founding of a new journal devoted exclusively to child behavior therapy which, indeed, is its name. Missing, thus far, has been a systematic textbook that integrated this diverse literature in a manner that lends itself to the teaching and learning of behavior therapy with children and adolescents. It is my hope that this book will serve this need.

My aim in writing this book is to provide a comprehensive review of the burgeoning field of child behavior therapy for readers whom I presume to possess some familiarity with psychological disorders of children. The principles on which behavioral treatment of children is based are briefly summarized, relevant research is extensively surveyed, and the behavioral treatment procedures that have been applied to the various problems of children and adolescents are presented in considerable detail. Citations of nearly 500 research and case studies should provide the reader interested in pursuing a given topic in greater detail with ready access to the pertinent literature. It is my hope that this coverage of principles, procedures, and research will make this book useful to students of child behavior therapy at all levels, whether they be advanced

vii

undergraduates, graduate students in clinical psychology or other helping professions, or professional practitioners seeking to update and expand their knowledge and skills.

My desire to make this book useful not only as a classroom text but also as a reference for the practicing clinician seeking a review of treatment approaches that have been used with a specific problem has led me to present the material in such a way that any chapter can be read by itself, provided the reader is familiar with the basic behavioral principles that are covered in the first chapter. This format also should enable an instructor to assign the various chapters in a sequence that differs from the one I have used or to omit any that are beyond the scope of a particular course. To achieve the aim of having each chapter capable of standing alone has necessitated a modicum of redundancy. For instance, those reading the entire book will find that comments about the implications of the technical meaning of time-out appear in more than one chapter. I trust that this repetition will serve to underscore the importance I attribute to such an issue, while it facilitates the process of learning.

A presentation of the psychological disorders of children is usually organized around such diagnostic labels as early infantile autism, mental retardation, or juvenile delinquency but such an organization would make little sense for a discussion of child behavior therapy because diagnostic labels are not the focus of treatment. When a behavior therapist sees a child who has been labeled as a case of early infantile autism, for example, the target of treatment is not that child's supposed early infantile autism. The treatment focus is instead on the various behavioral deficits and excesses this child manifests and that led to this diagnostic label being assigned. One child thus labeled may be engaging in self-injurious behavior and parrotlike speech while another, bearing the same label, may be totally mute and engage in repetitive body-rocking. For each of these children the targets of treatment and therefore the treatment method would have to be different. This makes it preferable to organize a discussion of behavior therapy under such headings as language deficits and self-injurious behavior and not around such categories as early infantile autism, particularly since such behaviors as body-rocking or self-injury are also encountered with children who bear other diagnostic labels, such as mental retardation. I have therefore organized this book around targeted behaviors and the treatment methods that have been applied to them, hoping that this will make it optimally useful.

As I reviewed the literature on child behavior therapy in the course of preparing this book I was repeatedly struck by the paradox that scientific rigor and clinical relevance usually stand in an inverse relationship. Well-controlled research studies are often concentrated on isolated fragments of disordered behavior or are based on analogues of clinical problems that bear only indirectly on the complex issues with which the clinician must deal. On the other hand, when a study deals with the treatment of complex clinical problems in actual clinical settings, essential experimental controls are often missing so that the report is an intriguing yet unconvincing demonstration of a given approach to treatment. The strict controls over variables that scientific standards demand are often impossible to introduce in a child's home or classroom where much of treatment has to take place. Even where a research design has been carefully planned, the vagaries of the clinical reality often require that these plans be set aside or modified in the interest of responsible therapy. The resolution of this paradox no doubt lies in our constructing the knowledge base of the therapeutic enterprise from both sources. The well-controlled laboratory research and the clinically sensitive case study each makes a valuable contribution. Taken together, they will ultimately provide us with a treatment approach that is both scientifically sound and clinically meaningful. With this goal in mind the chapters that follow draw as heavily on well-controlled laboratory research as on well-documented clinical reports.

I should like to credit Sol Garfield for unwittingly providing the original impetus for writing this book by his invitation that I contribute a chapter on behavior therapy with children to the second edition of the handbook he and Allen Bergin have edited for our mutual publisher. While working on that assignment I first realized how extensive the literature on this topic had become and that a chapter would only be a synopsis of a book that was clearly needed to do the subject justice. There are others who are no doubt unaware that they have indirectly contributed to the writing of this book and to whom I am therefore indebted. They are such friends and colleagues as Harry Kalish, Bob Liebert, and Susan and Dan O'Leary whose enthusiastic devotion to the science and profession of clinical psychology makes Stony Brook such a stimulating setting and gives it the atmosphere that I find so conducive to my work. Yet first and foremost in making life a joy and work rewarding is my wife, Ilse Wallis Ross, to whom I dedicate this book with sentiments to which she is privy but that would be inappropriate to publish because they are far too profound and personal.

Alan O. Ross

Contents

CHAPTER 1

Introduction

THE RANGE OF CHILD BEHAVIOR THERAPY

Child behavior therapy like behavior therapy, in general, is best defined as an empirical approach to psychological problems. It entails continuous evaluation of therapeutic interventions and thus calls for objectively defined terms and measurable procedures. Like other behavior therapists, those who work with children operate on the assumption that psychological disorders are forms of behavior that have been acquired or modified through the lawful operation of psychological principles of development, learning, perception, cognition, and social interaction and that the application of these principles can be used to bring about therapeutic change. They therefore seek to relate their treatment methods to contemporary knowledge based on psychological research. It can thus be said that child behavior therapy is the application of psychology to the alleviation of the psychological distress of children. As such, it is an open-ended, self-correcting, and constantly changing field of endeavor.

It should be apparent that behavior therapy, hence child behavior therapy, is not synonymous with any specific technique or theory and that it is not identifiable with any single person or "school." Although the approach to treating psychological disorders that has come to be known as behavior therapy is often exemplified by the historical case of Peter whom Mary Cover Jones (1924a) treated by the application of the principles of respondent conditioning, behavior therapy is more than the application of these principles. Nor is child behavior therapy the equivalent of operant conditioning, despite the fact that the work of Skinner (e.g., 1953) has been a major influence on those who approach their work with children from a behavioral point of view. Many have contributed to the growth and liberalization of child behavior therapy. Foremost among these has been Bandura (1969, 1977) whose social learning formulations and work on observational learning will be repeatedly cited in the chapters to follow. In recent years investigators like Meichenbaum (Meichenbaum & Goodman, 1971) and Kanfer (Kanfer, Karoly, & Newman, 1975) have demonstrated that verbal mediation can be put to constructive use in modifying the problem-solving and coping behavior of children, while Gibson and Levin (1975) have shown the relationship of perceptual development to reading and its relevance to working with children who have reading problems (Ross, 1976).

As the range of behavior therapy has been expanded, questions as to the limits of the field have invariably arisen. Not unlike other approaches to therapy that have their own purists, behavior therapy counts among its advocates some who would define it in such a way as to exclude any method that is not based on the principles of either operant learning or classical conditioning. Others would demand that behavior therapists limit their conceptualizations to overt behavior and eschew such mediating events as physiological arousal states or cognitive processes. Such arbitrary orthodoxy places unnecessary restrictions on those who seek to expand the effectiveness of behavioral approaches by employing empirically derived psychological principles that have, as yet, not found application in the therapeutic realm. The touchstone of a behavioral technique is whether it has objective, observable referents that permit one to put its validity to empirical test—not whether it fits neatly into the procrustean bed of one theory or another.

It would be folly to assert that everything a behavior therapist does in the course of a treatment program, let alone in an individual treatment session, is explicitly and directly derived from empirically supported psychological principles. The self-conscious rigidity this would demand would be unlikely to contribute to therapeutic progress. A behavior therapist is, after all, a person who interacts with a client as a human being. It is thus inevitable that in the course of a treatment session, a skilled clinician will do or say something that, at the moment, seems intuitive. What happens next is what differentiates the behavior therapist from therapists of a less rigorous persuasion. If the intuitive or serendipitous intervention appears to have the desired effect, behavior therapists will not blindly continue to use this intervention because it seems to work. Instead, they will ask questions about that intervention. Was the observed effect really due to that intervention? What aspect of that intervention was responsible for the effect? How does this intervention relate to other methods and what are the principles that underlie its effectiveness? Of course answers to such questions can only be found by conducting systematic research, and behavior therapists therefore take the questions derived from clinical practice back into the laboratory, just as they take methods evolved in laboratory research back to the clinic. In behavior therapy the relationship between science and practice is a two-way street and it is that aspect of behavior therapy which makes it an evolving, changing, dynamic approach to problems in human behavior.

Behavior therapists look to psychological principles for the conceptual framework of their activities but in so doing they are not denying the role of biological factors in human behavior. They recognize that genetically determined constitutional factors provide the matrix within which the psychological principles are operating to produce both adaptive and maladaptive behavior. At times, these biological determinants set limits on the skills a given person can learn and they certainly can make one mode of learning—hence of teaching—more effective than another. Ongoing assessment of treatment procedures is thus vitally important lest the therapist persist using an approach from which the client cannot possibly benefit.

Behavior therapists further recognize that a biochemical disorder or a physical disease can affect a person's behavior so that collaboration with specialists from these areas is often of paramount importance. Conversely, the behavior therapist expects that such specialists recognize the interaction between biological and psychological processes and that they are prepared to submit their procedures to the same objective tests of effectiveness behavior therapists demand of their own methods.

HISTORICAL BACKGROUND AND CURRENT TRENDS

Those who write about behavior therapy have a tendency to reach as far back as possible for their historical roots. The ability to claim Aristotle or, at least, John Locke as the intellectual forebear appears to lend respectability to an endeavor. We need not reach that far back but if behavior therapy with children consists of the application of psychological principles to the alleviation of children's psychological problems, then the ancestor of child behavior therapy is the same person who is viewed as the founder of clinical psychology: Lightner Witmer.

Witmer opened the Psychological Clinic at the University of Pennsylvania in 1896 and coined the term "clinical psychology." His focus on behavior, as opposed to inferred inner processes, is reflected in his definition of psychological diagnosis as "an interpretation of the observed behavior of human beings" (Witmer, 1907). Witmer's first case was a boy with a learning difficulty and he approached this child's problems by applying laboratory-derived psychological principles of perception and learning.

Witmer's psychological approach to children's problems seems to have been a historical oddity; he was several decades ahead of his time. One does not find a similar attempt to apply the principles established in the psychological laboratory to alleviating psychological problems of children until Mary Cover Jones (1924a, 1924b) explored a variety of methods for eliminating children's fears. Though her early work is best known for the oft-cited case of Peter (Jones, 1924a) whose fear of furry objects she treated through the application of the principles of respondent conditioning, Jones (1924b) had also explored the effect on children's fears of persuasion, of setting an example of fearless behavior, and of direct exposure. These methods, which behavior therapists would now call cognitive restructuring, modeling, and flooding, respectively, proved less effective than the conditioning approach that would now be called systematic desensitization or counterconditioning.

Despite the fact that Jones's (1924b) work with Peter had demonstrated the fruitfulness of applying conditioning principles to the elimination of irrational fears, the time was still not ripe for the adoption of such an approach by clinicians who worked with children. Even as influential a writer of those days as Arnold Gesell (1938) failed to have his message heard when he pointed to the relevance of Pavlovian conditioning to the treatment of psychological disorders. By then, the child guidance movement, strongly influenced by the work of Sigmund Freud, had become the dominant force in the treatment of children (Ross, 1959), leaving no room for other approaches. When Mowrer and Mowrer (1938) described the treatment of bedwetting by conditioning techniques, they had little or no impact despite the fact that their paper was published in the *American Journal of Orthopsychiatry* which was then the organ of the child guidance movement.

In view of the fact that much of child behavior therapy now involves children's school activities, it is noteworthy that parallel to the premature efforts to introduce the application of psychological principles in clinical work with children, similar events were taking place in the field of education. Graziano (1978) credits J. Stanley Gray (1932) with being the first to use the term *behavior modification* when, in an article directed at eduators, he urged them to focus on children's behavior and on the variables that control learning. In the same historical review, Graziano reminds us that, as early as 1919, Sidney L. Pressey had developed the prototype of what later became known as the teaching machine but that he abandoned this project in 1932 because it found no acceptance among educators.

It might be instructive to examine why these early voices went unheeded and to trace the historical trends and social changes that prepared the receptive ground on which the writings of Skinner (1953), Eysenck (1957), Wolpe (1958), and Bandura (1961) fell some 20 years later. Such an analysis is beyond the scope of this book but another interesting historical phenomenon is pertinent here because when behavior therapy did eventually find acceptance among clinicians, they used it primarily with adults, not with children. While the earliest attempts to apply psychological principles to clinical problems had taken place with children (Witmer, 1907; Jones, 1924b), some 20 years after Jones had treated little Peter one could find only occasional reports on work with children in the professional literature (Ross, 1964). Although some publications from South Africa (Lazarus, 1959) and Great Britain (Jones, 1960) carried reports on the behavioral treatment of children, it was not until operant methods were introduced into work with institutionalized, profoundly disturbed children (Ferster & DeMyer, 1962) that child behavior therapy became more widely used. It thus ensued that when Gelfand and Hartmann (1968) prepared the first review of this field, they were able to cite some 70 articles; by now the reference section of this book represents but a fraction of the available literature.

When behavior therapy first appeared on the clinical scene it occasioned considerable opposition on the part of therapists and writers who had been trained in the then dominant approaches to treatment. They viewed the newcomer with skepticism and questioned the effectiveness of what they saw as superficial and mechanistic approaches to treatment. Many considered behavior therapy but a fad and predicted that it would quickly join other faddish movements in oblivion. In reaction to this opposition, the early pioneers of behavior therapy spoke and wrote in rather arrogant and dogmatic terms, at times making hyperbolic predictions regarding the effectiveness and applicability of their form of treatment.

By now, with the early attacks from traditionally oriented adversaries abated and behavioral approaches widely accepted even in some of the most orthodox institutions, behavior therapists have entered a period of consolidation and circumspect exploration of new approaches. In a sense, the field has grown beyond its stage of missionary zeal and embarked upon a mature self-scrutiny which a securely established endeavor can afford. One now finds an increasing number of reports on research projects that explored the parameters of therapeutic methods and examined the conditions under which treatment-produced gains can be enhanced and maintained. There are promising publications whose authors reason that other therapeutic approaches cannot be completely wrong and who seek to discover the "active ingredient" of these approaches in hopes of incorporating them among their own procedures (Goldfried & Davison, 1976). In addition, one finds a liberalization in behavior therapists' perspectives of what phenomena can be legitimately included in the purview of a behavioral approach. Early behavior therapists had insisted on dealing solely with observable, overt behavior. In order to maintain this conceptual purity, however, they had found it necessary to ignore that their most extensively used method—systematic desensitization—entailed an inferred, covert process, the client's private imagery. Since that time it has become quite respectable for a behavior therapist to consider a client's cognitive processes and to seek influencing these while speaking unabashedly of self-control, self-instruction, and self-reinforcement.

Of the various aspects of human behavior that are the subject matter of psychology, some have been explored more thoroughly and for a longer time than others. Learning, in particular, has been the focus of laboratory investigations since the earliest days of the field. It is therefore not surprising that when the pioneers of behavior therapy sought to apply psychology in their treatment endeavors they turned to the knowledge that these studies had yielded and that they construed their efforts as helping clients learn, unlearn, and relearn critical aspects of their response repertoire. Had the primary focus of early laboratory investigations been on development, perception, or social interaction, it is conceivable that behavior therapy would have been based on research in one of these areas. As it is, the primary emphasis remains on learning but when the study of other aspects of psychology advances to the level that the study of learning had reached by 1960 one can expect that behavior therapists will find applications for more and more of psychology in their work. As we shall see, beginnings of this development have already appeared.

WHY "BEHAVIOR"—WHY "THERAPY"?

In tracing the historical background of behavior therapy with children, we pointed out that the early attempts to apply psychological principles to the treatment of children's psychological disorders had their counterpart in efforts to introduce these principles in the educational realm. Just as neither the clinic nor the school was ready to follow these recommendations in the 1930s, so both of these settings were ready to adopt them by 1960. Today, psychological principles find application not only in settings where children are treated but also where they are educated. In the school, these applications go considerably beyond the use of so-called teaching machines and programmed textbooks (which employ operant principles); such applications are also found in approaches to classroom management (O'Leary & O'Leary, 1977) and in working with the learning disabled (Hallahan & Kauffman, 1976). This raises the questions of the limits of behavior therapy and of the distinction between behavior therapy and behavior modification.

For purposes of this book, a very broad definition of behavior therapy has been adopted and the term *therapy* will here encompass considerably more than has traditionally been the case. Children encounter difficulties of a psychological nature in a great variety of areas having to do with their reactions and relations to the environment. These difficulties may involve interactions with parents, siblings, peers, and teachers and may entail the acquisition of skills and knowledge as well as the adoption of the norms society imposes on its members. The application of psychological principles can be helpful in any of these areas, both in overcoming difficulties a child may have encountered and in keeping such difficulties from arising. The word *therapy*, in its traditional use, applies to only a limited number of these potential applications; helping a child who has difficulty learning to read, for example, was not considered therapy but an aspect of teaching. Yet one must ask whether helping a child acquire more appropriate ways of interacting with peers or siblings is not also a form of teaching, particularly when one uses psychological principles of learning. As will be seen in the following chapters behavior therapy entails learning, unlearning, or relearning in one form or another, regardless of which of the various relevant psychological principles one may apply. Indeed, behavior therapy is an unfortunate term to use for all of this and we adhere to it in this book only because the term has found such wide acceptance by now that it would be folly to write on this topic using a different, though more appropriate expression, such as behavior change or behavior influence. Even the word *behavior* in these expressions is a somewhat unfortunate relic of earlier days. Learning to read, or to use language, or not to be afraid of school involves behavior only if the definition of that term is stretched to cover cognitive processes. Again, well-established usage precludes the introduction of a more felicitous expression with which to label the application of psychology to the varied problems of children.

Before leaving this issue, a word about the difference between behavior therapy and behavior modification. Since behavior therapy is used in attempts to modify behavior, behavior therapy may be subsumed under the more general term, behavior modification. But there are many ways by which behavior can be modified, including chemical means, as in the use of pharmaceutical agents; surgical means, as in psychosurgical interventions; and direct physical interference with a person's movement, as in the use of restraints. None of these is based on psychological principles nor, for that matter, are certain brutal approaches to disciplining children for which legitimization and respectability are sometimes sought by calling them programs of behavior modification. In order to differentiate the topics to be discussed in this book from all of these other approaches, we shall speak of behavior therapy, even when the application is in places far removed from clinic or hospital and when the target of the intervention is not a child's overt behavior.

THE THEORETICAL BASES OF BEHAVIOR THERAPY

Inasmuch as psychology is the science of behavior, all of its principles have relevance for the therapist who seeks to apply psychology in the treatment of psychological problems. As mentioned earlier, these principles include those of development, learning, perception, cognition, and social interaction. A comprehensive review of the theoretical bases of behavior therapy would require a review of all of psychology, a task that is clearly beyond the scope of this book. We shall therefore limit this review to those principles that, for reasons already stated, have had a dominant influence on the development of behavior therapy, the principles of learning. At the same time, we assume that anyone seeking to become a fully competent child behavior therapist will obtain a thorough background in psychology with a particular emphasis on developmental psychology.

Respondent Conditioning

As pointed out earlier, when Jones (1924a) treated Peter's fear of furry objects she used the principles of respondent conditioning (the details of this treatment will be presented in Chapter 11). Also called Pavlovian or classical conditioning, this involves changing the conditions under which an innate response takes place. An innate or *unconditioned response* is ordinarily elicited by an *unconditioned stimulus*. When conditioning takes place, this unconditioned stimulus is replaced by a *conditioned stimulus* which now comes to elicit the *conditioned response*. The conditioned response is essentially the same response as the unconditioned response except that it is now elicited by the conditioned stimulus while it had previously occurred only when the unconditioned stimulus was present. The prototype of this procedure is the well-known demonstration of Ivan Petrovich Pavlov who used a dog's salivation as the response that he conditioned to occur at the sound of a bell. Watson and Rayner (1920) attempted to demonstrate the operation of this form of conditioning in relation to emotional responses in humans. They used a 9-month-old child, who has come to be known as Little Albert, and conditioned him to make a fearful response when shown a white rat. At the beginning of the experiment the presentation of the rat had not elicited fear on Albert's part, but a fear response, manifested by startling, crying, and other indications of distress, could be elicited by producing a sudden, loud noise. Such noise is presumably an unconditioned stimulus that innately elicits the unconditioned emotional response we call fear. After the experimenters paired the presentation of the rat with the production of the noise seven times they found that Albert would manifest the fear response to the sight of the rat alone. In this case the noise had been the unconditioned stimulus that elicited the unconditioned response of fear while the rat, which up to then had been a neutral stimulus with respect to fear, had become the conditioned stimulus for eliciting the fear as a conditioned response. Needless to say, one cannot condone the kind of experiment that Watson and Rayner reported in 1920 and which, to the credit of psychologists, has never been repeated although, as Harris (1979) has pointed out, its content has often been distorted by later writers.

It is a distinctive aspect of respondent conditioning that a response or re-flex that a person is innately capable of making is *elicited* by a stimulus that *precedes* it and that the person is *passively responding* to that stimulus. As we shall see, this is distinctively different from the situation in operant learning where the individual is actively engaging in behavior to which the environment produces consequences. Lest it would seem that an individual who is exposed to respondent conditioning is entirely at the mercy of the person who presents the conditioned stimulus, it should be stressed that in the context of therapy such conditioning can only be carried out if the client is willing to cooperate with the procedure. Unlike Pavlov's dogs who were in a restraining harness or hapless, 9-month-old Albert behind whom an experimenter would sneak up to hit a steel bar with a claw hammer, clients of ethical therapists do not find themselves in such a helpless position. Children in treatment have such options as not looking at a stimulus that a therapist seeks to present, of covering their ears or making noise to keep from hearing a sound or, for that matter, of leaving the room. As we shall see in the later discussion of a frequently used conditioning method for treating bed-wetting, a child can readily avoid taking part in the procedure by unplugging the wake-up alarm, removing the device from the bed, or simply sleeping on the floor.

In respondent conditioning the conditioned response usually involves the autonomic nervous system and this form of conditioning is probably always implicated when emotional responses, such as fear, come to be attached to previously neutral stimuli. Various aspects of respondent conditioning have been extensively studied in the psychological laboratory and many of these have special relevance for the behavior therapist. Brief definitions of the most common of these phenomena should facilitate later discussion.

At the start of a conditioning sequence the conditioned response can be elicited only by a specific stimulus that has particular characteristics. When the response can later also be elicited by stimuli that are similar in some respect to the original one, the phenomenon is called *stimulus generalization*. In the classical Pavlovian example, a bell which at first had elicited salivation only at one tonal frequency or one level of loudness, could later serve the same eliciting function when frequency or loudness was slightly changed. The more similar the stimulus characteristic is to the original, the more likely is it that it will elicit the response at the same magnitude. When this similiarity is ordered along some dimension, the resulting continuum of response strength depicts a *generalization gradient*, on which response strength is greatest at the point most similar to the original stimulus and tapers off as dissimilarity increases.

When a conditioned response has been established by the repeated pairing of the conditioned stimulus with the unconditioned stimulus, the conditioned stimulus has acquired the capacity of eliciting the response that had previously appeared only when the unconditioned stimulus was presented. The conditioned stimulus will retain this capacity to elicit the response in the absence of the unconditioned stimulus for some time but after a while this capacity will diminish unless the unconditioned stimulus is occasionally brought back into the picture. This diminution of the capacity of the conditioned stimulus to elicit the conditioned response represents an *extinction* of the conditioned response. Extinction is manifested by a gradual diminution and eventual disappearance of the conditioned response. In the classical example of the salivating dog, when the sound of the bell, which had become a conditioned stimulus, is repeatedly presented without being paired with food the conditioned salivation response will gradually cease to appear. Yet, from time to time, the old conditioned response will momentarily reappear upon the ringing of a bell, a phenomenon called *spontaneous recovery*. When, on one of these occasions, the unconditioned stimulus is also present, the conditioned response is easily reestablished at its old strength. This suggests that a response that has undergone extinction is not lost or obliterated but is being actively held back upon the appearance of the conditioned stimulus. This process is called *conditioned inhibition*.

A conditioned stimulus such as a bell can be presented at varying levels of amplitude. By virtue of stimulus generalization a conditioned response can come to be elicited both when the bell is rung softly and when it is rung loudly. At the same time, it is possible to establish a differential response such that it takes place when the bell rings loudly but not when it rings softly. One way of accomplishing this is to pair the unconditioned stimulus with the conditioned stimulus only when the latter has the predetermined quality; only when the bell rings softly, for example. Conditioning of this kind is a form of *discrimination learning* and involves the process of *differential inhibition* in that the conditioned response is not produced (is inhibited) under only one of the stimulus conditions.

In using the example of the salivating dog we have thus far spoken only of the situation in which the conditioned response is associated with one conditioned stimulus, the bell. Once such conditioning has taken place and the bell has become a firmly established conditioned stimulus it is possible to pair it with a different conditioned stimulus, for example a light. The light would then also acquire the capacity to elicit the conditioned response, even when it is presented without the bell. This is known as *second-order conditioning*. It is possible to go even beyond this level to further *higher-order* conditioning.

In the course of a person's conditioning history many different responses will have come to be associated with many different stimuli. A flower, for example, may be capable of eliciting the positive emotion we call joy while a hornet may serve as a conditioned stimulus for the negative emotion we call fear. Under conditions of joy, we tend to approach the stimulus; under conditions of fear, we tend to avoid it. If we find a hornet inside a flower we are likely to avoid the flower. In such a conflict situation it can be seen that different conditioned responses can have different degrees of strength, based in part on the specifics of the original conditioning situation and the generalization gradient previously mentioned. The fact that two kinds of responses can be elicited at the same time led Wolpe (1969) and other behavior therapists to treat maladaptive emotional responses, such as fear, by what is variously called *counterconditioning* or *reciprocal inhibition*. Andrew Salter (1949), one of the earliest pioneers in this field, spoke of *conditioned reflex therapy*. This aspect of behavior therapy is now generally known as *systematic desensitization*. Derived from the Pavlovian principles outlined above, it operates, at least in theory, by substituting an incompatible emotional response, such as joy, for the maladaptive one, usually fear, that had come to be associated with a specific set of stimuli. To what extent systematic desensitization really works by the mere substitution of one response for another has been repeatedly questioned (e.g., Davison & Wilson, 1973) and, as we shall see, other processes no doubt enter the picture when a therapist seeks to help a child who is incapacitated by fear.

Operant Learning

In respondent conditioning, a stimulus elicits a response from a person who is relatively passive vis à vis the environment. The environment acts on the person and the person responds to the environment in an essentially reflexive manner (hence, "respondent" conditioning). In the case of operant learning the situation is reversed. Here the individual actively operates on the environment (hence, "operant"), emitting an action to which the environment reacts. The *response* is thus instrumental in bringing about an environmental event and for this reason the process is also known as *instrumental conditioning*. It is the environment's reaction to a person's response that determines what will happen to that response, whether it will be more or less likely to be emitted again under similar circumstances on future occasions. The key then to operant learning is the *consequence* of the response. Behavior, in Skinner's (1938) formulation, is a function of its consequences. We shall examine the components of operant learning in some detail because it forms the basis of most contemporary child behavior therapy.

   In a situation with identifiable aspects, that is, in the presence of a *discriminative stimulus* (often called *stimulus*, for short), a person emits a *response*. Assume that this response has a consequence that the person notices. When the discriminative stimulus is then presented again and one observes that this person again makes that response, the consequence that had been previously encountered is said to have served as a *reinforcer*. Having said that this consequence was something the person noticed and since something one notices is, in effect, a stimulus, the technical term for the reinforcer is *reinforcing stim-*

ulus. Note that we did not label the consequence "reinforcing stimulus" until we had observed its effect on the person's response on the occasion of the second appearance of the discriminative stimulus. We shall return to this point later.

Here we must underscore that the function of the discriminative stimulus in operant learning is *not* that of calling forth a response, as is the case in respondent conditioning. In the operant situation it is possible to conceive of the discriminative stimulus as a signal that indicates that the previously encountered consequence is likely to take place again if the same response were to be repeated. The discriminative stimulus is thus linked to the response consequence in an if–then relationship; *if* the response is emitted in the presence of the stimulus, *then* the previous consequence will again be forthcoming. This if–then relationship is known as a *contingency*; the consequence is contingent on the occurrence of the response taking place in the presence of the stimulus. When the likelihood of a response changes as a function of this contingency, *learning* is said to have taken place. It is in that sense that behavior learned under the operation of such contingencies—*operant behavior*—is a function of its consequences. To change such behavior one must change the contingency relationship; manipulating either the discriminative stimulus or the response consequence, or both. A systematic study of the relationship between the environmental antecedents and consequences of a response is known as a *functional analysis of behavior* because it asks what function a given response serves in its interaction with the environment. Such a functional analysis is necessary if one desires to bring about a change in operant behavior.

An example may serve to clarify the relationship between behavior and its consequences. Assume that a mother complains that every time she refuses to give her boy something he wants, he stomps his foot and has what she calls a "tantrum." To her it seems that saying "No" to the boy elicits the tantrum; that is, she speaks as if the "No" were a conditioned stimulus and the tantrum the conditioned response in the sense of the respondent conditioning paradigm. She is wrong. An observation of the sequence makes it apparent that when the boy emits a tantrum the mother capitulates almost every time by letting the child have the object he had demanded. The operant paradigm applies. The boy has been repeatedly exposed to the contingency that *if* he has a tantrum (response) in the face of his mother's saying "No" (discriminative stimulus) *then* her capitulation (reinforcing stimulus) will be forthcoming. The tantrum has thus come to take place with predictable regularity, the boy having learned this response under the prevailing environmental contingencies. This formulation could be tested by a functional analysis that would entail a systematic variation of the antecedents and of the consequences of the response while keeping a careful record of its frequency, intensity, and duration.

Removing either the discriminative stimulus (mother never refusing the boy anything) or the reinforcing stimulus (mother never giving in to a tantrum) should result in changing the tantrum, thus pointing the way to how this problem could be treated.

The Functions of Consequences. As was stressed earlier, a response consequence cannot be classified until one has observed what happens to the response on a subsequent occasion. If the response is more likely to occur, if it has been strengthened, the previously encountered consequence is viewed as having served as a *reinforcement*. If the response is less likely to occur, if it has been weakened, the previous consequence is viewed as having a *punishment* function. It is important to realize that the definitions of reinforcement and of punishment depend on the effect a consequence has had on the response it had followed and that this effect can be observed only at a later occasion. This means that it is impossible to speak of universal reinforcers or punishers so that the effect a given consequence has on specific behavior must be ascertained on each occasion and with each child. It is folly to make a priori assumptions about a particular consequence being either a reward or a punishment. Often a presumed reward turns out to be a punisher and what was thought to be a punishment turns out to be a reward.

Reinforcement and punishment can each be subdivided, based on whether they involve the response-contingent application or removal of an event. Since, as was pointed out, this event is something a person notices, one speaks of a *reinforcing stimulus* or a *punishing stimulus*, respectively. When the consequence involves the application of a reinforcing stimulus, as when a child is given a reward, it is called *positive reinforcement*. When the consequence involves the removal of a stimulus, as when relief is obtained from an irritation, it is called *negative reinforcement*. Negative reinforcement strengthens (reinforces) a response and should therefore not be confused with punishment.

Punishment can also take two forms. One involves the delivery of a stimulus, such as pain, and it is called *punishment by application*. This differentiates it from the situation in which a stimulus is removed, as when a child is deprived of a privilege, which is referred to as *punishment by removal*. In the behavior therapy literature, punishment by removal is usually called *time-out from positive reinforcement* ("time-out," for short) but since it has the effect of weakening the response for which it was a consequence it is more appropriate to view it as a form of punishment.

To summarize, any given response can have four possible consequences: Positive reinforcement and negative reinforcement, which have the effect of strengthening the response; punishment by application and punishment by removal, which have the effect of weakening the response. There is, of course, a fifth possibility, which is that a response will have no consequence at all. This will also weaken the response and the process is called *extinction*. As was the case with extinction in respondent conditioning, here too one finds occasional *spontaneous recovery* of the response and if, on one of those occasions, the response again encounters a reinforcing consequence, it can quickly become restored to the person's behavioral repertoire.

Schedules of Reinforcement. When the consequence of a response determines what will happen to that response in the future, whether it is going to be more or less likely to recur under similar stimulus conditions, it becomes important to consider the circumstances under which given consequences are presented. This aspect of the operant situation finds expression in the *schedule of reinforcement* (or of punishment), which states the qualitative and quantitative conditions under which a particular consequence will follow a response. Qualitative aspects of a response may entail such conditions as the inclusion of the word "please" in a child's request for a cookie. Here the child would receive reinforcement (the cookie) only if the response had the required quality. The reinforcement is thus contingent on that particular response. Quantitative variations in a schedule of reinforcement deal with how many responses must be emitted before a reinforcement is forthcoming. This is the *ratio of reinforcement*. Such a ratio would be in effect when a child is required to complete three pages in a workbook or to do two hours of homework before being given permission to watch television for half an hour.

Another aspect of a schedule of reinforcement is whether reinforcement is intermittent or continuous. If the completion of *every* three pages in the workbook earns a half hour of television-viewing, the child is on a continuous schedule; if the privilege is earned on some occasions but not on others (the ratio may be fixed or variable), the schedule is intermittent. When a new response is to be learned, continuous reinforcement (a reinforcement for each response) is the most effective but intermittent reinforcement is preferable when one wishes to assure that the newly learned response will be maintained (will resist extinction) in situations in which reinforcement is not always forthcoming. The schedule of reinforcement must therefore be adjusted over time. At first, reinforcement is given on a continuous basis but once the response is established, an intermittent schedule should be introduced; the schedule is thinned out. Similarly, the required response might at first be of fairly gross quality; a nonverbal child, for example, might be required to say no more than "cookie" before receiving reinforcement. Later on, however, more refined responses might be required until, finally, only the phrase, "I would like a cookie, please" would earn the reward. This is a case of *shaping* a response by reinforcing *successive approximations* of the goal response.

Yet another aspect of a schedule of reinforcement is the time that elapses between the emission of the response and the delivery of the reinforcement. In general, the effectiveness of the consequence is greater the sooner it follows the response. This is true of both reinforcement and punishment. Delay of either reduces its potency.

When one seeks to strengthen one response while weakening another, one resorts to a schedule under which the desirable response is reinforced while the undesirable response is placed on extinction (is never reinforced) or suppressed through punishment. An example of such *differential reinforcement* might be a situation where a parent seeks to teach a child to employ the socially preferred mode of asking for a cookie. Here the parent would place "Gimme a cookie" on extinction by consistently ignoring a request phrased in this manner while acceding to the request when worded as, "Please give me a cookie," thereby reinforcing that expression. Such a procedure is known as differential reinforcement of other behavior (*DRO*). Similar designations are used for schedules where behavior is differentially reinforced only when it is emitted at a high and never at a low rate (*DRH*) or, conversely, when only low and never high rates are reinforced (*DRL*).

An approach to teaching appropriate behavior that is closely related to differential reinforcement is represented by a schedule in which reinforcement is available only under one set of environmental circumstances but not under another. This is called *discrimination training* and the appropriate stimulus conditions are symbolized by $S+$, the inappropriate ones by $S-$. For example, "Please give me a cookie" might be reinforced only when this response is made as the child comes home from school ($S+$) but never as the family is about to sit down to dinner ($S-$).

"First You Do Your Homework." Reinforcers need not be limited to tangible objects that the child receives in consequence of a response he or she has emitted. There are situations where one response reinforces another. This hinges on the fact that any given response has a certain probability of occurring and that this probability may be greater for one response than for another. A child coming home from school may be more likely to turn on television than to do homework, the former having a higher probability than the latter. As first formulated by Premack (1959), the so-called *Premack Principle* holds that a response of higher probability can reinforce a response of lower probability. Thus, parents who require that homework be completed before television may be turned on, can be said to be employing this principle by making the more likely response contingent on the emission of the less likely one, thus reinforcing completion of homework. Although the empirical foundation of Premack's principle in use with humans is somewhat tenuous (Knapp, 1976), its application permits an expansion of potential reinforcers to include a wide range of activities in which children are likely to engage when left to their own devices. In order to be able to apply this principle it is of course necessary that a parent or whoever else wishes to use it be able to control when a child will engage in a given activity. In the foregoing example, television-viewing can only be used as a reinforcer if the parent can prevent the TV set from being turned on until the contingency of homework-completion has been met. This is no different, however, from any other application of operant principles where the ability to control the contingencies under which another person is operating is always a prerequisite, making such application far more feasible in the case of young children than with more independent adolescents or adults.

The Nature of Stimuli. Mention of the stimulus conditions under which a particular reinforcement contingency is operating raises the question how a stimulus is to be defined. Just as a reinforcer can only be defined in terms of its effect on the response it had followed, so can a stimulus only be defined in terms of its function in the operant sequence. In a summer camp, the ringing of the dinner bell is a stimulus that controls running to the dining hall only for those children who can hear the bell. For those too far away to hear it, the bell is not a stimulus. Neither is the bell a stimulus for the running response when the children have just come out of the dining hall after a meal. The stimulus, it must be recalled, serves to signal the fact that reinforcement would be available if a given response were now to be emitted. Whether a signal has the function of a stimulus, that is, whether it has an effect on the person, will depend on that person's condition and this condition, in turn, is a function of such *setting events* as prior deprivation or satiation for the reinforcer that has come to be associated with the stimulus.

In the application of operant principles the focus is often on the manipulation of the response consequences; reinforcements are given or withheld, punishments meted out or withdrawn. This neglects the important role of the discriminative stimulus because it too is subject to manipulations that will lead to changes in behavior. Once a stimulus has come to control a certain response, removing that stimulus should eliminate the response. Similarly, a signal that is ineffective as a stimulus can be made more distinctive or its impact enhanced by the addition of other stimuli. Among these, verbal statements can serve as potent stimuli. Being told, "It's dinner time," for example, will help a child discriminate between appropriate and inappropriate conditions under which to ask for a cookie.

As in respondent conditioning, the term *stimulus generalization* stands for the fact that not only the discriminative stimulus under which a response was first learned, but also a range of similar stimuli can become capable of controlling that response. Again there is a generalization gradient; the more similar the other stimuli are to the original one, the greater is the probability that the response will take place. Furthermore, generalization occurs not only for the discriminative stimulus but also for the reinforcing stimulus. The reinforcer for a given response need not always be the same; similar objects may also serve that function. It is in fact possible to make previously neutral stimuli into reinforcing stimuli by the paired presentation of the two. If the cookie, used to reinforce "please" is consistently paired with the statement, "That's a good boy," this statement may acquire reinforcing potential in its own right. The neutral stimulus has become a *conditioned, secondary,* or *acquired reinforcer.* It is thus possible to reinforce a child's responses not only with such *primary reinforcers* as food but also by such secondary, *social reinforcers* as approval, attention, praise, or smiles or by such intrinsically worthless objects as coins, tokens, or grades on report cards.

Just as neutral stimuli can become reinforcers by being paired with already effective reinforcing stimuli, so can neutral stimuli become punishers through pairing with aversive stimuli. Examples of *acquired punishers* are verbal reprimands, frowns, scolding, or threats. To make them effective in the suppression of responses, these would have had to be paired with the administration of more direct, physical punishment, deprivation of privileges, or withdrawal of such social reinforcers as attention or affection. This formulation should explain why verbal reprimands are effective punishing stimuli for some children but not for others and why some children can be reinforced with smiles and praise while others remain unaffected by them.

Punishment. Repeated reference has been made to punishment as one of the consequences that can be brought to bear in the course of applying the principles of operant learning. Because the use of punishment is deservedly controversial it calls for a discussion of its implications, especially where punishment entails inflicting physical pain.

Pain, when delivered in consequence of a response, serves as a punishing stimulus in the operant sequence when it results in reducing the likelihood of that response's recurring under the same or similar circumstances. At the same time pain is an unconditioned stimulus in the respondent conditioning sequence because it elicits the innate physiological arousal state that we usually call fear. While the theoretical status of the role of punishment in human learning is unsettled (Johnston, 1972; Parke, 1975), it is likely that this arousal state can become conditioned to the stimuli that are associated with the appearance of the unconditioned pain stimulus. In fact, the reason children tend to refrain from engaging in behavior that has been punished may well be that the stimuli associated with that behavior have come to arouse fear that they can reduce by not engaging in the punished activity. This would be an instance of *avoidance learning*. It is equally likely, however, that among the stimuli that have acquired the capacity to elicit fear may also be the person who delivered the punishment so that this person too may be avoided. Depending on who that person is, this may or may not be a desirable side effect of punishment.

Another consideration in the use of punishment as a device for changing children's behavior is that punishment does not actually eliminate the behavior in question. It simply results in a suppression of that behavior while the conditioned aversive stimuli, such as the punishing agent, are present. Once these are removed, the punished behavior is likely to reappear especially if other consequences stand to reinforce it. For this reason, as Lichstein and Schreibman (1977), among others, have pointed out, when using punishment for influencing child behavior it is important that one pair it with procedures that will strengthen desirable alternatives (Lichstein & Schreibman, 1977).

In considering the use of punishment as a procedure in child therapy it must be remembered that the definition of punishment is any stimulus that reduces the likelihood of the response for which it has been a consequence. This includes among punishing stimuli a wide range of objects or events among which the infliction of pain is the least desirable because of the emotional and interpersonal side effects mentioned. Time-out from positive reinforcement, social isolation, deprivation of privileges, fines, and required low-probability responses should be tried before, as a last resort, recourse is taken to inflicting pain. In fact, inflicting pain can only be condoned in cases where the alternative is a distinct danger to the child's health or safety. Admittedly, this statement represents a value judgment; it is not based on empirically established psychological knowledge.

Observational Learning

It is possible to learn complex responses via the reinforcement principles of operant learning when the behavior is shaped through a sequence of successive approximations. This, however, is a rather slow process which is so inefficient that it may lack survival value in natural settings. For the socialization of its young, a species needs a more efficient method and this, as Bandura (1969) has pointed out, is provided by the process of observational learning.

In analyzing observational learning one speaks of an *observer* who watches a *model* engage in some behavior; hence, the process is also known as *modeling*. When this takes place, three effects are possible. The observer may acquire new response patterns which had not previously been in that person's repertoire. This is traditionally and popularly known as imitation and as such has been of interest to psychologists for some time (Miller & Dollard, 1941).

A second effect that may result from observing a model is that the consequences of the action to the model strengthen or weaken the observer's inhibitory responses. This can be seen in cases where a child acquires a specific fear, not from a direct experience with the feared object but from observing another child having an untoward experience with that object. Conversely, a fearful child who observes another child having a positive experience with a feared object may be able to approach that object with reduced fear following that modeled exposure. This was demonstrated by Jones (1924b) and studied by Bandura, Grusec, and Menlove (1967).

The third possible effect of modeling is that the observer's previously learned behavior in the same general class of responses as those displayed by the model may be facilitated. This effect might be involved when a child, who already knows how to use a particular toy, acquires a new way of employing it by watching another child engage in such behavior.

Unlike respondent conditioning and operant learning, which have been analyzed into defined components, the observational learning paradigm is discussed on a more global level. Bandura (1969; 1971) differentiates between the *acquisition* of a response and its *performance*. This means that an observer may acquire the capacity to make a response that has been modeled without necessarily emitting that response until some later time. It is in whether and when the response is emitted that observational learning principles interact with the principles of operant learning because reinforcement becomes involved. Thus, a child who has observed a model engage in a given behavior may not perform that behavior until there is a likelihood that such performance will be reinforced (Bandura, Ross, & Ross, 1963).

Although a wide range of responses, ranging from motor acts to attitudinal statements and emotional reactions, can be learned through observation, the mere exposing of an individual to a model is not sufficient for such learning to take place. When such an individual does not perform the modeled response following such exposure, this may be due to the observer's failure to have attended to the relevant stimuli, failure to have retained what had been learned, a motor or intellectual deficit that makes it impossible for the response to be performed, or conditions of reinforcement that militate against the performance of the response.

There are, however, several conditions that can enhance performance of behavior acquired through observation of a model (Bandura, 1977b). An observer is more likely to perform behavior when the model received reinforcement rather than punishment as a consequence of the behavior. It has also been shown (Kornhaber & Schroeder, 1975) that similarity of the model to the observer enhances observational learning so that children may learn better when the model is another child rather than an adult. Learning is also enhanced when the model is high in status, prestige, power, or expertise and the effect is greater after observation of several models than after watching only one.

It has been mentioned that aspects of operant learning become involved when observational learning is taking place. This should underscore that the various modes of acquiring new responses that are here discussed under discrete headings do, in fact, occur together and interact whenever more than the simplest reflex learning takes place. The cookie given to a child as an operant reinforcer for a desired response is likely to elicit an emotional reaction that fits into the respondent conditioning paradigm and the parent who is presenting the cookie models a behavior that the child is observing. Furthermore, the child is without doubt experiencing something else while all this is taking place and whether we call this inner speech, thinking, or a cognitive process, it cannot be ignored if one wishes to gain a comprehensive picture of human behavior.

Cognitive Processes

Attention to cognitive processes is a relatively recent development in the field of child behavior therapy. Partly because these processes had not been studied as intensively in the psychological laboratory as had those of respondent conditioning and operant learning, partly out of an overreaction against the vague formulations of therapeutic approaches that focus almost exclusively on internal events, but largely because what people think cannot be directly observed, early behavior therapists sought to avoid working with cognitions because these must be inferred from overt behavior. There is no denying that people think, have fantasies, ideas, expectations, and memories, and there is is no reason why these cognitive processes should not be put to use in behavior therapy. In so doing it is necessary, however, that one keep in mind (yes, "in mind") that the behavioral orientation requires all terms and concepts to have ultimate referents in observable behavior so that their validity can be put to empirical test.

If the terms used in discussing observational learning lack the rigor of those of classical conditioning and the specificity of those of operant learning, a discussion of cognitive processes, as these relate to behavior therapy, must be even more imprecise. This reflects the present state of this area, which provides many demonstrations of the role cognitions seem to play in behavior but few if any formulations of how they function.

In what has somewhat paradoxically come to be called *cognitive behavior modification* (Meichenbaum, 1977), the emphasis is primarily on inducing the client to make verbal statements that either serve as self-instructions ("The dark is nothing to be afraid of") or enhance the distinctiveness of the stimuli being presented ("The b has the bulge on the right"). Verbal self-statements have been shown to improve the performance on laboratory tasks of hyperactive, impulsive children (Meichenbaum & Goodman, 1971) and this has led to the use of such statements in various forms of self-control training (Thoreson & Mahoney, 1974).

In a behavioral framework, self-control can be construed as a situation in which an individual has learned to emit responses that serve as discriminative or reinforcing stimuli for that individual. These stimuli then come to be relevant to other responses that prevent or alter behavior that must be changed because of the operation of environmental consequences. Thus, to avoid the strictures that a boy has almost invariably encountered when he got into a fight with another child, he may learn to say to himself when another makes him angry, "I must count to 10" and, doing so, replace hitting by counting. Then, having avoided a fight, he might say something like, "That was smart of me" thereby reinforcing himself. As will be seen in later chapters, self-control training always takes the form of teaching self-instruction, self-monitoring, self-rewarding, self-punishing, or combinations of these. In every instance, these behaviors are environmental events that children learn to produce themselves and by which they bring about changes in their own behavior. As Rachlin (1970) has pointed out, "*self*-control really refers to certain forms of environmental control of behavior" (p. 185).

In the study of observational learning it can be shown that children's performances can be enhanced if they are instructed to describe in their own words what they see the model doing (Bandura, 1971). It seems that these verbal statements highlight for the child what he or she is observing. This is similar to the function verbal statements appear to serve in recognizing the distinctive features of stimuli that are involved in learning to read (Gibson, 1969, 1970). In fact, such *verbal mediation* may be an important aspect of any learning and it may well enter into child behavior therapy at numerous points, often without being an explicitly stated part of the therapist's procedure.

From Principles to Practice

In presenting this review of the theoretical principles that contemporary behavior therapists apply in their work it was necessary to examine respondent condition, operant learning, observational learning, and the operation of cognitive processes separately but, as pointed out before, these usually occur together and probably interact in nearly all instances where behavior is learned. In the actual planning and conducting of behavior therapy one is rarely working with one isolated set of principles even though a given approach to a problem might be formulated in operant, respondent, or cognitive terms. Jones (1924b) recognized this long ago when she studied various methods for eliminating children's excessive fears and wrote:

> It should be noted that apart from laboratory analysis we have rarely used any of the procedures in pure form. Our aim has been to cure the fears by the group of devices most appropriate at any given stage of treatment (p. 390).

THE IMPORTANCE OF ASSESSMENT

A detailed discussion of the principles and methods of assessment is beyond the scope of this book but before we begin the presentation of treatment methods behavior therapists use with children it is essential to stress that any attempt to intervene in a child's life must be preceded by careful assessment. It is grossly irresponsible, if not unethical, to attempt influencing a child's behavior for ostensibly therapeutic purposes without first studying the particulars of the specific situation. This point is especially pertinent in the case of behavior therapy where many aspects involve well-defined, easily learned procedures that lend themselves to "treatment packages" that can be heedlessly applied even by people with little training or experience or can be dispensed as standard prescriptions for intervention solely on the basis of parents' or teachers' complaints.

The first question any assessment must seek to answer is whether the child who has been referred for help does indeed have a problem for which behavior therapy might be appropriate. We shall return to the issue of who decides when a problem is a problem that calls for treatment as we discuss noncompliant behavior in the last chapter. Let it be said here that assessment cannot be limited to the second-hand information provided by the child's parents or teachers and that the child must be directly observed in more than one setting. The totality of the child's current life situation must be taken into consideration. This is so not only because behavior is often situation-specific so that a child who is a problem at school may be a model child at home, or vice versa, but also because the feasibility of a plan for intervention often depends on the nature of the situation in which it is to be carried out and on the kind of people on whom the therapist may have to rely for support in the implementation of the plan.

Once the problem has been correctly identified, assessment must answer questions as to the antecendents and consequences of the target behavior and which of them lend themselves to manipulation. Measures of response frequency or intensity must be decided upon, schedules of reinforcement must be determined, and treatment goals must be specified. Where appropriate, available models must be identified or the child's ability to employ self-instruction must be ascertained. The methods used in such assessment have been outlined in several comprehensive handbooks (e.g., Ciminero, Calhoun, & Adams, 1977; Hersen & Bellack, 1976; Mash & Terdal, 1976) which the reader is urged to consult.

Careful assessment not only precedes an intervention; it must also continue while the intervention is being conducted. Only such continuous, objective monitoring of the targeted behavior can reveal whether the intervention is having the desired effect and alert the therapist to change ineffective procedures. Once intervention is terminated because the treatment goal has been reached, assessment should continue for an extensive period of follow-up evaluation. It is a part of responsible therapy to ascertain whether the changes brought about during treatment are maintained and that the child's development continues in the desired direction.

The Single-case Experimental Design

In assessing the effectiveness of their treatment, behavior therapists often turn to the single-case experimental design, thereby increasing the level of confidence with which they can draw conclusions from their clinical observations. This design fills the gap between the traditional, uncontrolled case-study method and the group-comparison approach to research that is rarely appropriate in a clinical setting. Since many of the studies that will be discussed in the following chapters employed the single-case (or $N = 1$) design a brief overview of the basic features of that design will facilitate this presentation. For more detailed discussion, books such as those by Hersen and Barlow (1976) or Kazdin (1980) should be consulted.

It is customary to identify the various stages or phases in a single-case design by capital letters. The letter A stands for the so-called *baseline* condition that exists before an intervention is undertaken while the letter B symbolizes the intervention (treatment). If other forms of intervention follow, these are labeled C, D, and so forth. When pretreatment, baseline conditions are reinstituted following treatment, these are again identified as A. A typical case study without experimental manipulations in which treatment follows an initial assessment can thus be said to use an AB design. A comparison of whatever data may have been gathered on the client's status during these two phases would reflect changes that occurred in that status in the course of treatment but in the absence of a control it would be impossible to say whether these changes were due to the treatment or to some other variable. It is this ambiguity of the case-study method that the single-case experimental design resolves by providing an answer to the question whether the treatment was indeed responsible for the changes in the client's behavior.

The ABAB or reversal design is the simplest of the single-subject designs. Here the investigator obtains quantitative data on the client's behavior during the baseline (A) phase while the client is still exposed to the contingencies that were in effect before the therapist was contacted. In the case of a preschool girl to be discussed at the beginning of the next chapter, baseline data were gathered while the nursery school teachers used the approach they would usually employ with a child who showed very limited interaction with other children, that is, while the teachers would solicitously encourage the girl to go and play with the others whenever she was alone. Following this baseline phase, the treatment, phase B, is put into effect. In the example, the teachers were instructed to ignore the child while she was playing alone and to attend to her when she approached other children. Once the behavior in question changes in the desired direction (when the nonexperimental treatment case is usually terminated), the experimental design calls for a return to the conditions that obtained during baseline (A). In the case of our example, the return to baseline entailed having the teachers once again devote their attention to the girl whenever she was alone, just as they had before the intervention was introduced. In other words, the contingencies were reversed; hence the term *reversal design*. The fact that under those conditions the girl's behavior reverted to her old pattern provided the basis for concluding that the behavior was indeed under the control of the independent variable, in this case the teachers' attention. At that point condition B was again instituted and, as expected, the girl's behavior changed back to increased interaction with her peers. Figure 1 (see p. 32) shows the graphic representation of data gathered in the course of such an ABAB design. Confidence in the conclusions drawn from such an experiment can of course be increased by using repeated reversals, as in an ABABAB design.

There are many situations where the use of a reversal design is inappropriate, undesirable, or impossible. With dangerous behavior, such as self-injury, for example, one would not want to reinstate baseline conditions after having found a way of reducing such behavior. When an ABAB design cannot be used, a *multiple baseline design* may provide a useful alternative for testing the effectiveness of a treatment procedure.

Multiple baseline designs may be employed across behaviors, across individuals, or across settings. To use a multiple baseline design across behaviors, an investigator identifies several changeworthy responses each of which is separately observed, measured, and recorded, first during baseline and later during treatment. The treatment, however, is instituted for the various behaviors in a sequential fashion. At first only one behavior is targeted for treatment while the others continue under baseline conditions and data continue to be gathered on all behaviors. Once the first behavior that has been targeted for treatment reveals a change, treatment is introduced for the next behavior while the rest continue in the baseline condition. This strategy is then pursued until treatment has been instituted for all behaviors of interest. Given this time-lagged procedure, the duration of the baseline condition will differ for the different behaviors and the results are analyzed to see whether the change in each of the behaviors coincided with the beginning of treatment for that behavior. If that is the case, one can have some confidence in concluding that it was indeed the treatment and not some other variable that had produced the desired effect. An example of data obtained with a multiple-baseline design can be found in Figure 4 (p. 77) which reflects the results of a study in which a child was sequentially trained to respond to different verbal stimuli.

A multiple-baseline design across individuals is used when different individuals with similar problems are treated with the same procedure. Here, baseline measures are obtained on each participant and treatment is then introduced with one of them at a time, while the others remain under baseline conditions (see Figure 11, p. 121). In a multiple-baseline design across settings, one individual's behavior is observed in different settings and treatment is instituted in a sequential order, one setting at a time. A child's disruptive classroom behavior might thus be treated first during the reading and then during the math period (see Figure 9, p. 113 where this design was used with several children).

In single-case experimental designs individuals serve as their own controls and the design, sometimes called a within-subject design, thus provides a substitute for the control group that is traditionally employed in group comparison studies. Whether it is an adequate substitute depends a great deal on the nature of the conclusion one seeks to draw from the study in which the $N = 1$ design is employed. If one wants to know whether the treatment one has employed was indeed the effective variable, the single-case experiment can provide a satisfactory answer. If one wants to know whether that treatment would also be effective in the hands of other therapists, with other cases, and in different settings, that is if one wants to generalize from one's results, the approach has limitations.

Recapitulation

Child behavior therapy, a specialized form of behavior therapy, was defined in terms of the empirical approach that makes child behavior therapy the application of psychology to the alleviation of the psychological distress of children. The historical background of the field and its current trends were briefly sketched, leading to the recognition that both the word "behavior" and the word "therapy" must be taken in their broadest sense if the term behavior therapy is to describe its contemporary scope.

A summary of the most important principles of learning that currently enter into child behavior therapy was provided, outlining respondent conditioning and its implications for emotional responses, operant learning with its ramifications for a wide range of behavior, as well as the more recent additions to the therapeutic armamentarium, which employ observational learning and cognitive processes. Finally, and in preparation for the treatment-oriented chapters to follow, the importance of assessment was stressed and research designs frequently used for this purpose were briefly sketched. A detailed presentation of these topics, however, is beyond the scope of this book.

THE TREATMENT OF
BEHAVIOR DEFICITS

CHAPTER **2**

Social Deficits

SOCIAL ISOLATION AND WITHDRAWAL

In the discussion of the principles of observational learning mention was made of the useful distinction between acquisition and performance of a behavior. Bandura (1969) had pointed out that the observation of a model may lead the observer to acquire (learn) the modeled response without necessarily demonstrating this by performing the behavior in question. When considering social and other behavior deficits it is well to keep the distinction between acquisition and performance in mind. Casual observation of a child who fails to use a particular skill does not permit one to conclude that the child lacks that skill; it may be that the child possesses the skill but fails to perform it while being observed. Before any intervention can begin it is necessary to differentiate between a *skill deficit* and a *performance deficit* and such differentiation requires careful assessment.

Children who fail to interact with their peers when they are in a setting, such as a nursery school, where such behavior is expected and encouraged have been called withdrawn, shy, or isolated children and their parents frequently voice concern because their child has no friends. Such a phenomenon may reflect either a performance or a skill deficit. A performance deficit in the area of social skills may be entailed when a child has the skills needed for interacting with other children but, like Ann who will be discussed shortly, finds alternate activities more rewarding. A different kind of performance deficit is involved in the case of children who avoid engaging in social interaction not because they lack the required skills but because fear of other children leads them to avoid such interaction (see Chapter 11). Social skill deficits can also find a variety of expressions. One child, lacking appropriate skills, may be approaching others in an inappropriate fashion, as by attacking them or otherwise engaging in such aversive behavior as to be rejected or avoided. Another child may lack the specific skills needed for coping with a particular social situation. For example, a deficit in appropriate assertive behavior may prevent a child from interacting with an excessively aggressive peer group. Still other children may have more pervasive social skill deficits, leaving them unable to interact with their peers. Each of these instances calls for a different focus of intervention.

Adult Attention Reinforces Child Behavior

A frequently cited demonstration of the application of operant principles in the development of peer interaction was reported by Allen, Hart, Buell, Harris, and Wolf (1964). A four-year-old girl, referred to as Ann, who was enrolled in a nursery school spent almost no time with the other children but engaged in a variety of behaviors that resulted in her gaining or prolonging the attention of adults. She did not appear frightened or severely withdrawn. In fact, she had well developed physical and intellectual skills that, though fascinating the teachers, failed to gain the interest of other children.

Since adult attention seemed to be the consequence that maintained Ann's adult-centered activities, it was decided to make adult attention contingent on her interacting with another child and to withdraw such attention from isolate behavior and contact with an adult. A system was introduced that permitted the recording of Ann's proximity to and interaction with adults and with children at 10-second intervals.

> After five days of baseline data had been secured, teachers were instructed to give attention to Ann whenever and only when she interacted with children. To begin with, any approximations to social interaction, such as standing near another child or playing beside another in the sandbox or at a table, were followed by teacher attention. As soon as Ann interacted with a child, an adult immediately gave her direct individual attention. A sample interaction was, "Ann, you are making dinner for the whole family." When she played alone, Ann was not given attention, and when she contacted an adult she was given minimum attention unless she was with another child.
>
> It was immediately apparent that a direct approach to Ann tended to draw her away from the play with children and into interaction with the adult. Original procedures were amended as follows: the teacher made comments and directed other attending behaviors to Ann, not individually, but as a participant in the on-

going group play; whenever possible, the adult approached the group prepared to give Ann an appropriate material or toy to add to the joint play project. A sample amended operation was, "You three girls have a cozy house! Here are some more cups, Ann, for your tea party." Whenever Ann began to leave the group, the teacher turned away from her and became occupied with some other child or with equipment. This procedure, which extended over six days, seemed to bring Ann into interaction with other children more frequently and for longer periods.

In order to substantiate whether the behavior changes effected by the above procedures had indeed been produced by the application of reinforcement principles, procedures were reversed for five days. Solitary pursuits and contacts made solely with an adult were once more made discriminative stimuli for adult attention. Ann was disregarded by adults whenever she interacted with children, and given only an unavoidable minimum of attention when she, in the company of another child, contacted them.

After this reversal, the previous contingencies were reinstated. For the next nine days teachers again gave (a) a maximum of attention for all play with children, (b) no attention when Ann was alone, and (c) a minimum of attention when she contacted adults, unless she was with a child. When she began spending longer periods in continuous interaction with children, adult reinforcement of interaction was gradually made more intermittent until she received adult attention in an amount normal for the group.

Following the last day of systematic reinforcement of interaction, the observers recorded Ann's behavior on four days spaced at irregular intervals during the last months of school (Allen, Hart, Buell, Harris, & Wolf, 1964, pp. 514f).

The results of this intervention are shown in Figure 1, where the data points reflect the percentage of time during approximately 2 hours of each morning session which Ann spent in interaction with adults (top half of figure) and with children (bottom half of figure). Open dots represent data gathered during baseline and reversal; closed dots represent those data obtained while interaction with children was being reinforced by the teachers.

As can be seen from these data, Ann spent little more than 10 percent of the time interacting with children and 40 percent of the time with adults while the baseline condition was in effect. The rest of the time her play was solitary.

Analysis of the data indicated that her isolate behavior was being maintained and probably strengthened inadvertently by adult social reinforcement. Using traditional nursery school guidance techniques, the teachers responded warmly to Ann whenever she contacted them and remained in conversation with her for as long as she desired. When she stood about alone, they usually went to her and tried to get her into play with children. All too frequently Ann was "out" again as soon as the teacher left, standing on the periphery, soliciting teacher attention, or playing alone.

On day 6, when Ann was first given teacher attention only when she was near children or interacting with them an immediate change in her behavior took place.

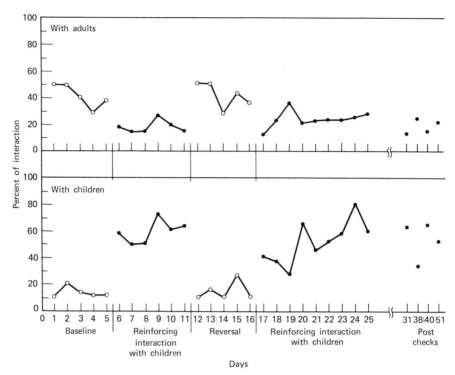

Figure 1. Percentages of time spent in social interaction during approximately 2 hours of each morning session. (Allen et al., 1964. Copyright by The Society for Research in Child Development, Inc.)

She spent almost 60 per cent of that morning first in approximations to interaction, and then in active play with children. Adult–child interaction, which was not followed by attention, dropped to less than 20 per cent. These levels of interaction varied little throughout the six-day period of continuous reinforcement of child–child interaction. Over the period, Ann spent increasing time in play with other children.

When procedures were reversed (12th day), Ann's previous pattern of behavior immediately reappeared. She spent the first few minutes after her arrival in close one-to-one interaction with a teacher, which was, of course, continuously reinforced. With this beginning, she spent the remainder of the morning much as she did during the baseline days. Over the five days of reversal she averaged less than 20 per cent of mornings in interaction with children and about 40 per cent in interaction with adults. She repeatedly ignored the contacts of other children and remained in some solitary activity where a teacher could attend to her. When she did enter play with children, she nearly always broke away after a few minutes to contact and remain with a teacher.

On the 17th day the final shift in contingencies was initiated and Ann was given adult attention only when she interacted with children. An immediate change in her behavior again occurred. Less than 20 per cent of that morning was spent interacting with adults and 40 per cent interacting with children. Interaction with adults was for the most part adult-initiated, as when the teacher reinforced her play or gave routine instructions. Over the ensuing eight days of the study her interactions with adults stabilized at about 25 per cent of mornings; interactions with children rose to the previous level of about 60 per cent. During the last days of this reinforcement period, teachers gave increasingly intermittent (nonsystematic) attention for interaction with children. The schedule of nonreinforcement of adult contacts was similarly relaxed.

Six days after the last day of reinforcement (25th day), the first post check of Ann's interactions with children and adults was made. . . . The data showed Ann to be spending more than 60 per cent of the mornings in interaction with children, and only 12 per cent in interaction with adults. Further checks taken on the 13th, 15th, and 26th days subsequent to the last reinforcement day (25th day) indicated that Ann was maintaining an average interaction rate with other children of about 54 per cent per morning. Interaction with adults on these days averaged about 18 per cent per morning. On day 38, Ann's mother was present during school hours. Her presence seemed to influence Ann's behavior in the direction of less interaction with children, although the rate was higher than during either the baseline or the reversal period (ibid., pp. 516f).

The fact that Ann began to interact with other children as soon as the contingencies of reinforcement were changed from interaction with adults to interaction with children shows that this child had a performance deficit. She did not lack the skills necessary for interacting with her peers but simply found such activity less reinforcing than interaction with adults. Had this child not possessed the skills needed for playing with other children, the intervention would have had to take a different form as, for example, the approach used in the following case study.

In working with a 3-year-old preschool girl, Buell, Stoddard, Harris, and Baer (1968) found it necessary to help the child learn to use outdoor play equipment as a tactic to produce increased social contact with other children. This was done by a method called *prompting*. Prompting may involve instructions, gestures, physical guidance, or modeling, all designed to initiate a response. In the work by Buell et al. (1968) it consisted of having a teacher place the child bodily on the piece of play equipment, such as a climbing frame, a swing, or a rocking boat, and remaining nearby as long as the girl stayed on the equipment. While she was thus close to the child, the teacher would display interest, approval, and delight in the girl's activity, touch her as seemed appropriate, smile, and talk about her play. A few days' experimental withdrawal of these teacher reactions (an ABAB design) revealed that they constituted reinforcements. The percent of time that the girl spent on the play equipment drastically declined at this point, to return to a high level when the social reinforcement was reintroduced. Prompting had been necessary for only nine days. After this, reinforcement alone was sufficient to maintain the use of the outdoor play equipment.

At the beginning of the study by Buell et al. (1968) the little girl had shown limited participation in her preschool program. She engaged in very little cooperative play with other children, never used their names, and infrequently touched or addressed them. Her major form of social interaction was some parallel play. In relation to the teachers, the girl's behavior consisted of following them about and engaging "in a type of stylized monosyllabic prattling which was clearly a bright imitation of her infant brother's babytalk" (p. 168). Other aspects of immature or inappropriate behavior included hand flapping, repeatedly hopping from one foot to the other, and speaking in incomplete sentences. None of these social skill problems was made the target of systematic attempts at intervention. Instead, the use of outdoor play equipment was selected as the treatment target because it was reasoned that if the girl could be helped to use that equipment, her play with it would increase her interaction with other children and reduce the class of behaviors that had been labeled "baby behavior." Careful observations and recording revealed that her behavior indeed took this course. Over the period during which the use of play equipment increased, there was an accompanying increase in the frequency of touching or speaking to other children, of using their names, and engaging in cooperative play with them. Concurrently, the baby behavior underwent a marked decrease in frequency. In the course of the study which extended over 50 days, baby talk, hopping, and flapping disappeared as did the incomplete sentences so that, by the end of the study, that entire response class was at near-zero level of frequency.

The Social Behavior of Severely Impaired Children

The two preschool girls who had been involved in the studies just described were essentially normal with relatively minor social deficits for whom the interventions may have done no more than to accelerate a learning process that might have taken place even without the introduction of systematic reinforcement contingencies. These early pioneering studies thus provide evidence for the potency of adult attention as social reinforcers for children without necessarily telling us anything about therapeutic intervention with children who are identified as having a psychological disorder. Work by Romanczyk, Diament, Goren, Trunell, and Harris (1975) and by Strain and Timm (1974) speaks more directly to this point.

Romanczyk et al. (1975) recognized that the normal child develops many social skills in the course of toy-play interactions with peers and that the profoundly disturbed child, who lacks such social skills, also does not use toys appropriately. They therefore set out to study the feasibility of teaching appropriate play to a group of severely disturbed children as a means of increasing their social interaction. The first group with whom they investigated this approach consisted of four children, ranging in age from 5 years, 3 months to 7 years, 7 months, who had been diagnosed as neurologically impaired, childhood schizophrenic, or as cases of early infantile autism. They displayed little or no verbal or other social interaction with adults or peers, had high rates of self-stimulatory behavior, possessed only minimal self-help skills, and were generally characterized as functioning at a severely impaired level.

During daily half-hour sessions, these children were placed in a play area within their classroom which contained the following toys: blocks, telephones, puzzle, book, peg board, ball, form box, gym mat, blackboard, and a stuffed animal. The first 10 days were devoted to gathering baseline data. During this phase, the children were told that it was play time but no other instruction or intervention took place. Observers recorded the percentage of total time during which specified categories of behavior occurred. These categories included vocalization, isolate play, social play, offering or taking a toy, aggression, motion, and idleness.

Following the baseline phase, systematic reinforcement was introduced for isolate play, defined as the manipulation of a toy that no other child was simultaneously manipulating. The reinforcement consisted of food paired with verbal praise in the form of, "I like the way you are building a tower with the blocks." This was dispensed by undergraduate volunteers who followed a variable interval schedule that provided each child the opportunity for being reinforced on the average of once per minute for a maximum of 30 reinforcements per session. During this phase playing alone (isolate play) rose from a baseline level of 65.6 percent to 85.0 percent, while playing with others (social play), which had occurred a mean of 10.6 percent of the time during baseline, fell to 2.2 percent. Clearly, the reinforcement was having a differential effect.

The next phase was devoted to the reinforcement of social play, while isolate play was to be ignored. Because social play occurred with such low frequency, the investigators introduced a *passive shaping* procedure. This consisted of placing a child next to another who was playing with a toy so that the hands of both children would touch the toy. No verbal statement accompanied this procedure nor was reinforcement given when it was necessary to resort to passive shaping. Reinforcement was dispensed only when a child was manipulating a toy, together with another child. With this intervention, the mean percent of the occurrence of social play rose to 87.5 percent while isolate play fell to 19.5 percent.

After 10 days of this procedure, a second baseline phase was introduced in order to ascertain whether the play with toys would be maintained in the absence of systematic reinforcement. The data showed that the mean (27.3 percent) for social play remained above the mean recorded during the first baseline although it appeared to drop off after some nine days. Isolate play, on the other hand, which had been quite frequent (65.6 percent) during the initial baseline phase returned to that level with a mean of 62.5 percent and seemed to be on the increase when the study ended. It is noteworthy that of the various behavior categories that had been observed and recorded, only those that had been subject to the manipulations (isolate and social play) varied in any systematic manner, reflecting the fact that the interventions had a very specific effect. What is more, the effect held for all four children even though they were not homogeneous as to either age or nature of disorder. Nonetheless, the eventual deterioration of social play during the second baseline limits the clinical implications of this study, a fact its authors readily admit. They therefore undertook a second study in order to see whether a modification in their procedure would result in greater resistance to extinction of the social play.

In the second part of their paper Romanczyk et al. (1975) report on a study in which four older, equally impaired children participated. They ranged in age from 7 years, 10 months to 12 years and had diagnoses similar to those of the children in the first study. They also exhibited a high frequency of self-stimulatory behavior and were marginally competent in self-help skills though academically they were more advanced than the younger group. Using somewhat different toys, more appropriate for these older children, the research group essentially repeated the earlier study except that they added a phase during which the passive shaping procedure was gradually withdrawn. This was done in order to test whether the passive shaping had served as a prompt for the children's interactions so that when it had been abruptly terminated at the end of the intervention, these interactions could not be maintained.

The results of this second study revealed that the gradual withdrawal of passive shaping did indeed lead to better maintenance (greater resistance to extinction) of social play. When all reinforcement and shaping was withdrawn in a return to baseline conditions, social play seemed to stabilize at a level that was more than twice that recorded during the baseline phase prior to the intervention. Though, as these investigators recognized, their studies are essentially exploratory in nature, they consider their findings encouraging because they demonstrate that the social play of profoundly impaired children can be modified in a group situation by personnel with relatively little training.

The reinforcement potential of adult attention was again illustrated in the study by Strain and Timm (1974) who worked in a preschool class, designed to further the language development of 17 behaviorally disordered children aged from 3 years to 4 years, 4 months. The problems of these children ranged from mild language delay to severe language impairment, combined with extremely high rates of disruptive, oppositional behaviors. A 3 years, 8 months old girl, named Martha, viewed as the most isolated child in the classroom, was selected for an intervention designed to increase her social interaction with other children. Adult attention in the form of verbal praise and such physical contacts as pats on the back or stroking the hair were made contingent on positive contact between Martha and any other child. During the first eight days of observations, while no systematic reinforcement was provided, the frequency of Martha's initiating contacts with other children or their initiating contact with her was essentially zero. During the next nine days, the peers were reinforced for initiating and responding to contacts with Martha, and the frequency increased to a mean of 21.4, only to drop to near baseline level during a second baseline phase when again no reinforcements were provided for the behavior under study. In a second intervention, also lasting eight days, adult attention was given to Martha whenever she initiated or responded to interaction with her peers. Mean daily frequencies now reached 30.6 with most of these interactions being initiated by Martha herself. Unfortunately this effect was not sustained when, in a third baseline phase, contingent adult attention was again withdrawn. To what extent this procedure is a useful clinical device is thus not known. Longer periods of intervention with reinforcement at first continuous, then intermittent, and eventually faded might make it possible to establish more lasting peer interaction.

Peers as Auxiliary Therapists

The study by Strain and Timm (1974) just mentioned had demonstrated the potency of adult attention as a reinforcer. It also illustrated the operation of a performance deficit in that socially isolated children possessed peer relationship skills but failed to use them in the absence of potent reinforcement. Conceivably, such reinforcement would be available were such children to interact with *normal* peers but in company with other disturbed children their interpersonal approaches fail to receive peer-reinforcement and therefore require intervention by an outside agent. That such an agent need not be an adult was demonstrated by the following studies in which peers were used as confederates of the therapist with the aim of increasing the social interaction of withdrawn and isolated children.

Strain, Shores, and Timm (1977) worked with six withdrawn preschool boys who ranged in age from 3 years, 3 months to 4 years, 5 months. These children not only displayed marked social deficits but they were also delayed in language development, engaged in frequent tantrums, and had intelligence test scores in the defective range (IQ scores ranged from 25 to 58 with a mean of 42). These boys were brought to a playroom in groups of three. There they were joined by one of two boys of similar age whom the experimenters had trained to act as auxiliary therapists by initiating social play. This they were to do by issuing verbal invitations (e.g., "Let's play ball") while proffering a toy appropriate for the purpose. These auxiliary therapists or confederates were bright (average IQ 129) four-year-old boys from a day-care program. They had impaired siblings who were enrolled in the same treatment center as the six target children in this study but none of their siblings was among these six. Their training had consisted of four 20-minute sessions during which they had been told that they were to try their best to get the other children to play with them, that many of their attempts were likely to be ignored, but that it was important to keep trying. The person doing the training of the auxiliary therapists role-played the procedure and praised the boy's performance both during training and at the end of each experimental day.

Observations were made during a baseline phase when the auxiliary therapist was in the room but had been instructed not to initiate any social play. During this phase, the withdrawn children largely ignored the therapist's confederate and emitted very few social responses. When active intervention was begun, the positive social behavior of all target children increased dramatically. They not only responded to the confederates' initiations, but also initiated play behavior of their own, directed toward the confederate. After nine days of this procedure, the auxiliary therapists were instructed not to initiate social play but to respond in their usual fashion if they were approached by one of the other children. This reversal to the baseline condition revealed the power of the intervention in that the frequency of positive social behavior by all target children decreased markedly, increasing once again when intervention was reinstated during the last eight days of the study.

The report of the study just cited does not contain information about the effect of this intervention on the children's behavior outside the special playroom in which they had been treated in small groups of three. Strain (1977) addressed this question in another study where he worked in the same setting and used the same procedure but with three different socially isolated boys. These children's behavior was recorded not only in the special playroom where treatment took place but also in their classroom during free play periods. This revealed that the increased positive social responding generalized across settings for the two of these three children for whom the intervention had been most effective. Here, as in the study by Strain et al. (1977) individual differences were found in the degree to which the children responded to the intervention. In each of the experimental triads, the boy who had displayed the fewest positive behaviors during baseline responded least to the confederate-initiated interactions. Strain (1977) suggests that overcoming the skill deficits of isolate children with such extremely limited social repertoires may require the explicit teaching of social responses through such approaches as direct shaping and differential reinforcement. The following are examples of such programs.

Teaching Social Skills

A program specifically designed to teach social skills to isolated children was tested by Gottman, Gonso, and Schuler (1976). These investigators reasoned that before one can undertake to teach socially isolated children the skills needed for social interaction, one has to identify what the skills are that popular children have and isolate children lack. In an earlier study, Gottman, Gonso, and Rasmussen (1975) had found that third- and fourth-grade children with low peer-acceptance scores differed from popular children in their knowledge of how to make friends, the frequency with which they emit and receive positive interaction with peers, and the effectiveness of their verbal communication. These were therefore the skills that Gottman et al. (1976) sought to teach to two socially isolated third-grade children.

Each of the children was assigned to an undergraduate psychology student who had been trained to teach the three identified social skills. Child and coach worked together for 30 minutes a day for one week, with treatment progressing through three stages. During the first stage the child watched a 10-minute videotape showing children who first thought about, and then decided to join some others in an activity with ensuing positive consequences. The narration that accompanied these scenes verbalized the child's thoughts about wanting to participate in the activity, worrying about negative consequences, debating with herself, making the decision, approaching, greeting, and asking permission to join. These are the kind of coping self-statements Meichenbaum and Goodman (1971) introduced in their pioneering work with impulsive children. Similar training films have been used by O'Connor (1969, 1972), Jakibchuk and Smeriglio (1976), and Weinrott, Corson, and Wilchesky (1979).

The second stage of the Gottman et al. (1976) procedure had child and coach engage in role-playing of the friend-making sequences that are routinely used by socially effective, popular children. This entails greeting, asking for information, giving information, extending an offer of inclusion, and effective leave-taking. The coach would pretend to be a new student in the class whom the child wished to befriend. During this stage each child was also taught "how to distribute positive interaction" (p. 184). This included showing interest in what the other is saying by summarizing in one's own words what had been said, giving the other something, showing approval, complying with a request, and giving affection.

Lastly, in the third stage the child was given practice in "referential communication skills" (p. 184). This included a word game requiring the use of synonyms, giving instructions, teaching something, and in other ways being able to assume the perspective of the listener. At each point in the training program, the child was instructed to practice the skills being taught with someone from her class. While all of this was taking place, two other socially isolated children who served as controls, spent time in the company of an adult who talked and played with them but did not touch in any way on the topic of friends.

The effect of this intervention was assessed by a sociometric device and by direct observations of the quality, frequency, and distribution of social interaction with peers. A comparison of these measures taken before intervention had begun with those obtained at a follow-up nine weeks after it had ended revealed that the sociometric position of the treated children had undergone a significant change. Although the total frequency of peer interaction had not changed for either the treated or the control children, the interactions of the former had been redistributed in that they would interact more with some and less with other kinds of peers. The control children, on the other hand, continued their tendency to withdraw from all peers.

The results of this study are intriguing in that they suggest that fairly long-lasting effects can be obtained with socially isolated children by as little as five 30-minute sessions devoted to teaching critical social skills. As is the case with so much of the available treatment research, this is no more than an abbreviated analogue of therapy and therefore leaves unanswered the question whether such an approach would be effective if used in a clinical setting over a longer period of time. As these investigators themselves point out, the Gottman, Gonso, and Schuler (1976) study also has the drawback that it did not include a measure of the extent to which the trained children had actually mastered the social skills they had been taught. "Social skill training programs need to demonstrate two things: that they teach the target social skills, and that these skills make a difference on criterion variables such as sociometric position" (p. 195). A comprehensive program instituted by Weinrott, Corson, and Wilchesky (1979) carried the investigation of social-skill training for withdrawn children several steps further by training teachers to intervene in their own classrooms.

In the context of an in-service teacher-training program, Weinrott et al. (1979) used 25 pupil–teacher pairs from regular grade 1 to 3 classes in 17 different schools. The children had been identified on teacher-completed behavior checklists as socially withdrawn to the point where some professional intervention seemed indicated. They rarely or never volunteered in class nor initiated conversations with peers, spending much time daydreaming. Direct classroom observations of these children and their classmates substantiated these teacher judgments and provided a composite score for normal peers as a basis for comparison. Twenty of the children and their teachers were assigned to a treatment group while the remaining five pairs served as a control group. After 6½ weeks of a baseline condition that included a quasi-placebo control of 2 weeks during which the teachers were urged "to try to make the target child appear as outgoing as possible," the training of the teachers was begun. In weekly sessions, the teachers were taught increasingly elaborate intervention procedures, covering such methods as contingent attention, modeling, role playing, point systems, and group contingencies.

Classroom observations by trained observers were conducted through the baseline phase, the 10 weeks of intervention, and over a five-week follow-up period. The dependent measures of interest were the frequency of self-stimulation, looking about the room, appropriate peer-interaction, volunteering, and addressing the teacher. The most pronounced treatment effect was reflected by the measure of peer-interaction which had been the main target of intervention. Here the treated children reached the level of their normal peers by the end of the treatment phase and through follow-up while the control children had failed to improve significantly, continuing to interact at a level far below that of their peers. Though no objective data were available on this point, anecdotal reports from teachers suggested that the increased peer contact of the targeted children generalized from classroom to playground and lunchroom, that they had increased social interactions with others outside of school, that they were happier, more alert, and eager to assume tasks of greater responsibility.

It will be recalled that the teachers in the project just cited had been taught increasingly elaborate intervention procedures. The teachers continued to apply these for as long as they deemed the target child's social behavior unsatisfactory. The more time-consuming procedure was thus not instituted until toward the end of the 10-week training program. The first five weeks of the program had been devoted to intervention methods that involve the targeted child as an individual, such as contingent teacher attention and role-playing sessions outside of class. During the second five weeks the other children in the classroom became involved in the intervention by the introduction of group contingencies and of the reinforcement of peers for initiating interaction with their withdrawn classmate. The data presented by Weinrott et al. (1979) reflect the fact that all but three of the pupil–teacher pairs proceeded to the second set of procedures and that the most pronounced change in the withdrawn children's peer interactions did not take place until these were introduced. It is thus conceivable that a combination of the peer–therapist procedure used by Strain, Shores, and Timm (1979) and a teacher-mediated program such as Weinrott et al. (1979) described might provide a highly effective approach to the treatment of socially withdrawn children.

INAPPROPRIATE GENDER BEHAVIOR

In the discussion of social-skill deficits at the beginning of this chapter it was pointed out that one consequence of such a deficit might be rejection or avoidance by peers if a child, lacking appropriate skills, approaches others in an inappropriate fashion. One dimension along which society, including its children, labels behavior as appropriate or inappropriate is in terms of the gender stereotype. A child who lacks gender-appropriate social skills and approaches others in a gender-inappropriate fashion is likely to be rejected and avoided by his or her peers, and, thus isolated, appear withdrawn. In order to improve such a child's peer relations, one must teach the gender-appropriate social skills that are missing from his or her repertoire. Once these gender-appropriate responses have been learned, one can consider the child to have been given a wider diversity and choice in the range of behaviors and this, as Rekers (1977) has pointed out, is one of the goals of psychological intervention in childhood. In other words, the goal of treatment is not the elimination from the child's repertoire of gender-inappropriate behavior but the addition of the previously missing alternative. After this alternative has become available to the child one can assume that the social environment, particularly the peer group, will selectively reinforce the gender-appropriate responses so that the inappropriate responses will ultimately undergo extinction, without their having been the explicit target of treatment. This is the therapeutic approach that has been taken by Rekers who, alone or in collaboration, has done extensive work in this area (Rekers, 1975; Rekers & Lovaas, 1974; Rekers, Lovaas, & Low, 1974).

What is appropriate and what is inappropriate behavior is a matter of public opinion, social judgment, and contemporary, hence shifting values. There is no absolute definition of what is and what is not disordered, either in the topic here under discussion or in any other area of behavior. Because gender identity and sex-role behavior are especially sensitive issues, this relativity of definitions has raised issues of who is to say whether a child should receive treatment. We shall return to a consideration of this controversy after examining some examples of behavior therapy with children considered to manifest inappropriate gender behavior.

The Case of "Carl"

A boy, aged 8 years, 8 months, identified as Carl, though this is obviously not his real name, was treated by Rekers, Lovaas, and Low (1974), who sought to replace the boy's full repertoire of so-called feminine behaviors with a repertoire our society associates with masculinity. Carl's speech had pronounced, stereotypically feminine inflection and content and he made excessively "female" gestures. He was unassertive with his peers, preferred to play with girls and girls' toys, and often stated that he preferred to be viewed as a girl. His male peers called him "sissy" and "queer" and ostracized him. This led to increasing social isolation, ridicule, and chronic unhappiness.

Carl's problem was not confined to specific stimulus conditions, but was manifested at home and in school and at the clinic. This pervasiveness and the fact that the problem involved a variety of discrete behaviors made it possible to study the effect of treatment by a multiple-baseline, intrasubject design across stimulus conditions and across behaviors. As Gelfand and Hartmann (1975) have pointed out, such a design lends itself well to testing the effectiveness of an intervention when it is not feasible or desirable to use the typical ABAB reversal design or other experimental controls.

Following their assessment, the therapists decided to treat Carl in one environment at a time. This permitted them to test for the generalization of treatment effects across clinic, home, and school. In each of these settings trained observers recorded clearly specified behaviors. The boy's mother had been trained to use a behavior checklist at home and was thus able to contribute an additional, independent set of data.

The categories used for the observations were highly concrete and objective. Feminine-gesture mannerisms, for example, subsumed eight specific behaviors, such as feminine gait which was defined as "walking with a rhythmic side-to-side movement of the torso and hips, while extending the arms away from the sides of the body or with the elbow(s) flexed such that an angle formed by the forearm and upper arm is less than 90 degrees" (p. 102). Such specificity of target behaviors is an essential of behavior therapy. Vague targets, such as "effeminate behavior," "insecurity," or "identity confusion" do not lend themselves to systematic intervention.

For treatment in the clinic Carl's sex-typed verbal behavior was chosen as the target. After gathering baseline data on masculine and feminine speech content during six story-telling sessions, the therapist introduced differential social reinforcement. If Carl verbalized statements or questions with masculine or neutral content, the therapist would show positive interest, but following any references to feminine topics he would withdraw his attention. This contingency remained in effect for three sessions during which the boy's feminine speech content decreased from an initial level of 21 percent to a mean of 2.5 percent of his total verbal behavior during a session. A brief reversal of contingencies demonstrated that the therapeutic intervention had indeed been responsible for the change in behavior since the feminine speech content immediately returned to a level of 20.5 percent. Masculine speech content complemented the changes in feminine content, increasing to 12 percent from an initial 6 percent level and then falling to 9 percent when the baseline condition was reinstated during the reversal.

It is noteworthy that a distinct response generalization could be observed in that the boy's feminine speech inflections showed a decrease concurrent with the changes in content although no reinforcement contingencies had been specifically applied to inflections. On the other hand, there was no stimulus generalization of the treatment effect to other settings. In the home and at school Carl's speech continued to have feminine content and inflections. At this point treatment was shifted to the home situation.

Carl's mother was taught to administer a treatment program based on a system of token reinforcements. At the beginning of this program, the boy was told that he would earn blue tokens whenever he engaged in masculine play with his brother. These tokens could later be traded for such back-up reinforcers as candy and television-viewing time. After two weeks under that contingency a response-cost condition was added to the system. Whenever Carl made a feminine gesture he would be handed a red token, it having been explained to him that one red token would cancel out one blue token when it came time to obtain the back-up reinforcers. Under these conditions the continuously collected observational data showed an increase in Carl's masculine play with his brother and a concomitant decrease in feminine gestures, feminine speech content, feminine voice inflection, and playing with his sister. Again, however, the treatment effect remained specific to the setting in which treatment was being conducted, the home. There was no generalization to the school situation.

Treatment was now extended to the school where the teacher was taught to apply a response-cost procedure to Carl's feminine mannerisms and noncompliant disruptive behaviors. Under this system Carl automatically received ten points at the beginning of each school day. From this "credit account" he would lose one point each time he created a class disturbance, behaved rudely to the teacher, bossed or teased another child. When these problem behaviors had decreased, the system was extended to cover feminine-gesture mannerisms as well. The effectiveness of these interventions was once more demonstrated but the improvement again failed to generalize from the classroom in which the intervention had taken place. When, in line with routine school procedures, Carl's class was moved to a different classroom and teacher, his pretreatment behaviors reemerged until the new teacher also introduced the treatment contingencies. At that point the positive effects of the intervention manifested themselves immediately.

Formal treatment extended over a total of 15 months at which point the explicit token-economy contingencies were discontinued. Reports from various sources, including an independent evaluation by two clinical psychologists who administered a battery of personality tests and interviews, confirmed that Carl's previous feminine behaviors had markedly decreased to only rare instances and that there was no remaining evidence of a cross-gender identification. He had developed a masculine interest pattern and major improvements were observed in his overall social and emotional adjustment. When he was transferred to a different school in order to get away from his prior reputation as a "sissy or queer," the new teacher considered him to be as well-adjusted and well-accepted as any other child in her class.

In view of the fact that Carl had a major lack of gender-appropriate social skills, there now followed an additional 15-month period designed to teach him games and sports, considered appropriate for boys in our society. Because he lacked a stable relationship with his new stepfather, a young male undertook to establish a buddy relationship with the boy. A year later, a follow-up revealed that the therapeutic gains continued to be maintained by this boy who was now 12 years, 2 months old.

Implications. The multiple baseline design which Rekers, Lovaas, and Low (1974) had employed with Carl permitted them to conclude that their treatment had indeed been instrumental in changing the boy's behavior. At each point in the program, appropriate responses appeared only after the treatment contingencies had been introduced in a specific setting or targeted on a particular behavior. In a multiple baseline design a response is held in baseline condition while another response is made the target of intervention. Only when that target has shown a clear change in frequency does one bring the next response under the treatment contingency. If, in this stepwise approach, responses remain stable while in baseline and change only when targeted for intervention one can conclude that it is the intervention that is responsible for the change. The design thus hinges on the expectation that the treatment effect does not generalize across responses or (where this is the variable on which the design is based) across stimulus conditions. This represents a paradox. While such lack of generalization is desired in order to demonstrate treatment effectiveness, it is a problem from a clinical point of view since it implies that treatment must be conducted in the various settings where the maladaptive behavior is manifested or that it must be specifically targeted at every changeworthy response in the child's repertoire. In practice, treatment effects often do generalize from one response or one setting to another. In fact, there had been an instance of generalization in Carl's case when his speech inflections changed together with his speech content. In cases where generalization occurs spontaneously, a multiple baseline design would not be an appropriate vehicle for demonstrating the function of the independent variable.

The generalization of treatment effects is a critical issue in child behavior therapy. Many maladaptive child behaviors are limited to one setting; the child who is disruptive in the school may be a very compliant child at home or vice versa. In these cases, treatment can focus on the setting where the problem behavior takes place and once this behavior has been changed in the desired direction, treatment can be terminated. Many other problem behaviors, on the other hand, manifest themselves in a variety of settings, as was the case with Carl. Here it is not enough to work on the problem in one setting only. Helping Carl emit more gender-appropriate behaviors in the clinic had no effect on his behavior at home or school. The therapist thus had to plan explicitly to bring about a generalization of the treatment effect. When situational variables are seen as having major control over behavior, plans for behavior change must take these variables into consideration.

Another implication that the case of Carl has for child behavior therapy is the importance of parental participation in the treatment plan. Treatment has little chance of being effective if it is restricted to the intermittent contact between the professional therapist and the child. The traditional weekly 50-minute session can hardly be expected to carry the burden of changing behavior during the remaining 10,000 minutes of the week. Child behavior therapists often include in the treatment plan significant other persons who are in contact with the child in day-to-day living, such as teachers and parents. Involvement of such auxiliary therapists cannot be done casually, such as by asking a parent to read a manual on behavior change. As was the case with Carl's mother, an auxiliary therapist must be taught to discriminate the behaviors to be changed, to observe and record these behaviors, and to manage the reinforcement contingencies in a consistent and systematic fashion. In fact, child behavior therapists often find that their time is spent more effectively and efficiently in training and working with auxiliary therapists than in face-to-face contact with the child. It stands to reason that the same principles of learning that form the basis of the intervention with the child should also be employed in the training of the auxiliary therapist. Since success can be a powerful reinforcer for parents and teachers, it is well to select as the first target of intervention one of the child's behaviors that has high probability of responding quickly to a therapeutic regimen, thus reinforcing the auxiliary therapist's efforts.

Yet another implication of the treatment of Carl is the importance of making explicit efforts to strengthen desired responses and to teach the responses that are not in a child's repertoire when one undertakes to reduce the frequency of undesired responses. It was, for example, not enough to ignore Carl's feminine speech content, thus hoping to have these responses become extinguished. The therapist systematically attended to and thus reinforced desired verbalizations. Similarly, after Carl had ceased his interest in feminine play and companionship, he was helped to acquire masculine interests and skills which facilitated his interaction with same-sex peers.

Lastly, the case of Carl serves to highlight a phenomenon that can be observed in therapy about which we know relatively little. It is that certain discrete responses seem to belong to response clusters, forming *functional response classes*, so that, when one of these responses is modified, others in the same cluster also undergo change. In Carl's case, clinic treatment had been targeted on the content of his speech and while a record of his feminine voice inflection was kept by an observer, no contingency was applied to it. Nonetheless, the record showed that the increase in masculine speech content and the concomitant decrease in feminine speech content were accompanied by a marked decrease in feminine voice inflections. Content and inflection thus seem to belong to a cluster, facilitating response generalization. Most child behavior problems consist of many discrete and different responses but it is not necessary to set up explicit treatment procedures for each of these. Work on one response often generalizes to others but at this point we do not know how to identify these "key" responses and the clusters to which they belong. This issue represents a crucial agenda item for research in child behavior therapy and assessment.

Self-control

In speaking of the value of involving a child's parents and teachers in the treatment process, we made the point that such auxiliary therapists can be so effective because they are with the child for so much more time than any therapist can ever hope to be. There is of course someone who can be said to be with a child all of the time and that is the child who is the client. Treatment could probably achieve maximum effectiveness and efficiency if the child could be taught to be his or her own therapist. Steps in this direction are being taken by therapists who are studying techniques of behavioral self-control (e.g., Spates & Kanfer, 1976).

Rekers and Varni (1977a) reported work with a 6-year-old boy who, not unlike Carl, had gender identity problems. After they had been able to demonstrate that this boy's gender-typed behavior could be modified by social reinforcement delivered by the child's parents, they taught him to monitor his own masculine play, using a wrist-counter to record his own responses. This training was accomplished in the clinic where a special device ("Bug-in-the-ear") permitted the transmission of verbal instructions through a miniature FM receiver that is worn like a wireless hearing aid. As is often the case when people begin to make an explicit record of their own behavior (Broden, Hall, & Mitts, 1971), the child's masculine play increased in apparent reaction to the self-monitoring. This reactive effect diminished over time and the child was then instructed to give himself a small piece of candy for each point recorded on the wrist-counter. Assessment, using a reversal design, demonstrated that this reinforcement condition produced exclusively masculine play. Unlike reinforcement delivered by the parents, where the effect had remained highly situation specific, self-monitoring combined with self-reinforcement was shown to generalize across activities. When this boy was reassessed 12 months after termination of treatment, he was found to have abandoned the behavior that had initially led to his being viewed as exhibiting a gender disturbance and the independent interviewer saw him as a relaxed, generally happy boy. A similar combination of self-monitoring and self-reinforcement was used by Rekers and Varni (1977b) with a 4-year-old boy who had manifested stereotypic feminine gender-role behaviors. Here too these self-regulation strategies were effective in instituting gender-appropriate behavior that was maintained over a two-year follow-up period.

The limited number of cases for which this form of treatment has been reported and the (inevitable) lack of rigorous experimental controls would make it premature to say more than that therapy based on self-regulation of behavior holds an intriguing promise for maximizing the help that can be rendered by the relatively few available professionally trained therapists. It is also too early to tell whether behavioral treatment of gender problems in young children has long-range effects; whether, in particular, these children will engage in gender-appropriate social behavior when they become adolescents and young adults.

Is Intervention Justified?

As pointed out earlier, the topics of sex role and gender identity are sensitive issues, particularly so when one seeks to change gender-related behavior by therapeutic means. Whenever therapeutic intervention is contemplated one ought to ask whether such intervention is justified. Who is to say that a child who disrupts the classroom should be helped to "settle down"; that a child who attacks other children should be taught alternative, less aggressive forms of interaction; that a boy who wets his bed should be trained to remain dry? Somehow questions whether intervention is justified in such cases rarely reach the level of controversy (Winett & Winkler, 1972), yet when it comes to therapeutic intervention in the area of sex-role behavior such discussion frequently ensues (Davison, 1976). There seems to be a consensus that classrooms should not be disrupted, that attacking other children is undesirable, and that beyond a certain age bedwetting represents a disorder that calls for treatment. In the case of what constitutes appropriate sex-role behaviors for boys and for girls, however, the consensus that prevailed in the past has begun to dissolve and people are asking whether there is anything wrong with boys playing with dolls or girls with toy trucks. As our society has become more permissive regarding the life-styles of adults and as stereotypes of sex-linked occupational choices are being abandoned, we have come to ask whether children should be exposed to treatment when someone has decided that their behavior is not appropriate for their sex.

It was in this context that Winkler (1977) and others (Nordyke, Baer, Etzel, & LeBlanc, 1977) questioned the appropriateness of the therapeutic intervention Rekers and Lovaas (1974) had undertaken with a 5-year-old boy who displayed marked cross-gender behavior. The boy's parents had been greatly concerned about this and had sought treatment for the boy, wishing that his behavior might become more appropriate for a boy of his age. Of course they defined the appropriateness of behavior in terms of the norms of their social environment, according to which boys don't insist on wearing women's dresses, play with dolls, pretend to be a mother, walk with a feminine gait, and speak with feminine inflections. Nordyke et al. (1977) questioned these norms asking, in effect, what is wrong with a boy's playing with dolls and what defines a gait or an inflection as "feminine." Winkler (1977), in turn, raised the question to whom therapists owe their first allegiance: to the child's parents, to the prevailing social norms, or to the therapist's own values? Who is to say that the child does not have a perfect right to engage in the behavior described? Why oblige the parents in their moralistic notions about appropriate behavior? What is wrong with growing up as a potential transvestite or homosexual? Why could the therapist not have undertaken to help the parents become more accepting of their child's cross-gender behavior while, at the same time, helping the child to be more assertive in the face of the negative sanctions imposed by his parents and peers?

As Rekers (1977) points out in a carefully reasoned reply to these and other questions, they reflect a lack of appreciation for the world of the gender-disturbed child and completely ignore the fact that such behavior elicits social ostracism and ridicule from peers of both sexes, leading to depression, frustration, and negativistic behavior on the part of the child. He states that while the peer group's intolerance and rejection are morally wrong, "the most benevolent and direct strategy is to change the child's individual behavior to alleviate his suffering" (Rekers, 1977, p. 561). This goal alone, he views as sufficient justification for intervention.

Beyond this therapeutic rationale, which is based on trying to relieve a child's personal suffering, Rekers (1977) sees grounds for intervention in three other considerations. One is to prevent the severe psychological and social maladjustment in adulthood that accompanies transsexualism. Another is to prevent later sex-role identity problems which he sees as the most probable outcome in adulthood unless treatment is provided for the child. These points are based on the continuity assumption according to which gender-identity problems in childhood lead to similar problems when the person is an adult. This assumption rests on the relatively weak evidence provided by retrospective studies. If intervention could be justified by no more than the hope of preventing hypothetical later problems those who took issue with Rekers and Lovaas (1974) might have a point.

The third consideration Rekers (1977) advanced in justification of his approach is that the therapist is obligated "to respond to the parents' legitimate request for professional intervention" (p. 560). This raises such issues as the rights of children and the legal guardianship of parents. Do parents have the right to request that a therapist treat their child so as to change what they perceive as homosexual behavior? It is here that personal values and the contemporary standards of the community must be taken into consideration. As with other issues of an ethical or moral nature, there are no absolute answers as to what is right and what is wrong and a potential therapist must make judgments in terms of his or her own value system after seeking as much information and as many opinions as possible. When, as was the case in the instance reported by Rekers and Lovaas (1974), all considerations point in the direction of the desirability of treating a gender-disordered child, the therapists are fully justified, if not obligated to offer help.

Recapitulation

There are many social skills that children must possess in order to be able to interact constructively with their peers. Some children have never acquired the appropriate skills while others, having acquired them, fail to use them appropriately. It is therefore useful to distinguish between skill deficits and performance deficits. Studies have demonstrated that the contingent attention of adults can be a powerful source of reinforcement for child behavior and that such attention can be used to develop peer-relationship skills. Even severely impaired children can be taught to interact socially by such means as differential reinforcement, peer modeling, and passive shaping. Many of these procedures can be applied by auxiliary therapists, including children, college students, and classroom teachers.

Gender-appropriate behavior can be construed as a social skill, the lack of which can seriously interfere with a child's peer relationships. A successful behavior therapy program used with a boy who had such a problem was reviewed and its implications were discussed in some detail, including the question how such intervention can be justified.

3

Academic Deficits

READING AS OPERANT BEHAVIOR

Behavior therapy is construed as a process of learning, unlearning, and re-learning and the methods of behavior therapy are derived from the principles of learning. In view of this it is not surprising that behavior therapists have expanded their activities beyond the psychological problems usually encountered in clinical settings and have become involved with children who experience difficulties with the acquisition of such academic subject matter as reading.

Staats was among the first psychologists who conceptualized reading as an operant response and who applied operant principles in a systematic fashion to help children with reading difficulties (Staats, Minke, Finley, Wolf, & Brooks, 1964; Staats & Butterfield, 1965; Staats, Minke, Goodwin, & Landeen, 1967; Ryback & Staats, 1970). When a child looks at a word printed on a page and says that word aloud, one can construe that sequence as the presentation of a stimulus and the emission of a verbal response. If, in consequence of a correct response, the teacher says "Good" and correct responses thereafter increase in frequency, the teacher's praise can be seen as a positive reinforcer. The operant conceptualization of reading then leads one to the systematic use of reinforcement contingencies so as to increase correct, and decrease incorrect responses. Saying the correct word upon the presentation of a written stimulus is, of course, a necessary but not a sufficient condition for reading. As Lahey, McNees, and Brown (1973) have pointed out, a primary purpose of reading instruction is to teach students to answer accurately questions about passages they have read, that is, to demonstrate comprehension. It is this cognitive process that must be brought under effective stimulus control if reading is to be taught by the application of behavioral principles. For this reason it is important in setting up remedial reading programs for children who are deficient in that area that one select an outcome criterion that is relevant to the ultimate goal of obtaining meaning from written material. A child's ability to make a correct verbal response to the stimulus of a written word (decoding) is not an adequate outcome measure, nor is it sufficient to demonstrate that a child's sight vocabulary has increased or that the rate and accuracy or oral reading of single words or passages have improved. As will be seen in the following, those investigating various approaches to working with children's reading problems have dealt with this issue in a variety of not always entirely satisfactory ways.

THE REMEDIATION OF READING DEFICIENCIES

Reinforcement

The usual behavioral procedure for working with children who have a deficit in an academic skill such as reading is to begin by using some tangible reinforcers, such as tokens or checkmarks, which are delivered contingent on the desired response, usually accompanied by a verbal praise statement. Dalton, Rubino, and Hislop (1973) demonstrated that token reinforcement is superior to verbal praise in producing improvement in the academic performance of retarded children. In practice, however, it is probably best to combine the delivery of a token with a verbal praise statement, as Ryback and Staats (1970) had done. The tangible reinforcers and the verbal statements each have their own advantages and disadvantages. Praise statements are more likely to be available in a child's natural environment where the reading behavior must be maintained after the special remedial program with its tangible reinforcers has ended. Hence it is desirable to have the child encounter the contingent relationship between reading and praise. On the other hand, for some children praise may initially have no reinforcement value. Here the pairing of a tangible reinforcer with a social reinforcer can be an effective way of attaching reinforcement properties to the praise (Lovaas, Freitag, Kinder, Rubenstein, Schaeffer, & Simmons, 1966). In the case of retarded children it has been shown (Zigler & Balla, 1972) that different children respond to social reinforcement in different ways, depending on such factors as age (younger, are more responsive than older children), and the retarded child's history prior to institutionalization. In an institution, greater responsiveness to social reinforcement was found among retarded children who received few visits from relatives and who had greater deprivation prior to institutionalization. These findings should serve to remind one that no reinforcer can be deemed universally effective and that one must establish in each and every case which consequences strengthen and which weaken the preceding response since reinforcement can only be defined in terms of this function. In addition, the Zigler and Balla (1972) study highlights the fact that a social reinforcer, like any other reinforcer, is subject to the effects of deprivation and satiation, calling for the ongoing monitoring of reinforcer effectiveness even after the potency of a given reinforcer has been established for a particular child.

At the initial stages of a training program when acceptable responses should be on a near-continuous schedule of reinforcement, verbal praise has the disadvantage of potentially leading to satiation when used with great frequency. When the word "good" is said fifteen times in three minutes, the word will quickly lose its reinforcing potential. Dropping plastic chips into a child's cup or placing checkmarks in his record book, on the other hand, will remain effective for a long time particularly because these tokens can later be traded for a back-up reinforcer of the child's choice, a choice that may vary from day to day. Such selection of back-up reinforcers can be facilitated by the use of a so-called reinforcer menu, as was done by Dineen, Clark, and Risley (1977) in their study of tutoring procedures which will be discussed later in this chapter. The reinforcer menu, a list of available choices, was posted on the classroom wall and each child could select the back-up reinforcer for which he or she wanted to work that day prior to entering the tutoring session.

The use of a reinforcement menu places the choice of the back-up reinforcer in the hands of the child, thereby personalizing the reinforcer and enhancing its potential effectiveness. It has also been shown that when reinforcement contingencies are determined by the children themselves, the contingencies are as effective as when they are imposed by the teacher (Felixbrod & O'Leary, 1973). Similarly, as Lovitt and Curtiss (1969) demonstrated in working with a single child, a higher rate of academic performance can be achieved when the child manages the contingencies than when performance standards are set by the teacher.

Ferster (1967) has drawn the useful distinction between arbitrary and natural reinforcers, emphasizing that wherever they are available, natural reinforcers are to be preferred because their continuing availability will maintain the behavior beyond the termination of the systematic training program. In the case of reading, the natural reinforcement for proficient readers probably resides in the information they obtain by reading and from the ultimate benefits to which this information can lead. These are the consequences that have a natural, logical relationship to the behavior. Any consequence that is not logically related to the reading response must be classified as arbitrary. Thus the word "good" or other praise voiced by an adult is as arbitrary as a plastic chip, a checkmark, or a score on a test. Such arbitrary reinforcers may at times be needed in the early stages of reading acquisition before a child "gets something out of" reading, before reading has become "its own reward." It is in that sense that arbitrary reinforcers have to be used with children who experience difficulty and for whom reading may actually have become an aversive activity. Again, a child who is reinforced by the joy of discovery or the pleasure of learning something new needs neither explicit praise nor tokens to reinforce reading behavior. In fact, it may be the absence of these natural, intrinsic reinforcers that prevents some children from learning. It is they who must be helped by the use of arbitrary reinforcers but these should eventually be replaced by the natural reinforcers inherent in being able to read well and at that point the child will be "reading for the sake of reading."

It can be demonstrated that even children who do not have a pronounced reading deficit may progress more quickly in the *early* acquisition of reading when their performance is reinforced by tokens. Lahey and Drabman (1974) compared two groups of second-grade children whom they taught to read 30 new words. The children in one of these groups were given only a verbal consequence for correct responses (the word "right"). Those in the other group received this verbal consequence plus a token worth one-fifth of a cent. The reading words were taught in lists of 10 and each child was seen for three individual sessions. Reinforcement was given for every correct response and the session continued until the criterion of reading all 10 words correctly had been reached. Retention for all 30 words was tested immediately after the end of the third training session and again two days later. By then it was nine days after the first list had been learned. The results revealed that the children in the no-token group needed on the average twice as many trials to reach criterion on the three word lists as did the token group. What is more, the children in the token group displayed significantly better retention after the longer retention intervals and the differences between the two groups increased with increasing retention intervals. It thus appears that providing praise plus a token not only facilitates reading acquisition but that it also enhances retention of what has been learned. Moreover, the advantage of token-plus-praise over praise alone becomes more pronounced, the longer the newly learned material is to be retained.

Discrimination Learning

An application that derives from the view that reading acquisition is a form of discrimination learning was demonstrated by Staats and Butterfield (1965). These investigators report on work with a 14-year-old boy who at the beginning of their study was reading below the second-grade level, having continually received failing grades in all subjects. He came from a large, disadvantaged, Mexican-American family, had a long history of delinquent behavior and resided in a juvenile detention home while attending the local high school. Staats and Butterfield gave this boy a total of 40 hours of individual reading training over a period of 4½ months at the end of which his reading-achievement test score placed him at the 4.3-grade level. This student, who had never passed any course, now received passing grades in all of his subjects and his behavior in school, which had been described as "incorrigible," caused no further complaints. The procedure that led to this remarkable change bears detailed presentation.

In order to employ reinforcement procedures in a reading tutoring program, three conditions must be met: One must be able to monitor all of the student's responses; training trials must be so structured that they can be presented in discrete units; and response quality must be objectively defined. To meet these requirements, Staats and Butterfield (1965) modified the material contained in a commercially available reading kit. For each of the stories to be read, a list of all new words was prepared and each word was typed on a 3×5 card for individual presentation. Next, each paragraph in a story was typed on a separate 5×8 card so that the story could be attacked one paragraph at a time. Lastly, each story, together with the comprehension questions provided by the publishers, was typed on a separate sheet of $8\frac{1}{2} \times 13$ paper.

The reinforcer system involved plastic tokens of three different colors, each color representing a different value. A blue token was worth one-tenth of one cent; a white one, one-fifth of a cent; and a red one, one-half of one cent. These tokens could be used to purchase a variety of items chosen by the child ahead of time so that he always knew for what prize he was working. As the boy acquired tokens, a visual record was provided so that he knew at all times how many reinforcers he had earned.

For each story the procedure began with the presentation of the new words contained in that story. These were presented one at a time and the child was asked to pronounce them. A correct response was immediately reinforced with a midvalue token and the card was then dropped from the group to be learned. When the boy made an incorrect response or failed to respond, the teacher would provide the correct response as a prompt. The student was then to repeat the word while looking at the stimulus card which was retained in the stack for later presentation. When, on a later presentation, that word was read correctly the boy would earn a low-value token and the vocabulary presentation was continued until all words had been read correctly without prompting.

After all the new words appearing in a story had been learned by the procedure outlined above, the next step was the oral reading of each of the paragraphs in that story. This was attacked paragraph by paragraph, following their sequence in the story. When a paragraph had been read correctly, the boy was given a high-value token. Note that only midvalue tokens had been awarded for the correct reading of individual words while reading the word correctly in the context of the paragraph earned a high-value reinforcer. This underscores the idea that reading individual words is but a subskill of reading sentences. When the boy made an error in the reading of a paragraph he was given the correct response and asked to repeat the word correctly while looking at it. That paragraph was then put aside to be taken up again after all other paragraphs had been completed. It then had to be read correctly in its entirety and this earned a midvalue token. As had been true in the vocabulary phase, a correct response on the first try—being closer to the ultimate goal of independent reading—earned a higher value reinforcer than a response given correctly only after one or more prompts.

When all paragraphs in a story had been completed correctly, the last step in the training sequence was introduced. This entailed practice in the ultimate target skill, silent reading for comprehension. For this the boy was given the sheet on which the story and the comprehension questions had been typed. He was told to read the story silently and to write out and say his answers to the questions. During this phase there were two sources of reinforcement, one related to the silent reading, the other to answering the questions correctly. Since comprehension is the goal of reading, it earned high-value tokens; one token for each correct answer. If the written answer contained a spelling error, the boy had to correct it and then received a midvalue token. If an answer was incorrect, he had to read the relevant paragraph over and correct his answer before receiving a midvalue token.

Because silent reading is a covert response that cannot be directly monitored, the reinforcement contingencies were based on looking at the material, what the authors refer to as "attentive behavior" and "appropriate scanning" (Staats & Butterfield, 1965, p. 930). The inference that the boy was reading when looking at the story was strengthened by his ability to answer the comprehension questions correctly but there remains the possibility that he could have learned the answers to the comprehension questions from his previous exposure to the paragraphs during the oral reading phase. In that case, he might have been receiving reinforcement for merely directing his glance in the direction of the typewritten words on the page. While this is unlikely, given the fact that he made such remarkable progress and that in one-to-one tutoring a teacher may be able to tell genuine silent reading from staring at a page, it is worth recognizing the dilemma encountered when one is trying to deal with covert processes from a behavioral standpoint.

The reinforcement for attentive behavior during the silent-reading phase was given on a variable interval schedule because such a schedule is known to maintain behavior at a steady rate. As long as the boy was looking at the material he was given a low-value token an average of every 15 seconds. The exact time was determined by a table of random numbers and varied from 1 to 30 seconds. Whenever he did anything other than scan the material, reinforcement was suspended, to be resumed when he was once again engaged in silent reading. In order to discourage frequent stops and starts, no reinforcement was given sooner than 5 seconds after the resumption of reading so that, if an interval was less than 5 seconds long, no token was given until the next interval had also occurred. Lastly, in order to encourage silent reading without lip movements, the boy could earn an extra midvalue token at the end of stories that had been read in this manner.

During an average training session, which might last anywhere from 30 minutes to 2 hours, the time actually spent on reading was 35 minutes. The rest of the period was taken up with plotting the reinforcers the boy had earned, preparing the material, and recording his performance. About three days after one of the stories in the kit had been completed, the boy's retention for the vocabulary was tested. After 45 and again after 70 training sessions, he was given a standardized test of reading achievement, administered by outside examiners. These tests showed that this boy, who had read below the 2nd-grade level at the beginning of the training program, achieved at the 3.8-grade level after 45 sessions and at the 4.3-grade level when the program was terminated after 4½ months. Staats and Butterfield (1965) make the important point that the training procedure they had used is relatively simple and that, because it is very specific, it can be administered by people without a high degree of training in educational methods. In the case just presented, the tutor was a probation officer.

Behavioral Tutoring

Following the pioneering work just described, Staats and his colleagues have demonstrated that remedial reading training based on operant principles can be given by adult volunteers and high school seniors or by the parents of the reading-disabled children (Ryback & Staats, 1970; Staats, Minke, Goodwin, & Landeen, 1967). Others have reported on successful remedial programs that used college students as tutors (Heiman, Fischer, & Ross, 1973; Schwartz, 1977). In any such program it is important that reinforcers be used in a carefully planned and systematic fashion. The schedule of reinforcement to be used and the nature of the tokens and of the back-up reinforcers must be carefully individualized and it is here that the person with extensive technical training plays an important role. Sibley (1967) has demonstrated that tokens, initially delivered on a continuous or near-continuous schedule must be thinned out as training progresses until they may be given as infrequently as once for every 30 correct responses. What is more, according to Sibley (1967), less successful, less persevering children seem to perform best under low ratios of reinforcement (one reinforcement for every two responses) while more able readers do better when the ratio is higher (one reinforcement for every 30 responses).

The early work conducted under the direction of Staats had been designed primarily to discover effective ways of working with disabled readers by using minimally trained individuals as tutors. As such, no attempt was made to adduce proof that these procedures were indeed the crucial independent variables. Such proof requires the use of experimental controls, particularly if one seeks to establish whether the operant tutoring procedures are superior to some other method of helping reading-deficient students.

A Comprehensive Tutoring Program. Schwartz (1977) conducted a well-controlled study of the effectiveness of using college students as contingency managers (tutors) in a program designed to develop the reading skills of retarded readers who were attending seventh grade in four different high schools. From among 1,265 students who had taken the Gates-MacGinitie Reading Test, 260 who had scored between 1.5 and 4.5 years below grade level were selected for participation in this research. Matched pairs of these students were assigned at random to an experimental and one of four control groups. Those in the experimental group participated for 10 weeks in a remedial tutoring program that had three aims. It was to remediate specific deficiencies in the students' reading skills; to modify their negative evaluations of their own reading skills and their negative attitudes toward reading; and to motivate them to learn and practice new skills and strategies in reading.

Schwartz (1977) used four different control conditions. In one of these conditions the subjects received a letter telling them that they had been selected for special attention because they had the potential to improve and that their progress would be monitored by another test at the end of the semester. The classroom teacher of these students was told that they needed special help with their reading but the nature of this help was left up to the teacher. Under the constraints of the regular school situation, where no special reading program was available, this usually meant that these control subjects received only superficial assistance.

A second control condition, conducted in a different school, entailed giving all seventh-grade students in addition to their regular lessons in reading, the reading development program Schwartz (1977) had developed for use by the special tutors and which will be described below. This control condition had been designed to compare individual tutoring with the effect of the program when administered by the classroom teacher as part of the regular curriculum. In a third control condition the students continued in their regular reading program without change, thus providing a comparison between typical classroom instruction and the various experimental manipulations. Lastly, there was a control condition in which individual college students met with the reading-deficient subjects for one hour each week to help them with their homework but without employing any systematic skill-training or behavior management procedures. This served as a control for the individual attention that the students in the experimental group were receiving during the 10 weeks of the project.

The undergraduates who served as tutors were given training in applying the principles of reinforcement, contingency contracting, and behavior management. They also learned to use diagnostic materials, remedial workbooks, and a manual for reading tutors that the investigator had written for this purpose. This manual contains specific instructions and exercises for the various reading strategies, such as sequencing, generalizing, detailing, and organization. The entire training for the tutors took five weeks.

The tutors had the following distinct, but interrelated tasks in line with the aims of the program:

1. Tutors were to establish baselines in each of the basic reading-skill areas, using the diagnostic materials and approaches they had been taught. They had to decide on target behaviors and on the strategies best suited to reach these. During their contact with their student they were to model effective reading strategies and styles of productive thinking. The program was thus designed and conducted to meet the needs of each individual student.

2. As an important supplement to the one hour per week in which tutor and student met for the purpose of skill training, the tutor devised and entered into a reading contract with the student. In this contract all reading behaviors had specific consequences in terms of points that would ultimately be exchanged for a course grade on the school report card. Some of these points could be earned for specific behaviors during the tutoring sessions, such as arriving on time, paying attention, and making a good effort. Most points, however, were to be earned through reading at home in books that had been selected jointly by student and tutor. This homework was monitored by requiring the student to summarize what he had read and to answer questions about it. Reading assignments were introduced gradually, beginning with a minimum of 15 minutes each night and increasing 3 hours per week over the 10-week period of the program. In order to earn enough points to complete a contract, a student had to have read at least 500 pages of average difficulty.

3. The tutors systematically reinforced with praise and points all of the students' positive verbal statements about reading and about themselves as readers while ignoring all negative statements of this kind. This was intended to modify the students' negative attitudes toward reading and their poor opinions of themselves in relation to reading.

4. In order to enhance the probability that improvements would be maintained beyond completion of the program, each tutor entered into a summer contract with his or her student according to which the students were to read as many books as possible during the summer while recording their progress and awarding points to themselves. They were to aim at earning at least as many points as they had achieved during their original contract but no back-up reinforcement was promised. Instead, the tutor stressed the student's

achieved level of success, the importance of reading well for future success in school, and the pleasure of reading.

In the week following the termination of the program and before the summer vacation, all students were retested, using an alternate form of the Gates-MacGinitie Reading Test and 74 percent of the subjects were tested once more six months later. Comparisons with pretest scores revealed that the treatment procedures had accelerated the rate of growth of the experimental subjects three times the expected rate for average students and four times their own previous rate. The controls, on the other hand, had advanced only 1.4 times the average expected rate and twice their previous rate. The tutoring program was thus clearly effective and superior to the other approaches but as Schwartz (1977) points out, singling out poor readers for special attention seems generally beneficial, whatever form that attention might take.

The follow-up six months later showed that all subjects had consolidated their gains and that they had continued to make progress. The rate of increase expected for average students between the pretest and the follow-up test is 1.0 grades. For the experimental subjects in this project, this increase was 2.6 grades; for the control subjects it was 1.6 grades. Treatment procedures had thus accelerated the rate of growth of the experimental subjects to 3.7 times their previous rate which had been 0.7 of a grade per year and to 2.6 times the expected yearly rate for average students. For the control subjects the rate of growth was 2.3 times their previous rate and 1.6 times the expected rate for average students. The impressive results of this study might be even more striking had they not been attenuated by the fact that some of the lowest scoring students had, by chance, been assigned to three of the control groups. Error of measurement and the regression-to-the-mean effect resulted in these students showing the greatest improvements, thus masking somewhat the changes of the experimental subjects.

In addition to the data based on the standardized test of reading achievement, Schwartz (1977) presents other information that reflects the success of the tutoring project. Completion of the reading contract required reading a minimum of five books. This was done by 40 of the 42 experimental subjects. Of these, 37 received an A in the course, which means that they had earned more than 200 points. To earn 250 points, which was accomplished by 27 students, they had to read an average of 8.9 books. One student, who earned 499 points had read 18 books, improving in his reading scores by 3.6 grades. At the onset of the program, many students had indicated that they could not concentrate on reading for more than one-half to three-quarters of an hour at a time. Yet by the end of the program some reported that they were able to read for two to three hours at a stretch. Attitudes toward reading also improved. By the seventh week, tutors reported that students were choosing books on their own, browsing in book stores and libraries, and taking the initiative for choosing extra books. Teachers noted that participants in the program demonstrated greater self-confidence in other academic subjects and parents told of lessened tension regarding homework and school achievement and of having discussions with their child about books both of them were reading. Some noted that their youngsters were carrying books around the house and reading under the bed covers after they were supposed to have their lights out. Librarians reported that subjects in the project were now visiting the library, a place they had not frequented before. The changed attitude about reading was also reflected in the fact that the 13 students for whom the effect of the summer contract could be checked, had read an average of 6.3 books (1026.6 pages) between May and August, a considerable amount even by the standards of an adult reader.

The Training of Tutors. Schwartz (1977) has thus demonstrated the effectiveness of a relatively brief remedial tutoring program carried out by college students with minimal technical training. Since these students had previously taken psychology courses to satisfy the prerequisites for the class in developmental psychology as part of which they participated in the tutoring program, it might be argued that they possessed more than minimal technical training. To counter this, one can point to the successful work of Ryback and Staats (1970) who used the parents of poor readers as "therapy-technicians" in remedial reading programs after having given them only four hours of training. Even children can serve as tutors for their peers as has been demonstrated by Harris and Sherman (1973), by Johnson and Bailey (1974), and by Dineen, Clark, and Risley (1977).

The amount of special training given to the peer tutors has varied from none to three half-hour sessions. In the study by Harris and Sherman (1973) the arrangement was very unstructured and, although they refer to their procedure as peer tutoring, it was really more an arrangement of having several children work on mathematics problems cooperatively than tutoring in the traditional sense of having a person who possesses a certain skill teach another who is less advanced. At any rate, whatever it might be called, Harris and Sherman demonstrated that when students worked on math problems in groups of two or three for a period of 15 minutes per class period, the later performance of all was better than under a control condition in which they worked independently. The group approach improved both speed and accuracy not only on the problems on which the students had worked together but also on related problems, reflecting a generalization of skills. Because these fourth- and fifth-grade students were, on the average, one year below grade level in their mathematics performance, this group approach can be viewed as a remedial procedure that is very easy to implement.

A slightly more involved procedure, and one that entails tutoring in the traditional sense, was introduced and assessed by Johnson and Bailey (1974) who taught fifth-grade students to tutor five kindergarten children in basic arithmetic skills. The program extended over 7½ weeks and the tutors ranged in age from 10 years, 4 months to 11 years, 3 months. Their assignment was to teach their students the following basic arithmetic tasks:

1. Recognizing the numbers 0 to 10
2. Naming the numbers 0 to 10
3. Counting objects from 11 to 20
4. Recognizing the numbers 11 to 20
5. Naming the numbers 11 to 20
6. Counting by tens from 10 to 100
7. Recognizing the numbers 10 to 100
8. Naming the numbers 10 to 100

To prepare the five tutors for their assignment, they received three 30-minute sessions of training on consecutive days. On the first day the tutors were given a description of the program and the experimenter modeled such teaching behaviors as speaking clearly, praising appropriate and ignoring inappropriate academic and social behavior, correcting incorrect responses, and repeating a stimulus after correcting an incorrect response. These teaching behaviors were reviewed during the second session which also contained an introduction of the tutoring materials and the data recording sheets. For each task in the tutorial program, the tutors were furnished specific verbal instructions that they were to use with their students, such as "How many squares are there? Point to each square as you count them aloud." The trainees then paired off and role-played being tutor or student, each of them having at least one opportunity to practice handling the materials, interacting with a student, and recording the data.

The third training session was devoted entirely to role-playing, special emphasis being given to providing social reinforcement contingent on appropriate academic and social behavior on the part of the surrogate student. The tutors-in-training were in turn given social reinforcement by the experimenter for emitting appropriate tutoring behavior.

When the actual tutoring began, Johnson and Bailey (1974) randomly assigned each tutor to one of the five kindergarten children who had been selected because they could not count or name the numerals up to 10 and who had been matched for arithmetic ability with another five children who were to serve as a control group. The tutoring program extended over 26 daily sessions, lasting 20 minutes each. Before the end of each session, the tutor was to go over all of the tasks worked on that day and to record the student's responses. These responses were then scored and graphed, thus giving the student immediate feedback on the day's progress. As soon as a student received a perfect score on any task for three consecutive days, work on that task was discontinued and a new task begun. In addition to the feedback provided at the end of the sessions, each of them was followed by a 10-minute period of play activity, intended to serve as reinforcement.

In most studies of tutoring, tutors are trained in a given approach and then assigned to a student with whom they are supposed to use the tutoring procedures they have been taught. The effect of the intervention is then evaluated in terms of the students' progress but usually little or no effort is made to ascertain whether the tutors' activity, the independent variable in such studies, actually conformed to the procedure they had been taught. The study by Johnson and Bailey (1974) represents an exception to this in that they were as interested in the behavior of the tutors as in the progress of the students with whom these tutors had worked. In order to obtain data for this analysis, they used trained observers who recorded relevant tutor behaviors such as giving praise for correct responses and correcting wrong answers. Because the tutoring took place in the school conference room, the observers were able to sit relatively unobtrusively at the end of a long table without interacting with either tutor or student during the session. Another person in that room at the same time was the experimenter who handed out the material at the beginning of the session, reviewed for the tutor what he was to do that day, and was available to answer any questions that arose. Occasionally she would give social reinforcement to both the tutors and the students. It is of course not known to what extent the presence of these adults affected the effectiveness of the cross-age peer tutoring.

The results of the Johnson and Bailey (1974) study showed that cross-age tutoring as here conducted by fifth-grade students is capable of teaching basic arithmetic skills to kindergarten children. As a group, the tutored children who, like the controls, had responded correctly to only 26 percent of the items on the pretest, showed an increase of 40 percentage points on the posttest where they got 66 percent of the items correct. The children in the control group, on the other hand, increased only 12 percentage points, getting 38 percent of the items correct. Proficiency tests given at two midpoints, one after approximately two weeks and another after approximately four weeks of tutoring, revealed that the largest gain (to 48 percent correct) was made at the beginning of the program. After that these gains were consolidated, increasing less precipitously over the next four or five weeks. These changes are shown in Figure 2.

Johnson and Bailey (1974) also present an analysis of the progress of each of the five children, showing a wide range of individual differences. One child mastered each of the tutored skills within the first 15 sessions, while another, who required many more repetitions to gain mastery, ended up being tutored in only three of the eight skills by the time the seven and one-half week project came to its end.

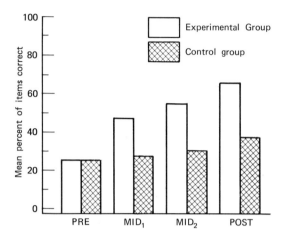

Figure 2. The mean percentage of items correct on the arithmetic tests at pretest, midpoint tests 1 and 2, and posttest. (Johnson & Bailey, 1974. Copyright by the Society for the Experimental Analysis of Behavior, Inc.)

When the observations of tutor behavior were compared with the progress made by the individual children, it emerged that the tutors of the children who had made the least progress were those who had given the least praise for correct responses. These tutors had praised fewer than 20 percent of their students' correct responses and one of them also had prompted his student considerably more often than had the other tutors. Johnson and Bailey (1974) correctly conclude that the tutor-training procedure they had used bears refinement. Instead of giving all tutors the same number of training sessions, it would probably be desirable to establish a criterion behavior that a tutor must reach before being permitted to engage in tutoring inasmuch as student progress appears to be a function of tutor competence.

Tutoring As a Learning Experience. What is the effect of a tutoring experience on those who are doing the tutoring? Johnson and Bailey (1974) reported the impression that participation in their tutoring program had been a positive and rewarding experience for the tutors. Data on this issue are provided by Dineen, Clark, and Risley (1977) who investigated the educational benefits a tutor derives from the experience of tutoring. They selected three children, ages 9 to 10 years, who attended an ungraded, open classroom for children with normal intelligence who were two years below grade level in reading and one year retarded in mathematics. The task of these three children was to tutor each other on lists of spelling words. An ingenious triadic design in which each of the three children took turns serving as tutor, being tutored, or remaining a control permitted a large number of comparisons over a short period of time.

Each of the children in the Dineen et al. (1977) study was given 20 to 30 minutes of training for the tutoring task which consisted of saying a word from the word list and having the tutee write it down and spell it. If the word was spelled and written correctly, the tutor praised the performance, recorded it, and proceeded to the next word. Misspelled words were to be corrected, spelled out by the tutor while the tutee wrote it down, and then spelled again, until both verbal and written spelling were correct. Any word that had not been spelled correctly on the first presentation was set aside for review at the end of the list. The adult teacher taught this tutoring procedure to each child, using modeling and role playing, until the child was able to carry it out consistently over several training trials.

Prior to the beginning of the tutoring, the three children were given a spelling test, covering 45 of the words to be used during training. This test was repeated one day after the last of eight tutoring sessions each of which lasted 20 minutes. The results showed that on 1 percent of the words on which they had been in the role of neither tutor nor tutee the children had become less accurate in their spelling. On those words that they had used as tutors they showed a gain of 47 percent in spelling accuracy, while on the words on which they themselves had been tutored the gain was 50 percent. Thus, as the investigators concluded, being tutor to a peer increased a child's spelling accuracy nearly as much as being tutored by a peer. The tutors' improvement may well have been a function of the fact that in the role of tutor a child listened to the verbal and examined the written version of each spelling word and frequently spelled a word as part of the correction procedure. In addition, the tutors may have been especially careful in evaluating their students' work because reinforcement for taking part in the tutorial session was contingent on the tutee's performance on a spelling test given at the end of each session.

Not only did the tutors learn nearly as much as the children whom they had tutored, thus making this kind of peer tutoring a beneficial method of individualizing education, but anecdotal reports from the children's teachers suggest that participation in the tutorial sessions promoted an increase in the children's cooperative social behaviors in other school settings and that they expressed a preference for tutoring over independent study. Meanwhile, the classroom teacher had more time for helping other students with academic problems because monitoring the tutoring took less time than individually checking each student's work. Whether these benefits would hold up once peer tutoring became a classroom routine or whether one is here dealing, at least in part, with the effect of novelty remains a topic for further investigation.

Recapitulation

Academic deficits, here largely exemplified by difficulties in the acquisition of reading, are among the targets of the interventions provided by behaviorally oriented psychologists whose focus on learning, unlearning, and relearning logically places learning difficulties within their scope. Defining reading as a response to the stimuli represented by the printed words leads one to inquire into the nature of available reinforcers. Remedial programs employ both verbal praise and tangible objects as reinforcers. Each has its advantages and disadvantages. A useful distinction can be made between arbitrary and natural reinforcers. In reading, the natural reinforcer is the information inherently available to the reader but for individuals who are not yet competent readers this reinforcer is not available. Arbitrary reinforcers must therefore be employed until the goal of the remediation is reached. Investigators have demonstrated that reading can be taught by approaching the task as one of discrimination learning, by using college students as tutors for individual children, and by having children tutor one another. This last approach has the distinct advantage that both tutor and tutee improve the skill on which they are working.

4

Language Deficits

LANGUAGE AS OPERANT BEHAVIOR

The remarkable human ability to communicate by what we call language has occasioned the development of a variety of theories and a good deal of mystique. We like to think of language as a uniquely human accomplishment and are, in fact, inclined to see it as the characteristic that defines the difference between human and nonhuman animals. It is thus not surprising that a conception of language as verbal operant behavior that follows the same principles of reinforcement as any other operant behavior, as Skinner (1957) has proposed, continues to be the source of much and often impassioned discussion. Surely, it is argued, "the human's gift of language" is qualitatively different from the rat's bar-press or the pigeon's disk-pecking. Highly sophisticated nativistic counter-theories are offered which propose an innate capacity for language that is independent of experience and unfolds as a part of human development (e.g., Chomsky, 1965).

From the standpoint of the clinician who encounters children who require special help in order to learn what other children seem to acquire as a "natural" aspect of their development, the issue of the nature of language reduces to the question: Which theory provides the best tools with which to help children who have not acquired any language or whose language is, in some way, deficient? Again, as was true in the case of reading difficulties, the issue is not how the skill is normally acquired but how a child who has failed to acquire the skill in the normal course of growing up can be helped to compensate for and overcome that deficit. In this pragmatic test, the principles of reinforcement are clearly superior to any other formulation that deals with the development of language.

The most extensive application of the view that language is a form of operant behavior is found in the work of O. Ivar Lovaas (1977) and his students and colleagues, who have sought to develop the language of profoundly impaired, autistic children in a project that was initiated in 1964. In a comprehensive summary of his approach, Lovaas (1977) points out that language acquisition entails two interrelated processes. The child must first learn to emit certain vocal responses. These are the sounds of our language, including the phonemes (vowels and consonants), the morphemes (words), which must be ordered in proper sequence into grammatical sentences. Since learning these components of language involves the elimination of incorrect responses and the strengthening of correct responses, the process is a form of *discrimination learning*. Soon after the child has learned to vocalize phonemes correctly and when these phonemes are combined into words, the second process begins. Here the task is to relate the words being formed to the objects or concepts for which they stand. That is, the child must learn the meaning of the words and sentences he or she is acquiring. There are two aspects to this: One has to do with the relation of the word or sentence to the internal or external stimulus that it expresses. The other aspect has to do with the effect the utterance has on the social environment. For example, the sight of an inaccessible ball and the presence of an adult will come to control the response, "I want that ball" only if the child has found in the past that these words result in the adult's complying with that request. We are dealing here with the stimulus function of the object in relation to the words and with the stimulus function of the words in relation to the consequence. Learning to associate the correct verbal response to a given stimulus and to its effect on the environment is again a form of discrimination learning. The child must learn that the sentence, "I want that bear" is not the correct response to the stimulus of a ball or that "I have that ball" will not result in the adult's taking the ball off the shelf and handing it to the child. It should be noted that if the adult, inferring from "I have that ball" that the boy wants the ball, were consistently to give him the ball in response to that sentence, the child could never learn correct usage. The adult must see to it that only the correct response is followed by reinforcement and such *differential reinforcement* in the context of discrimination learning forms the basis of the approach applied by the Lovaas group.

Steps in Language Training

Lovaas (1977) describes a series of programs (steps) in which his approach to language training for autistic children is organized. While these programs are arranged in a hierarchy from the easiest to the most difficult, there is no firm dividing line between them and many run concurrently as the child's progress continues. The following is merely a sketchy summary of these programs; they are described in considerable detail in the work (Lovaas, 1977) from which this is taken.

Program 1. With children who lack language altogether, training begins with the production of speech sounds or words. The vehicle for this is to have the teacher model the sound that the child is to imitate. In some instances it may even be necessary to precede this by teaching the child to imitate an adult (Hewett, 1965). A great deal of prompting and shaping enters into Program 1 which relies heavily on the use of continuous positive reinforcement and close physical contact. The child learns to match the verbal productions of others but at this level vocalizations are without meaning. Once the child can produce 10 recognizable words, Program 2 is begun and run concurrently with the continuation of Program 1 with the goal of developing a large range of complex verbal behaviors.

Program 2. Here the goal is to teach the child to use the words he or she has already learned and to produce them as labels for discrete events, such as everyday objects and activities. Once a few such labels are mastered, they are to be used to answer questions like, "What is it?," to state simple requests, and to respond to simple instructions.

Program 3. The child must now add labels for abstract concepts to the labels for objects and activities learned in the previous program. Pronouns, prepositions, time concepts, colors, shapes, and sizes are all abstractions in that they are related to many different objects which share the same quality. Among the terms to be taught in this program are also such concepts as fast and slow, more and less, same and different, as well as yes and no. Lovaas (1977) points out that in order to function at even the most minimal level in society, a child must know a large number of these abstract concepts. Yet it is these very concepts that are the most difficult to teach because they do not have concrete referents in the environment that could be used as a training stimulus. As a result, training on only one of these concepts requires from one to two hours of concentrated practice per day. With up to 10 trials per minute, this may add up to anywhere from 600 to 1200 trials on a single day.

Program 4. Progress in Programs 2 and 3 merges gradually into the task of Program 4 which Lovaas refers to as Conversation. Here the interaction between teacher and child becomes a verbal exchange in which questions are asked and answers are given. This begins with such simple exchanges as the teacher asking, "What's your name?" and the child responding, "Billy." Much later, such an exchange may take the form of the teacher's question about the child's experiences at school that day, leading to a detailed and lengthy recounting of the day's events, a transcript of which reads like a tale told by a typical child that age. But before that point can be reached, several other steps must be mastered.

Program 5. This is designed to teach the child to seek information, such as what is going to be served for dinner or when school will be over. At the same time this program aims at developing the skill of providing information in response to a question and learning to say, "I don't know." To accomplish this, Lovaas places the child in a three-person situation where Person A asks the child a question, for the answer to which the child has to turn to Person B. Once B has provided the answer, the child has to transmit the information back to A.

Program 6. This again is not a step that awaits completion of the earlier programs before it is initiated for it deals with the development of grammatical skills. This must start as early as the labeling training in Program 2 where, for example, singulars must be discriminated from plurals and it obviously continues during the conversation training of Program 4. Largely through modeling, drill, and correction, the teacher conveys to the child certain basic rules for how to combine words into grammatical sentences.

Program 7. Under an earlier heading (Program 4) mention was made of a child's ability to respond to a question about his experiences at school that day. This requires that the child can recall aspects of the past. It too is a skill that must be taught before a child can use it. Program 7 makes this instruction explicit. It begins by teaching the child to tell what had transpired just a few seconds before and leads, by gradual steps, to descriptions of the previous day. This skill permits a child to communicate with another person in an interesting fashion in that the other person can now find out about events he or she had not directly experienced. As such, it is an interpersonally enriching ability that makes the child a more interesting and rewarding person with whom to interact.

Program 8. Here one is concerned with helping the child learn to use language for making statements that are not the direct answer to a discrete question. Whereas earlier programs concentrated on getting the child to name or describe specific objects or events, the aim now is to use language in a more spontaneous fashion. To accomplish this, the teacher initiates a conversation with an open-ended question such as, "Tell me about yourself," prompting elaborations by asking, "What else?" By now, the tangible, arbitrary reinforcers such as food which were used in the early programs have long given way to the natural reinforcers that maintain the conversational use of language, namely the attentive interest and encouraging comments of the other person and that person's reciprocation with information of his or her own.

Program 9. This is a direct extension of the preceding program. Lovaas (1977) refers to it as Storytelling. Here the aim is to have the child communicate ideas that are not directly related to immediate and concrete stimuli but involve a combination of different experiences. Making up stories touches on fantasy and serves to express private ideas and images. It is the creative use of language and not all of the children with whom Lovaas and his colleagues worked had reached that level.

Outcome and Implications. The level of receptive and expressive speech reached by the autistic children treated by the Lovaas group seems closely related to the child's age when intervention is first begun and the nature of the child's verbal development at that point. As Lovaas, Young, and Newsom (1978) pointed out in a summary of this work, treatment of autistic children is likely to be most effective when work with them is started before they are 40 months of age. With such children, improvement occurs within the first year of treatment, covers the full range of social, affective, and intellectual behaviors, and appears to be quite permanent. With older children, on the other hand, and particularly those who are mute, progress is much slower and they rarely reach the highest level of language development. What is more, the effect of treatment is reversible unless the reinforcement contingency used during the treatment can be maintained in the child's posttreatment environment (Lovaas, Koegel, Simmons, & Long, 1973). In order to facilitate this maintenance of treatment effect and to enhance generalization across settings, the Lovaas group routinely teaches the child's parents to participate in the treatment program so that the skills the child learns in the specialized clinical setting can be practiced and reinforced at home where the skills must ultimately become a part of the child's behavioral repertoire.

Following the detailed explication of the language development programs he had evolved while working with a number of older autistic children, Lovaas (1977) discusses some of the implications of his work. He points out that while his group had succeeded in teaching expressive and receptive language to varying levels of sophistication, they were disappointed in that the children did not seem to use language to "control their own behavior." This is a behaviorist's circumlocution of the question whether language helped the child to be aware of himself as a person; whether he became intellectually curious, whether, in ordinary formulation, language enabled the child to think. For the children with whom this language training program had been developed, the answer to this question appears to be generally negative and Lovaas wonders whether the programs he and his team had evolved were inadequate to that task. This, in turn, leads him to speculate about what it is that reinforces the covert use of speech (i.e., "thought") which occurs at an extremely high rate in the normal human, seemingly in the absence of extrinsic reinforcers. It may be, he ponders, that self-directed thought is reinforced by its self-stimulatory function, a function that might be filling an innate need of the nervous system for fairly continuous stimulation. Conceivably, the self-stimulatory rhythmic rocking, twirling, or hand-flapping so typical of autistic children is the nonverbal child's alternative to the self-stimulation others achieve through the use of internal language. To follow these considerations would lead us far beyond the topic of language deficits and into realms where speculations are plentiful and research-based data scarce.

Echolalia

Profoundly disturbed children sometimes engage in a form of verbal behavior that, although employing real words in appropriate combinations, fails to serve as a basis of communication. Such a child, for example, may respond to the question, "Do you want some milk?" with "Do you want some milk?" or "Want some milk." This is echolalia. It may take one of two forms. In immediate echolalia the child repeats all or part of the phrase as soon as it is heard. In delayed echolalia the child repeats a phrase after a considerable interval. In neither case do the words serve the function of communicating with a listener although parents or caretakers sometimes try to guess what the child might mean and to respond accordingly.

While echolalia generally fails to communicate and must thus be viewed as speech and not language, the fact that a child who engages in such behavior is using words permits one to begin a language training program several steps above the rudimentary teaching of speech sounds and individual words. Furthermore, as Harris (1975) observed in her extensive review of studies dealing with the teaching of language to nonverbal children, this is more easily accomplished with a child who is echolalic than with one who is totally mute.

As is usually the case when a description of observed behavior comes to be used as a label for children who engage in that behavior, it is likely that so-called echolalic children do not form a homogeneous group. An analysis of echolalic speech conducted by Goren, Romanczyk, and Harris (1977) revealed that it is not a unidimensional response pattern but varies as a function of the individual child and of the antecedents and consequences of the behavior. It is not unusual, for example, for a child to use primitive expressive language at one time but to resort to echolalia at another. What are the variables that control this behavior? This question has not only theoretical but also practical import because as long as a child merely echoes the teacher's instructions it will be difficult or impossible to establish functional language.

A valuable contribution to the understanding of immediate echolalia in psychotic children was furnished by Carr, Schreibman, and Lovaas (1975) who conducted a functional analysis of this behavior. They started with the assumption that echolalic speech represents a general response strategy to which these children resort in situations where they are incapable of producing a more appropriate response. Since echolalia occurs both in response to questions and in response to instructions, Carr et al. (1975) suggest that the child's strategy is, "When you can respond, do; when you can't, echo the stimulus."

In order to put their assumption to a test, Carr et al. (1975) studied five echolalic and five normal children by presenting them with neutral and discriminative stimuli. Neutral stimuli were defined as those to which no appropriate response can be made, like the nonsense words "Tas poo grot." Discriminative stimuli, on the other hand, were sentences that set the occasion for an appropriate response. Five of these discriminative stimuli called for a verbal response, such as the question "What's your name?" and five called for a motoric response, such as the instruction "Clap your hands." Each of these 10 discriminative stimuli was matched with a neutral stimulus on the basis of the number of words in the phrase and the distribution of syllables among the words. "What's your name?" for example was paired with "Gin ra moo." All sounds used in the neutral stimuli were already in the children's expressive repertoire.

The study proceeded in two phases. The first was designed to assess the amount of echolalia that the children produced in response to the two kinds of stimuli. Each child was tested in two sessions during each of which 40 stimuli were presented. The stimuli for the verbal response tasks were presented during one session, those for the nonverbal response tasks during the other, with the sequence counterbalanced across children. In confirmation of the investigators' hypothesis, the psychotic children tended to echo the neutral nonsense stimuli while responding appropriately to the discriminative stimuli. The normal children, on the other hand, (who ranged in age from 2.1 to 3.7 years) typically echoed neither type of stimulus, usually remaining silent or asking "What?" when a neutral stimulus was presented. Figure 3 presents these results in graphic form and highlights some interesting exceptions from the general trend of the data.

In the left half of Figure 3, which shows the results for the nonverbal response tasks, it can be seen that one of the psychotic children, Gary, echoed the neutral stimuli (hatched bars) only 80 percent of the time while the other four responded with echolalia 100 percent of the time. The record showed that when Gary did not echo the nonsense sentence, he simply remained silent. Ruby is the other exception, for unlike the other four psychotic children, she not only echoed all of the neutral stimuli but also 50 percent of the discriminative stimuli. Ruby, it turns out, functioned in her everyday environment at a level markedly below that of the other children. While the others were able to respond appropriately to such simple commands as "Pick up your clothes," Ruby obeyed only the most rudimentary requests, such as "Come here" or "Sit down." For her, it seems, half of the instructions for the motoric tasks were, in effect, nonsense words to which she responded in the same way as she did to the meaningless neutral stimuli.

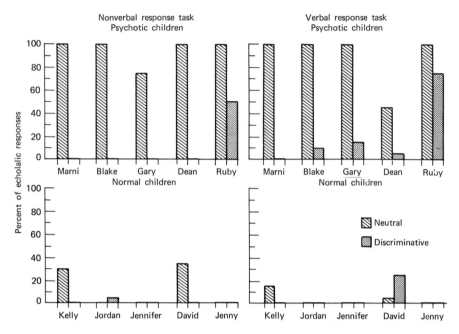

Figure 3. Percentage of echolalic responses for the psychotic and normal children on the non-verbal response task (left half) and verbal response task (right half) as a function of type of stimulus presented. The hatched bars are the data for the neutral stimuli and the filled bars are the data for the discriminative stimuli. (Carr, Schreibman, & Lovaas, 1975. Copyright by Plenum Publishing Corporation.)

When one turns to the right half of Figure 3, which displays the data for the verbal response tasks, neutral stimuli are again echoed 100 percent of the time by all children except Dean, who simply remained silent 55 percent of the time. Ruby again echoed a large proportion (75 percent) of the discriminative stimuli but now she is joined by three of the other children who also engage in some echolalia to these, for us, meaningful questions. The fact that these children had not echoed the stimuli for the nonverbal response tasks would seem to reflect the phenomenon that language-impaired children usually have better receptive than expressive language. They are able to respond to such instructions as "Touch your head" although they are unable to respond to such questions as "How are you?" If, as these investigators had speculated, echolalia is a strategy for responding to verbal stimuli to which impaired children have no other response, then these data may mean that to Blake, Gary, Dean, and Ruby some of the discriminative (meaningful) stimuli were the functional equivalent of neutral (nonsense) sentences. Incomprehensibility of words, as Carr et al. (1975) point out, may well be one determinant of echolalic speech.

Turning now to the data for the normal children, shown in the bottom half of Figure 3, we see that they gave echolalic responses to only a very small percentage of stimuli. Jennifer and Jenny echoed none of the stimuli, while Kelly and David echoed some of the neutral stimuli. David and, to a minimal extent, Jordan also echoed discriminative stimuli. It turns out that Kelly and David were 25 and 26 months old, respectively, and as such were the youngest of the five normal children. The other three ranged in age from 36 to 44 months. Carr, Schreibman, and Lovaas (1975)) cite reports that suggest that occasional echoic utterances are a normal aspect of early speech development. If this is the case, the behavior of Kelly and David would not be unexpected. Indeed, one might speculate that psychotic children who are echolalic when they are 10 to 15 years old, as were those in this study, function at the level of very young normal children, having failed to develop beyond that stage.

Before presenting the second of the two experiments conducted by Carr, Schreibman, and Lovaas (1975), it may be well to consider for a moment the complicated issue of the meaningfulness of language. How does one know whether a sentence spoken to a child has meaning to that child or, conversely, how does one know whether a child who utters a given sentence knows the meaning of what he or she has said? In the terminology of the operant approach to verbal behavior, meaning is a stimulus function that can only be inferred by observing behavior. If I say to a girl, "Sit down" and she responds by sitting down, I can assume that she has understood the meaning of my words. If I ask a boy, "What time is it?" and he tells me, "Three o'clock," I infer that he knows the meaning of my question. In both instances, my words function as stimuli that control specific responses, motoric in the case of the girl, verbal in the case of the boy. As with other inferences, trouble ensues when the child fails to respond or responds by echoing my words. Does that reflect that the child does not know the meaning of what I have said? Or could it be that the girl prefers not to sit down; that the boy does not know what time it is? In the absence of a verbal response from the child, such as "I don't want to sit down" or "What do you mean?" or "What did you say?" or "I don't know," I have no idea why I did not receive a response to my request. There is a difference between not knowing the meaning of a question and not knowing the answer to the question, but psychotic and other language-impaired children cannot tell us. All we know is that, for some children, much of our verbal behavior is not discriminative for an appropriate response; this may have many reasons. These reasons would have to be investigated separately before the answer could be known. An investigation along this line was the burden of the second phase of the study conducted by Carr et al. (1975).

Carr, Schreibman, and Lovaas (1975) reasoned that if echolalia represents psychotic children's response to verbal stimuli for which their repertoire does not contain an appropriate response, then teaching them an appropriate response to these stimuli should elminate the echolalic response. Put another way, if such children give echolalic responses to incomprehensible words, making these words comprehensible should make the echolalic response unnecessary.

Three psychotic children who gave echoic responses to neutral stimulus phrases participated in the second phase of the Carr et al. (1975) experiment. Two of these children, Blake and Marni, had also participated in the first study; the third child, Jimmy, aged 9½ years, had not been involved in the previous work. The stimuli were divided into those to which a verbal response would be appropriate and those to which a nonverbal behavior was going to be expected. Neutral stimuli, defined as those to which the child had no appropriate response, differed for the three children. For Marni these were the same nonsense sentences used in the first experiment but for the two boys they were genuine questions or requests to which they had not responded appropriately on five consecutive trials during preliminary testing. They were such phrases as "What is a rose?" "What is baseball?" and "Feel the cloth."

Once it had been established that the child gave echolalic responses to each of the neutral stimuli, training sessions began during which the child was taught an appropriate response. In the case of Marni, for whom neutral stimuli were nonsense words, an appropriate response was arbitrarily defined. Thus, she was taught to say "juice" to the phrase "min dar snick" and to tap the table when the experimenter said, "blat ver shot." For Blake and Jimmy, for whom the neutral stimuli were real phrases ("What is a rose?"), the appropriate response exists in the language ("Flower"). The children were taught these responses by prompting and the delivery of reinforcement in the form of praise and food. The prompts were gradually faded and reinforcement became intermittent as training progressed.

The experimenters employed a multiple baseline design, training on one stimulus while leaving the other stimuli alone until responses to the stimulus being trained reached a criterion for learning. This design provided a control for the effect of the training procedure. As can be seen in Figure 4 which shows the data for Marni, echolalic responses did not cease until she had been trained to give an "appropriate" response to the neutral stimuli. On two phrases ("gin ra moo" and "fop vit gerpy") this girl received no training and whenever these were presented she continued to respond with echolalia while on those stimuli for which she had been trained to give a specific response she rarely resorted to that behavior. In the few instances when she did use echolalia again, she received additional training (indicated by arrows). It is of interest that the appropriate responses generalized to different experimenters who had not been involved in the training and were naive as to the conditions (indicated by asterisks).

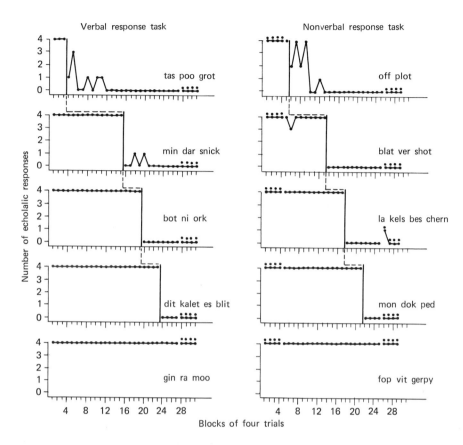

Figure 4. Number of echolalic responses made by Marni to several phrases before and after training over blocks of four trials. The left half of the figure presents the data taken from the verbal response task and the right half presents data from the nonverbal response task. Arrows beneath abscissa show temporal position of later training sessions. Data collected by naive experimenters are indicated with asterisks. (Carr, Schreibman, & Lovaas, 1975. Copyright by Plenum Publishing Corporation.)

Similar results were obtained with Blake whose training had aimed at teaching him such responses as to say "Flower" in answer to the question "What is a rose?" and to feel a cloth when given that instruction. Jimmy, who was the most profoundly disturbed child in the entire series, also learned to give appropriate verbal responses instead of echoes to the questions on which he had been trained. Nonetheless, on one of the nonverbal tasks ("Indicate the eraser") he would touch the eraser *and* echo the instruction after first having made the appropriate nonverbal response alone during four test trials. Here the experimenters assume that they had inadvertently reinforced the combination, echo-and-touch, underscoring the great care one must exercise in a training program of this type.

Jimmy's mixed result notwithstanding, the experiment by Carr et al. (1975) demonstrated that children who echo a stimulus phrase can be taught to give up that inappropriate response when they are taught to make an appropriate response. It should be stressed that the children in this study were at no time presented with negative consequences when they echoed a response. That response dropped to zero frequency as soon as the alternative response had been acquired so that it seems that echolalia and appropriate verbal behavior are mutually exclusive response classes. When one occurs, the other does not and vice versa. The clinical implication of this finding is that when children display echolalia this behavior can be eliminated through teaching them appropriate alternative behaviors via positive reinforcement; that timeout or other forms of punishment are unnecessary. In view of this, one might question whether it is efficient to begin language training of echolalic children by using their echolalia as a starting point, a procedure that had been employed in a pioneering study by Risley and Wolf (1967).

Carr, Schreibman, and Lovaas (1975) had undertaken their investigation on the assumption that echolalia is a response to verbal stimuli that are incomprehensible or meaningless to the child. While they are careful to stress that their experiments should not be construed as a test of that hypothesis, it would seem to have much merit. On the other hand, one still does not know whether a child's echolalic response is the equivalent of "I don't understand," or "I can't do (or say) it," or of "I don't know." Not being able to make an appropriate response may be due to the fact that the words being presented do not have a stimulus function or to the stimulus not being discriminative for the specific response society considers appropriate. In order to bring an echolalic girl's verbal behavior to the point where it is like that of a normal child, one would have to begin by teaching her to say "I don't know" to all questions that she could not answer and "What?" to all commands that she could not carry out. Carr et al. (1975) had suggested this approach and Schreibman and Carr (1978) as well as Tucker, O'Dell, and Suib (1978) have demonstrated that it is feasible. Beyond this stage, however, one would also have to teach such a child to discriminate between questions to which she does not know the answer ("I don't know") and those she does not understand ("What do you mean?"). One would further have to teach her to differentiate between commands she does not understand, where "What?" would be an appropriate response, and those she cannot carry out to which "I can't do it" would be more appropriate than "What?" All of which of course underscores how difficult it is to establish functional language in a child who, for whatever reason, has missed acquiring that ability in the normal course of development.

A Nonverbal Approach

Language is a means of communication but the verbal mode is only one of several ways that permit communication. From a developmental perspective, in fact, nonverbal communication precedes verbal language both phylo- and onto-genetically. If one assumes that the behavior of profoundly impaired children, like those with early infantile autism, represents a developmental disability then teaching language to such children might well have to begin at a nonverbal level. The work of deVilliers and Naughton (1974) stands as an example of such an approach, although their reason for using it was somewhat different.

Working with two language-deficient, autistic children deVilliers and Naughton (1974) used a so-called particle language to teach the rudiments of communication. This approach permits the teacher to retain strict control over the alternatives presented to the child, thus facilitating errorless learning. It was this consideration that led these investigators to adapt for their use the nonverbal symbol language used by Premack (1970) in his work with a chimpanzee. The medium of communication was a metal-covered display board on which magnetized particles could be affixed. These particles, each with a different color and design, were labeled with printed words which, when properly combined on the board, could be used to form such telegraphic sentences as, "Joe give pretzel Adam" or "Who has cracker?"

The children with whom deVilliers and Naughton (1974) worked were labeled autistic but they had, at other times, also been diagnosed as brain damaged. The older boy, Adam, was nine years old and his speech consisted primarily of echolalia. He engaged in such autistic behaviors as twirling, spinning, toe-walking, head-banging, and other forms of self-stimulation. The younger child, Bobby, was six years old. He had no speech other than an infantile babbling and while he did not engage in such atypical behavior as Adam, he would spend most of his day running or walking around the ward without an apparent aim. Also unlike Adam, who was generally attentive, Bobby was highly distractible.

Working with one child at a time for two 15-minute sessions over a period of about nine months, the investigators sought to teach the boys to communicate by means of the particle board. In the early stages of training, the experimenter would place a sentence on the board, leaving blank one space that the child was to fill in with a word selected from among five or six available choices. For example, when the examiner ("Joe") held up a small pretzel and displayed the phrase, "Joe give _____ Adam," the child was to select the word pretzel from among six names of edibles that were displayed on the board just above the incomplete sentence. When the child had placed the correct word in the blank space, the examiner would present a pretzel to the child and read the completed sentence aloud. Adam would echo the spoken sentence and he was soon able to "read" the sentences without the examiner's prompt so that reinforcement could be made contingent on the completion of the display plus the appropriate vocalization. With this procedure, Adam was able to advance from simple requests to simple questions and equally simple answers. By the time the project drew to an end he could verbalize such sentences in the absence of the particles, thus being able to produce and comprehend four-term statements where he had previously produced no more than a two-term utterance in spontaneous speech.

The work with Bobby did not progress this far. He needed considerably more trials at each stage before reaching the criterion of 80 percent correct responses in two successive sessions and he did not get beyond the stages of simple requests and descriptions. As had been observed with other autistic children (Lovaas, Koegel, Simmons, & Long, 1973), the total absence of speech, even to the exclusion of echolalia, makes the development of language extremely difficult.

The use of a particle language in training language-deficient children would seem like a complicated detour to verbal communciation but it has several advantages over the more usual manner of language training. If one remembers that children with severe language impairment or a total absence of language form a heterogeneous group, it stands to reason that a therapist's armamentarium must include a variety of methods and approaches. A symbol language, either in the form just described or like the sign language Gardner and Gardner (1969) used to communicate with a chimpanzee, represents one such alternative. Another advantage is the fact that the particles that are physically manipulated on a display board require that the child pay close attention to the behavior of the other person. With a visual display it is easier to monitor and thus to reinforce attentive behavior than it is when the stimuli are limited to the auditory sphere where one cannot tell whether the child is listening. Yet another advantage, pointed out by deVilliers and Naughton (1974) lies in the fact that the concrete stimuli on the display board remain present for constant reference so that the need to remember what the teacher has said is not a handicap for children who might have difficulties with immediate memory or attention. In addition, the experimenter can control the alternatives available for the required answers. This may be the greatest advantage of the particle approach to language training because it facilitates errorless learning. If, as was the case with Bobby, the child has difficulty selecting the correct word from among several choices, the experimenter can remove all but the correct choice from the board or move the correct choice directly above the blank space thereby making an error nearly impossible and guaranteeing an occasion in which reinforcement can be presented. The situation can then be made gradually more complex and cues can be faded until the child has reached the desired criterion. As deVilliers and Naughton (1974) pointed out, the degree to which the procedures are errorless depends on the ingenuity of the instructor.

Extending Rudimentary Speech

Language impairment can take many forms. A few children are totally mute, others resort to echolalia, and some possess a rudimentary repertoire of speech. With the latter, the therapeutic task is to expand this repertoire with the goal of developing age-appropriate language. Wheeler and Sulzer (1970) reported on their work with a speech-deficient 8-year-old boy who spoke in what they called "telegraphic" English which was characterized by his leaving out most articles and auxiliary verbs. At one time this boy had been echolalic and he had been variously labeled as brain damaged, autistic, and retarded. After two years of speech training, he had gained a repertoire of a large number of individual words but failed to combine these into complete sentences.

The primary purpose of the study conducted by Wheeler and Sulzer (1970) was to examine whether language training based on operant principles would generalize from specific responses thus taught to other responses that had not been the object of training. This question has important theoretical implications. It is improbable that in the process of normal language acquisition every combination of verbal responses that eventually becomes a part of a person's language has at one time been emitted in the context of a reinforcement contingency, thus having been explicitly taught. Some form of generalization has to be taking place if the acquisition of language follows the principles of operant learning. Similarly, a language training program for impaired children that is based on operant principles would have to depend on such generalization if it were ever to reach its goal of establishing normal language.

The generalization involved in language acquisition is a special case, known as *generalization of a functional response class*. A functional response class is composed of a number of discrete responses that bear the same functional relationship to the environment. The existence of a functional response class can be demonstrated when all responses in the class show the effect of a consequence that is brought to bear in relation to only some members of the class. Physical aggression is an example of a functional response class. It contains such components as hitting, kicking, scratching, and biting, yet under certain circumstances it can be demonstrated that when one of these components is placed on an extinction schedule, the frequency of the other components will also be reduced. Imitation is another example of such a response class as Baer and Sherman (1964) demonstrated when they showed that if one reinforces a child for imitating some of a model's behavior, the child will also begin to imitate other aspects of the model's behavior without ever having been explicitly reinforced for imitating these. In the case of language, aspects of grammar and syntax can be construed as functional response classes. The meaning of adjectival inflections, for example, need not be trained for every word in the vocabulary, but a child having been trained to use these correctly on some exemplars will generalize this correctly to words on which no such training had taken place (Baer & Guess, 1971; Schumaker & Sherman, 1970).

Since the boy with whom Wheeler and Sulzer (1970) worked had a well-established imitative response, this could be used in the training program they sought to test. They selected a series of pictures to serve as stimuli. Each showed a person engaged in a specific activity. The boy's vocabularly contained the words needed to describe each picture but in the baseline phase of the study he failed to put these together to form appropriate descriptions, such as "The man is smoking a pipe." Seven such pictures served as training stimuli, two were used to test for generalization during training, and six were reserved to perform a before-and-after test for generalization.

The procedure, here reproduced in somewhat condensed form, consisted of the experimenter's presenting a picture and asking, "What do you see?" Except during baseline, where no instructions or reinforcement were given, the experimenter would provide prompts and reinforce correct responses with tokens. No prompting or reinforcement followed the two pictures used for the generalization test which was interspersed between training trials. An examination of the data reveals that as correct responding increased to the training pictures, correct responses to the generalization pictures, for which no training had been provided, increased correspondingly, though at a somewhat lower level. When the six pictures that the boy had seen only during the baseline phase were presented again 30 sessions later, his responses revealed substantial improvement in the ability to produce correct sentences descriptive of the pictures' content. Wheeler and Sulzer (1970) interpreted their results as evidence for the generalization of a complex verbal response and concluded that it is feasible to use an operant approach to teach language to a speech deficient child without having to give training on every specific linguistic response that the child will eventually employ, to establish, what linguists call, generative language.

Generative Language. The question whether verbal responses taught to one set of stimuli would transfer to other stimuli also concerned Stevens-Long, Schwarz, and Bliss (1976). Following an earlier study conducted by Stevens-Long and Rasmussen (1974) that had demonstrated the feasibility of using operant procedures to teach an autistic child to use compound sentences, the later work was specifically addressed to the question of generalization. The investigators chose a 6-year-old autistic boy whose speech consisted almost entirely of partial sentences and echolalia. The stimuli were a series of commercially available teaching pictures that depict two or more people engaged in a variety of easily identified activities. Some of these pictures were used as training stimuli, others as tests of generalization.

There was a total of 31 half-hour teaching sessions, held at least twice a week just before lunch. During the first two sessions (Step 1) a baseline was obtained of the boy's spontaneous production of simple and compound sentences in response to the presentation of a stimulus card and the statement, "Look at the picture. What do you see?" No prompts were provided and any response, regardless of content, was reinforced with praise, a pat on the head, or other social reinforcement.

During the next seven sessions (Step 2) the boy was trained to produce simple sentences to describe the elements of stimulus cards (e.g., "The boy is playing ball. The children are running."). This was accomplished by having the teacher model correct responses and reinforcing these with bites of food and verbal praise. A correct response was defined as the reproduction of the complete sentence with all grammatical elements in proper sequence. A form of time-out was used when the boy failed to imitate a prompt. It consisted of the teacher placing the stimulus card face down and turning away for 10 seconds. This procedure was apparently effective since the production of correct, unprompted responses rose from 10 percent in Step 1 to 75 percent during Step 2 (see Figure 5).

In order to test whether the teaching procedure was responsible for the increased production of simple sentences, baseline conditions were reinstated during the next five sessions (Step 3). Because correct responses fell to 23 percent during this condition, with rapid and complete recovery in the next five sessions (Step 4, when the intervention was once again in effect), it seems that the teaching was indeed the critical variable. During session 18 the first probe for generalization was introduced. It consisted of the interspersed presentation of the seven pictures on which no training had ever been given. A correct response to such a picture was defined as a complete sentence that was grammatically correct and semantically relevant. As shown by the open triangle in Figure 5, the boy gave correct responses to 50 percent of these generalization probes.

Up to this point, the child had never produced a compound sentence to any of the pictures (e.g., "The boy is playing ball and the children are running."). In session 19 Step 5 was begun. It entailed the teaching of such sentences by prompting the boy to say "and" between the two simple sentences that described the picture. By the sixth session, correct production of such compound sentences had risen to 78 percent and the boy produced no further simple sentences in response to training pictures. During the final sessions, compound sentences were correctly produced 91 percent of the time. Generalization probes (shown as closed triangles in Figure 5) revealed that the boy was also able to make correct compound sentences to pictures on which he had not received any training.

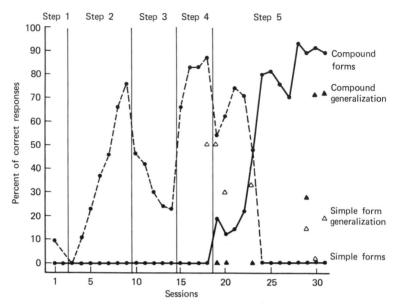

Figure 5. Percentage of correct unprompted responses for training cards and generalization cards for Steps 1 through 5. (Stevens-Long, Schwarz, & Bliss, 1976. Copyright by Academic Press, Inc.)

The controlled and carefully documented training sessions had clearly shown "that differential reinforcement can produce the generative use of simple and compound sentence structures, i.e., that with training, a child can come to use simple and compound structures to describe novel stimuli as well as stimuli directly trained" (Stevens-Long, Schwarz, & Bliss, 1976, p. 403). While these authors do not present objective data for this, they also report that this boy used the new sentences on which he was being trained in both classroom and playground conversations. During the last phase of the training, his teachers reported that he had begun to describe everyday objects and events in compound sentences. That, of course, is the ultimate test of generalization. Effective language training must be shown not only to generalize from one set of pictures to another set of pictures but also from the training sessions to everyday life. Documentation of this is difficult to obtain because it requires the introduction of observers into the typical, everyday situation.

Planned Generalization

As in every form of treatment, generalization from the treatment setting to the child's natural environment must be a planned aspect of the intervention. When a child has learned some phrases that have a high degree of social utility in that they elicit reinforcing responses from people to whom they are addressed, such speech has a high probability of generalizing beyond the immediate training situation. It is therefore important to include such phrases as early as possible in a language training program. Among these phrases are simple requests which people to whom they are addressed are highly likely to meet, inquiries that are easily answered, and greetings which most people will return (Stokes, Baer, & Jackson, 1974). Another means of facilitating generalization, as Harris (1975) has pointed out, is to prime key persons in the child's natural environment, such as the parents, to reinforce appropriate responses at home and in the various places the child visits so that the newly acquired responses do not remain specific to the stimuli present in the original training situation. On the other hand, where a problem is present in the classroom it is best to conduct treatment in the classroom rather than in a different locale from where the treatment effect would then have to generalize to the classroom. In such instances the teacher becomes a crucial auxiliary therapist. Such an approach was demonstrated by Bauermeister and Jemail (1975) in the case of a child with so-called *elective mutism*.

Unlike the language problems of autistic and retarded children discussed thus far which represent a skill deficit, elective mutism is a performance deficit in that the child fails to emit verbal behavior only under specific stimulus conditions. The boy treated by Bauermeister and Jemail (1975) is a case in point for he spoke freely at home with members of his family, but remained totally silent in school where he would address neither his teacher nor his peers. Intervention was designed to be carried out by the boy's teachers in the classroom in such a manner that it would not interfere with normal classroom activity. After preliminary observations, four behaviors were selected as targets for the therapy program. These were hand-raising, answering questions from the teacher, reading aloud, and completing classroom assignments. Treatment was carried out by the homeroom teacher and the English teacher and consisted of four phases. During Phase I, baseline data were obtained by having the teachers record the occurrence of any of the target behaviors. In Phase II, the teachers were instructed to encourage active class participation and to reinforce the boy with praise for the occurrence of any target behaviors or any reasonable approximations thereof. Because reliability checks revealed that the teachers were not being consistent in praising the occurrence of the target behaviors, more specific criteria were established for the third phase. The homeroom teacher was now asked to set goals for each class period, to give social reinforcement for each target behavior every time it was emitted, and to award the boy a star at the end of the class period if he had met the specified goal.

At this point in the treatment, the child's parents were brought into the plan in that for every 15 stars the boy brought home, he was given a "super star" by his mother. For three such big stars a back-up reinforcer was established; it took the form of a bicycle. While all this was going on, the English teacher continued the Phase II contingencies. Only with the beginning of Phase IV did the English teacher also introduce the procedures that had been followed in the homeroom during Phase III. This multiple baseline design enabled the investigators to demonstrate the effectiveness of the more systematic Phase III. After this program had been carried out for approximately 20 school days, the boy's behavior showed dramatic changes. He now raised his hand when questions were addressed to the group, answered questions from the teachers, and read aloud whenever asked to do so. His grades improved, he requested help instead of sitting passively when unable to complete a task, and his peer interactions during recess increased considerably. Follow-up observations one year later revealed that the boy had maintained his increased verbal communication in the classroom despite the fact that he now had five different teachers for each of his fourth-grade subjects.

As Sanok and Ascione (1979) pointed out in their review of behavioral interventions in childhood elective mutism, the study by Bauermeister and Jemail (1975) shares with similar work in this area a number of methodological shortcomings that limit the conclusions one might draw from it. Like many other case reports, this one lacks the refinements one would demand from a more rigorous research study. Interobserver reliability data, for example, are available only for the hand-raising behavior. Nonetheless, Bauermeister and Jemail's case does demonstrate that when treatment takes place in the settng where the problem is manifested the issue of generalization from treatment to real-life setting becomes moot.

Recapitulation

The verbal behavior we call language follows the principles of all other behavior. They can thus be applied in efforts to overcome the language deficits often manifested by profoundly impaired children such as those called autistic or mentally retarded. These efforts usually proceed from the paradigm of discrimination learning and make use of differential reinforcement. The steps used in such a program were outlined and the outcome of the program was examined. Language deficits can take a variety of forms, some children being totally mute while others will parrot the words they have heard someone else say, a behavior called echolalia. Such echoing can be used as a starting-point in a language training program but a detailed functional analysis of this behavior reveals that the echo is emitted by a child when he or she has no other, more adaptive response available. Once more adaptive responses have been taught, they can be shown to displace the echolalia. One approach to teaching language, deserving further exploration, begins with a non-verbal form of communication via signs or symbols. These have the advantage over words that their presentation can be standardized and controlled. Beyond the rudimentary speech that can be established by teaching specific words, the learning of a functional language requires that such linguistic rules as those of grammar and syntax must be generalized over a wide range of exemplars. It has been demonstrated that syntax operates as a functional response class that does indeed generalize beyond the specific word combination on which a child may have been trained. Another generalization that is essential if the child is to be able to use the language established in a specialized treatment setting involves the transfer of the learned behavior from that setting to the natural environment. Such generalization must be planned as part of the treatment program and it can sometimes be facilitated if the treatment takes place directly in the child's natural environment.

5

Deficits in Attention

THE CONSTRUCT "ATTENTION"

Cognitive processes, whether they be memory, information processing, or attention, are constructs whose existence can only be inferred by observing behavior. It can be argued whether one such construct is preferable to another and one can question whether constructs contribute anything to the study of behavior. Ultimately, these issues must be resolved in terms of the usefulness of a construct; whether, like a theory, it permits one to generate questions that can be put to the empirical test and whether it enables one to order disparate facts into coherent formulation. From this heuristic perspective the construct *attention* has shown some merit and it is on this basis that it will be used in the following.

Attention is a particularly useful construct when one seeks to analyze a child's failure to emit an expected response. Suppose a child has been instructed to make a response when a given signal appears on a display panel and this child is then observed to make that response when the signal is presented. The simplest way to describe what has been observed is to state that the response was under the control of the stimulus. This avoids inferences that invoke internal constructs though it begs the question how the functional relationship between stimulus and response came to be established. Such an inference would be involved if one were to reason that the signal served as a discriminative stimulus because the child attended to it since without such attention the response would not have taken place. Attention is then viewed as a link or mediator between stimulus and response; it is a mediational construct. Whether to invoke such a construct in the situation we have described is largely a matter of theoretical predilection.

Take now the situation in which a child has been given the same instruction but when the signal appeared no response was forthcoming; the stimulus did not control the response. In fact, the signal did not seem to serve the function of a stimulus. What happened? Could it be that the signal was too weak or indistinct; that the child had not understood or not remembered the instructions or that the child was not capable of emitting the response because it was too difficult? Could it be that the child did not find it worthwhile to make the response, did not feel like following the instructions, wanted to annoy the experimenter by being unresponsive? To say merely that the stimulus failed to control the response makes it very difficult to decide what steps to take in order to change the child's behavior so that the stimulus will indeed control the response on future occasions. In order to plan an intervention, such as treatment, response failure must be analyzed, not merely described, and for such an analysis constructs like attention can be very useful guides.

In the foregoing example, one must first ascertain that the child can indeed understand the instructions, that the signal is in a perceptible range, and that the response is within the child's capacity. One must then make sure that sufficient incentives in terms of response consequences (reinforcers) are available. If all of these requirements are met and the response is still not emitted in a consistently predictable fashion, it helps to ask whether the child is attending to the signal.

Let us now take the situation in which the child is presented with one of two different stimuli, such as an arrow pointing up and an arrow pointing down, with the instruction to press a button only when the downward-pointing arrow appears. In other words, the child must discriminate between the two arrows and learn to make the response to only one of them. It is a case of discrimination learning. If the child has difficulty learning this discrimination, makes the response to the wrong stimulus or to either of the stimuli indiscriminately, what is going on? After again disposing of questions about stimulus quality, response capacity, motivation, and comprehension of instructions, it is useful to construe the problem as one involving the child's failure to attend to the distinctive feature (the position of the arrows' point) that differentiates the two stimuli. Not only must the child be attending to the appearance of the stimulus but once it has appeared, attention must be selectively deployed (focused on) the position of the point; is it on top or is it at bottom of the vertical line?

This focusing of attention on the distinctive feature of a stimulus is called *selective attention*. Since almost all learning is a matter of discrimination learning, between telling the right stimulus from the wrong stimulus or the right response from the wrong response, the ability to deploy attention selectively is an exceedingly important capacity and any deficit in this skill will materially interfere with a child's ability to benefit from opportunities to learn.

The Development of Attention

If selective attention is conceived of as a skill, it is possible to examine how this skill develops and to what extent it can be learned or a deficit in it overcome. A review of the available research on the development of selective attention reveals that there are important changes with age in the ways children regulate and direct their own attention (Pick, Frankel, and Hess, 1975). One way of conceptualizing this development and of relating delays in such development to certain psychological disorders has been presented by Ross (1976). According to this formulation, the very young child attends to stimuli primarily in terms of their salient characteristics, such as novelty and movement. Once their attention has been "captured" by a given stimulus, infants seem to remain "riveted" to it but even at this early age one finds individual differences in the degree to which this *overexclusive attention* is maintained. With increasing age, the mode of attending to the environment undergoes gradual changes. By the time a child enters school he or she will be attending to a great many different aspects of the environment. One can now speak of *overinclusive attention* in the sense that the child seems to attend to many more aspects of the stimulus field than are necessary for efficient coping with situational demands. With continuing development and exposure to teaching, the child learns that stimuli such as letters can be differentiated by focusing on the distinctive features of similar objects (Gibson, 1975). At this point, the child will be actively directing attention at selected aspects of the environment in such a way that irrelevant and redundant features are ignored, thereby making processing of information highly efficient. *Selective attention* has now emerged in its mature fashion, permitting the young person to shift attention as the requirements of changing tasks might demand.

Developmental changes in the manner children at different ages deploy their attention have been demonstrated by various investigators (Adams & Shepp, 1975; Shepp & Swartz, 1976; Smith, Kemler, & Aronfreed, 1975), with different methods (Conroy & Weener, 1976; Hale & Taweel, 1974), and in different sense modalities (Geffen & Sexton, 1978; Hallahan, Kauffman, & Ball, 1974; Henek & Miller, 1976). All of these studies point to children's increasing capacity to deploy attention selectively as they get older.

With any capacity that undergoes developmental changes one finds individual differences both in the rate at which the development takes place and in the level of competence to which it ultimately advances. The same individual differences can be expected to exist in the case of the development of selective attention. Some children are bound to develop more slowly, others more rapidly than others, and some will end up with a more highly developed skill at selectivity than others. Furthermore, and again in line with other developmental phenomena, it is to be expected that a few children will fail to advance beyond a certain immature level, remaining fixated, as it were, at an early stage. As will be seen in the following, fixation or delay in developing age-appropriate deployment of attention appears to play a role in certain psychological disorders and a focus on this role can facilitate the treatment of children with such disorders.

THE TREATMENT OF CHILDREN WITH ATTENTIONAL DEFICITS

Overexclusive Attention

The tendency of the very young child to focus on only one aspect of a complex stimulus environment has been observed in mentally retarded and autistic children (Wilhelm & Lovaas, 1976). Schover and Newsom (1976), who refer to the phenomenon as overselectivity, have demonstrated that when autistic children are matched with normal children on the basis of mental age, overselective attention is present in both groups, reflecting a developmental lag on the part of the autistic. The original demonstration of overexclusive attention in autistic and mentally retarded children by Lovaas, Schreibman, Koegel, & Rehm (1971), can serve to illustrate the problem and highlight the severity of the handicap that a fixation at this level of development can entail. These investigators trained autistic, retarded, and normal children to respond to a complex stimulus consisting of simultaneously presented auditory, visual, and tactile components. All of the children eventually learned to make a simple motor response to the presentation of the stimulus complex, giving the appearance that the stimulus complex had come to control the response. When the separate elements of the stimulus complex were presented alone, however, (for instance, when the auditory cue was presented in the absence of the visual and tactile cues that had accompanied it during training) it became obvious that the autistic children had actually been responding primarily to only one of the three elements of the complex. The nature of this element varied from child to child, some children having responded to the visual, some to the auditory, and some to the tactile part of the complex. Unlike the autistic children, the normals responded uniformly to all three of the components when they were presented singly, while the retarded functioned between these extremes. To test whether the atypical responding of the impaired children was due to a defect in any sense modality, Lovaas et al. (1971) trained each child on the stimuli to which he or she had not previously responded. This showed that the children were able to learn the required response when the stimuli were presented alone; that their previous failure had indeed resulted from these children having overexclusively attended to only one of the three components of the stimulus complex.

Since that pioneering demonstration, overexclusive attention by autistic children has also been shown to occur in two-stimulus situations (Lovaas & Schreibman, 1971), and when all stimuli are in the same sense modality (Koegel & Wilhelm, 1973; Reynolds, Newsom, & Lovaas, 1974). What is more, the existence of the same pattern of responding to only a part of a stimulus complex has been demonstrated when autistic children are presented with social stimuli (Schreibman & Lovaas, 1973).

Nearly all learning involves the presentation of several stimuli, whether this be the contiguous appearance of conditioned and unconditioned stimulus in respondent learning, the juxtaposition of discriminative and reinforcing stimuli in operant learning, or the pairing of an effective reinforcer with another stimulus that is to be established as a conditioned reinforcer. A child who attends to only one of these simultaneously or contiguously presented stimuli would be severely handicapped in any such learning. On this basis Rincover and Koegel (1977) have reasoned that overexclusive attention or, as they call it, stimulus overselectivity, interferes with the acquisition of social reinforcers, the learning of language, the development of appropriate affect, and the establishment of interpersonal responsiveness. It is thus possible to construe most if not all of the characteristic deficits of autistic children as related to their failure to have developed an age-appropriate mode of attending to the complex stimuli emanating from the environment. If this is the case, the important question to ask is whether such development can be enhanced or how, at the very least, the difficulty can be taken into account in working with autistic children from a therapeutic–educational point of view.

Establishing Discriminations. Working with autistic children, Schreibman (1975) attacked one of their learning problems by accommodating the teaching strategy to the children's inability to respond to multiple elements of a complex stimulus. She accomplished this by taking a task that required a difficult discrimination and breaking it down into single component elements that were presented to the children one at a time. Those who attended in an overexclusive manner were thus helped to focus their attention. A task involving the discrimination between two stick figures can exemplify this approach.

An inspection of Figure 6 shows that it would be impossible to differentiate between the two figures if a child were to attend overexclusively to either the head or the body or the arm at the left, inasmuch as these are redundant features, common to both figures. The sole distinctive feature is the arm at the right which is raised in the figure identified as S+ and lowered in the one marked S−. It is an indication of the inordinate difficulty autistic chilren have with discriminations of stimuli composed of multiple elements that those par-

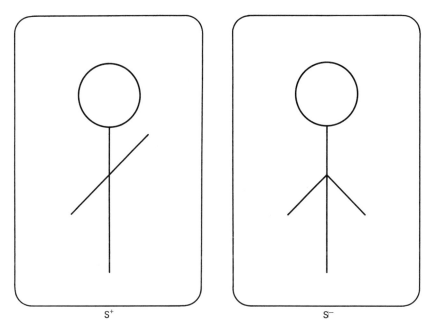

S^+ S^-

Figure 6. Stimuli like those used by Schreibman (1975) in teaching a discrimination to autistic children.

ticipating in Schreibman's study usually failed to learn this simple discrimination without special help.

The help Schreibman (1975) provided entailed taking only the diagonal line representing the arms of the S+ figure, showing this in exaggerated form on one card while the second card was blank. When a child was now asked to point to "the correct card," acceptable responses were easily forthcoming and could be reinforced. In subsequent presentations, the distinctive feature of the S− stimulus was faded in on the previously blank card, first in vague outline and gradually in more pronounced form until one card displayed a large, heavily drawn diagonal and the other an equally large, heavily drawn chevron. At every step of this fading-in procedure children were asked to point to the correct card and reinforced for doing so. The exaggerations in size and thickness of line were then gradually faded out and in the last step of the training sequence the redundant components, "body" and "head," were faded in until both figures could be presented in their entirety, as shown in Figure 6. With this method, the children were usually able to learn the discrimination. Significantly, when the experimenter had attempted to help the child learn the discrimination by pointing to the correct stimulus, this "help" turned out to be a hindrance probably because a child who attends in an overexclusive manner may focus attention on the pointing finger and not on the cue to which the finger is pointing.

Schreibman's (1975) approach to the problem of overexclusive attention required no modification in the child's mode of responding to available cues because the teaching strategy had been modified to facilitate learning by taking advantage of that mode. Such modification can be introduced where a child is in a special learning environment where the discrimination of letters, for example, might be taught by focusing on the distinctive features of the various characters in the alphabet (Gibson & Levin, 1975). In nonspecialized situations, however, such as those represented by the natural social environment, it is rarely if ever feasible to learn by attending to only one stimulus element at a time. For helping autistic children acquire a more adaptive response repertoire, it would therefore be extremely valuable to have a method for teaching them to respond to simultaneously presented, multiple stimulus elements. Such a method would entail a modification of these children's mode of attention, helping them adapt to multiple-cue learning rather than a modification of the learning situation, accommodating it to the children's mode of attention.

Some beginnings have been made in finding ways to modify the overexclusive mode of attention manifested by autistic children. Schreibman, Koegel, and Craig (1977) worked with 16 autistic children in a study designed to demonstrate overselectivity (overexclusive attention). When they continued to present the same stimuli to these children beyond the point where their overselective mode of attention had been ascertained, these investigators observed that 13 of the 16 children eventually became less overselective. This seems to suggest that autistic children can learn to respond to the multiple cues of complex stimuli but that in order to do so they need considerably more exposure to the cues than is necessary for normal children of the same chronological age. This may be the reason why those who employ the principles of operant learning in working with autistic children are able to establish new responses only by means of large numbers of trials (Lovaas, Young, & Newsom, 1978).

A direct attack on teaching autistic children to respond to the simultaneously presented, multiple cues of complex stimuli was reported by Koegel and Schreibman (1977). These investigators worked with four autistic boys whose mean age was 6 years, 9 months and a comparison group of normal children with the same mean chronological age. These children were taught to press a bar, using food as the reinforcer. The cues were visual (a red light) and auditory (a white noise). The first series of sessions involved single-cue training in which the child was to respond to the presentation of each of the stimuli when they appeared alone. Once this response had been reliably established, conditional-discrimination training was begun in which the simultaneous presentation of the two stimuli together was interspersed with the presentation of either stimulus alone. Now reinforcement was forthcoming only when the child responded to the multiple cues, never when a response was emitted to either cue alone. The discrimination was considered to have been learned when a child reached a criterion of two consecutive test blocks of 30 trials with no response to the single cues and 100 percent response to the cue complex. Although they required up to 990 trials, all of the autistic children eventually learned to discriminate between the single-cue and the multiple-cue situations. As might be expected, the normal children learned this discrimination in relatively few trials. What is more, when single-cue responding was placed on extinction, the normal children ceased responding to both single stimuli simultaneously, that is, when they showed extinction to one of the single cues, they would also no longer respond to the other. The autistic children, on the other hand, tended to cease responding to one of the single cues considerably earlier than to the other, a form of "stimulus-bound" responding that appears to be characteristic of children who attend to the environment in an overexclusive fashion.

The study just discussed had demonstrated that autistic children could learn to respond to a stimulus complex when alternative responses are on an extinction schedule. The question now arises whether such children can be taught a strategy or set to respond to complex stimuli; that is, whether they can learn to respond in the manner similar to that used by normal children. Koegel and Schreibman (1977) present some preliminary evidence, based on work with one autistic child, which suggests that this is indeed possible. They trained an autistic girl to respond to a visual stimulus, containing two redundant components (e.g., color and form, as in a green square). They then tested the girl to determine whether she had been responding on the basis of one or both of these components. On the first two of such discriminations it was clear that the child had been overexclusively attending to only one of the two stimulus components. As new sets of stimuli were introduced for further discriminations, however, the girl began to respond to both components, suggesting that she had acquired a learning set to respond on the basis of multiple cues. Her performance was now similar to that shown by normal children, except for the fact that she continued to require an inordinate number of trials to learn the original discrimination.

Research of this nature points to a direction that might be taken in work with profoundly disturbed children whose difficulties in the realm of attention are of the overexclusive kind. As Koegel and Schreibman (1977) point out, "if the autistic child can learn to respond to multiple cues as a general set, perhaps he can then respond to his environment in a manner more similar to normal children" (p. 310).

Overinclusive Attention

In the normal course of development, children leave behind the immature overexclusive mode and begin to attend to their world in an overinclusive manner. This has been most clearly demonstrated in studies using the incidental learning paradigm (Crane & Ross, 1967; Hagen & Hale, 1973). In this paradigm, a child is shown a series of stimuli that have two aspects to them, cards displaying an animal and a household object, for example. The experimenter calls attention to one of these aspects by instructing the child to remember its position on a subsequent sorting task (e.g., "Remember that the horses go on this pile, the cows on this pile, etc."). That aspect (animal) is thus central to the task; the other aspect (household object) is not mentioned and, not being essential for performing the task, it is considered as incidental. Upon completion of the sorting task, the child is asked questions relative to the previously unmentioned, incidental aspect of the stimuli ("What household object went with the horses?") in order to determine the extent to which the child had also attended to it.

When the stimuli used in a learning task have both relevant (central) and irrelevant (incidental) features, the most expeditious way of learning the task is to attend only to the relevant feature. The amount of information a child acquires about the incidental features, the incidental learning, reflects the degree to which his or her attention had been overinclusive. Research with the incidental learning paradigm (Hagen & Hale, 1973) has shown that high incidental learning takes place at the expense of efficiency on the central learning task. There is, so to speak, a trade-off effect in that the child learns a lot about the irrelevant, incidental aspects but relatively little about the central aspects. Conversely, as the child begins to be able to concentrate attention selectively on aspects of the task that the situation defines as central, he or she comes to learn relatively less about the incidental aspects. Studies with reading-disabled children (Pelham & Ross, 1977; Tarver, Hallahan, Kauffman, & Ball, 1976) have demonstrated a relationship of high incidental learning to poor reading and Siegel (1968) has found that good readers show less incidental learning than normal readers. It is to be expected that children who overinclusively attend to a lot of material that is irrelevant to the task at hand have more difficulty learning task-relevant information than those who are able to attend selectively to the central aspects of the stimulus material. In the case of reading, the task defines as the central material the letters, words, phrases, and sentences on the chalkboard or printed page. If, in addition to attending to these, the child also attends to many irrelevant stimuli, learning to read will be impaired and special help is called for. Such help would have to take the form of enhancing the child's ability to attend selectively to the task-relevant material.

The Role of Distinctive Features. With the beginning and disabled readers one frequently encounters a confusion of similar letters, particularly the reversal of letters like *b* and *d*. This can be construed as a failure to attend selectively to the distinctive feature (Gibson, 1975), which, in the case of *b* and *d* is the position of the circular portion relative to the vertical line. Help for children who have difficulties with this and similar discriminations would have to take the form of teaching them to focus their attention on this distinctive feature. As will be illustrated, this can be done by modifying the stimuli so as to make them more distinctly different, by teaching the child an information-enhancing strategy such as verbal labeling, or by following correct responses with positive reinforcement which may well have the function of providing additional information.

Koenigsberg (1973) demonstrated that children between the ages of 4 and 6 who had not yet acquired the ability to discriminate between _b_ and _d_ can be taught to do so by helping them focus their attention on the essential difference between the two graphemes. This experimenter would present to the child paired stimuli that differed in spatial orientation and ask whether these were the same or different. To teach the discrimination, she would then place a transparent copy of the stimulus over both the standard and the comparison thereby highlighting the similarity or difference which she would then verbalize and explain. That demonstration was sufficient to teach the children the discrimination they had previously been unable to make.

A similar approach of highlighting distinctive features in teaching children the discrimination between easily confused letter pairs was used by Egeland and Winer (1974) and by Egeland (1975). Working with prekindergarten children who were unable to identify any letters of the alphabet, Egeland (1975) employed a highly effective method to teach them to discriminate between the letter pairs _R-P, Y-V, G-C, Q-O, M-N,_ and _K-X_. As Gibson (1969) had pointed out, each of these pairs contains letters with a number of similar distinctive features, making them difficult to tell apart. In order to teach the necessary discrimination, Egeland (1975) highlighted the distinctive feature that differentiates the two letters, the diagonal stem of the _R_ in the _R-P_ discrimination, for example. Highlighting was accomplished by making the distinctive feature appear in bright red. That color was gradually faded on succeeding training trials until both letters were shown in black only. When two stimuli that are to be discriminated are so distinctly different at the beginning of training, errors are unlikely and learning can thus progress in an errorless manner.

Errorless discrimination training, originally demonstrated by Terrace (1963) in work with pigeons, has many advantages over the usual procedure used with young children. As Egeland (1975) pointed out, the common procedure used in the classroom is to ask the child to identify a letter and to provide positive or negative feedback, depending on the child's response. When the answer is wrong the teacher may be able to tell that the child attended to an irrelevant cue and provide some elaboration so that the child will know why the answer was wrong. If the answer is right, however, the child will usually not be told what made it right. It is thus possible that children learn to make correct responses without recognizing the salient cues that differentiate one letter from another. Teaching children to discriminate letters by allowing them to respond to an irrelevant cue and then seeking to extinguish that incorrect response would seem to be an inefficient method. Errorless discrimination training is a means of avoiding that wasteful detour by maximizing the production of correct responses.

Egeland (1975) undertook to compare three training methods. One group of children was given errorless training in a condition where the distinctive feature of the letter to be discriminated was highlighted in red. A second group was also given errorless training but for them the red color was used to underline the "correct" letter. A third group of children received the traditional reinforcement–extinction approach in which they were told after each trial whether their response had been correct. When the learning of the three groups was assessed on both an immediate and delayed posttest, the first errorless training group proved to be making significantly fewer errors than the other two groups. It is noteworthy that the supplementary red color facilitated learning only when it was used to highlight the relevant distinctive feature, not when it merely assisted the differentiation between the two letters, as in the underlining. In both instances the color provided a redundant cue, that is to say that during the early training trials the letters R and P can be discriminated either from the presence of the extra stem on the R or from the presence of the color. Yet only when the color is used to highlight that stem does it call attention to a relevant feature. In that case, as the color is gradually withdrawn, the stem continues to serve as the distinguishing feature. When color is used to underline the R it is not clear to what a child's attention is drawn. A correct answer may well have been given, based on the presence of the underlining, but when that extra cue is then gradually withdrawn the child is left without a distinguishing feature on which to base a response.

The results of Egeland's (1975) research suggest that a redundant cue that is not part of the relevant stimulus can hinder learning if the child selectively attends to that cue and not to the relevant distinctive feature. Similar findings were reported by Koegel and Rincover (1976) who speak of the detrimental effect of using extraneous stimuli to guide the discriminations of both normal and autistic children. When one wishes to modify stimuli to help focus children's attention, one must use care when increasing the difference between stimuli that this difference is relevant to the ultimate discrimination that is to be learned. If the difference is irrelevant to that discrimination, attention may come to be focused on that irrelevant aspect, thus making learning more instead of less difficult.

Another method for helping the overinclusive child to focus attention selectively on the distinctive feature of stimuli that are to be discriminated is to provide a strategy for approaching the task, such as using verbal labeling or rehearsal of the material to be learned. Learning-disabled children do not seem to use such strategies as readily as normal children (Torgesen & Goldman, 1977). On tasks that assess incidental learning, learning-disabled children, as was pointed out earlier, tend to devote attention to incidental, task-irrelevant stimuli to the detriment of their performance on the task that has been defined as central. Tarver, Hallahan, Kauffman, and Ball (1976) have shown that when such children are instructed to label the central stimuli and to say these labels to themselves by way of rehearsal in the course of the testing, their performance can be markedly improved. A similar facilitating effect of labeling was reported by Dusek (1978) who worked with normal children in third, fifth, and seventh grade. Like others, he showed that as the ability to deploy attention selectively improves with age, central learning increases while incidental learning decreases. When he taught children to label the stimuli, Dusek (1978) was able to show that this enhanced selective attention, that is, it raised the children's learning scores. It seems that such labeling not only aids to focus the child's attention but that it also facilitates the encoding of information which is an important skill, particularly on such a memory task as the incidental learning experiment.

A third method for enhancing the selective attention of children who are still predominantly overinclusive is to provide positive reinforcement for emitting responses that require selectivity. This represents a direct teaching of selective attention and it can be used either in isolation or in combination with the methods of enhancing distinctive features and providing a task strategy. Heiman, Fischer, and Ross (1973) gave children enrolled in a remedial reading program supplementary reinforced practice in focusing attention on printed material. They found that the scores of these children on standardized reading tests improved significantly more than those of children in a control group. Similar evidence that it is possible to improve selective attention by training was reported by Clifton and Bogartz (1968) who used the auditory task of dichotic listening to assess that skill. In dichotic listening two different words or digits are simultaneously presented over two earphones and the child is instructed to attend selectively only to the messages coming in on one side. Using this method with preschool children, Clifton and Bogartz (1968) provided positive reinforcement for responses to the attended channel and found that this improved the children's performance.

Impulsive Behavior

One of the characteristics often attributed to learning-disabled children is difficulty with impulse control (Douglas, 1972). Whether the construct *impulse* contributes anything to the understanding and treatment of learning-disabled children is open to question (Ross, 1976) because all of the observations that lead one to infer poor impulse control can also be construed as the result of inadequately developed selective attention. Nonetheless, because research has been focused on the impulsive behavior of learning-disabled children some discussion of the treatment methods that have been employed would seem indicated.

Impulsive behavior is characterized by a response style in which when asked a question or presented with a task, the child initiates a response after only minimal delay. The responses thus produced are frequently wrong or inappropriate. Because children who produce their answers less rapidly often arrive at correct responses it has been assumed that the impulsive style causes the response to be wrong. Based on this reasoning, therapeutic interventions have frequently taken the form of seeking to increase the child's response latency. Douglas (1972), for example, has spoken of the need to teach such children to "stop, look and listen" and Palkes, Stewart, and Kahana (1968) sought to teach impulsive children to "stop, look, listen, and think" before giving an answer or responding to a task. There is evidence that suggests that the key to helping impulsive children improve their performance does not lie in the "stop" part of these instructions but in what is implied by the injunction to "look, listen, and think," that is, one must do more than tell a child, "Take your time." One must also provide specific instructions as to what the child is to do with the time thus taken. Merely exhorting the child to "think" may also not be enough.

A popular measure of impulsivity is the Matching Familiar Figures (MFF) test developed by Kagan (1966). On this test, the child is instructed to select the exact match to a standard stimulus from among a series of highly similar exemplars. Performance is measured by two scores. One reflects response time, the other the number of errors. Impulsive responding is then defined by the combination of high-error scores and short-response time, while low-error scores and relatively long response time defines the so-called reflective child. From a psychometric standpoint this instrument has several shortcomings (Block, Block, & Harrington, 1974) but a child's performance on it can serve as an operational definition of impulsive or reflective response style. Using this instrument, several studies have demonstrated that inducing impulsively responding children to delay their answers by a fixed amount of time will not, in and of itself, result in a reduction in error scores (Kagan, Pearson, & Welch, 1966). More is needed and that seems to be to provide the child with a specific strategy regarding what to do during the delay between stimulus presentation and response emission.

Teaching Response Strategies. Palkes, Stewart, and Kahana (1968) addressed a study to the question whether impulsive children can be helped to improve their performance by teaching them to use self-directed verbal commands designed to induce them to approach a task with deliberation and reflection. As is regrettably true in many such studies, learning disability, impulsivity, and hyperactivity were confounded and the authors speak of the children with whom they worked as "under psychiatric care for hyperactive behavior disorder" (ibid., p. 818). Their emphasis, however, was not on the children's level of motor activity but on their precipitous (and inadequate) test responses. The criterion task, which served both as a basis for matching experimental and control groups and as a measure of outcome, was the Porteus Maze Test. This test furnishes not only an estimate of general intelligence but also a qualitative score, which has been shown to distinguish between groups differing in impulsiveness (Porteus, 1942). The children in the study by Palkes et al. (1968) approached this task in a slapdash manner, cutting corners, crossing lines, and moving in the wrong direction in the mazes that make up the test.

For training the children in the experimental group to use self-directed verbal commands, Palkes, Stewart, and Kahana (1968) employed visual training aids that combined written instructions with cartoonlike illustrations of the injunction to stop, listen, look, and think before answering. These training aids, printed on four "reminder cards" were arranged on the desk in front of the child and the experimenter directed attention to them, pointing out that the cards were to serve as a reminder of what the child was to say before beginning any work. The children were given two 30-minute training sessions on two successive days during which they were presented with paper-and-pencil tests that are frequently used to assess impulsive behavior; Kagan's (1966) Matching Familiar Figures Test, the Embedded Figures Test, and the Trail Making Test. Each of these tests requires deliberate care and attention to detail for optimal performance.

Before presentation of a task, the child was asked to read aloud the instructions on the first reminder card which carried the legend "This is a Stop!, Listen, Look, and Think Experiment." When the task was placed before the child, the experimenter again asked that the injunction to listen be said aloud. The task was then exposed and the relevant instructions were presented but before the child was permitted to begin, the self-directed command, "I'll look and think before I answer," had to be read from one of the reminder cards. Before turning the page in the test booklet, the child again had to say aloud, "Stop—listen" after which the experimenter would present the next figure, give the appropriate instruction, and insist that the child say "I look and think before I answer." This procedure was followed for each of the training tasks. If the child failed to use the appropriate self-command, the experimenter would point to the respective reminder card and insist that the child state the command before continuing. When a command had been produced spontaneously, the experimenter praised the child with, "Good, you remembered the commands."

Palkes, Stewart, and Kahana (1968) used this procedure with 10 boys between the ages of 8 years, 2 months and 9 years, 11 months. Ten other boys, comprising a matched control group, were given the same tasks but instead of

receiving training in the use of self-directed commands they were given additional work with embedded figures. When, after the two training sessions, all
children were given an alternate form of the Porteus Maze Test, on which the
groups had not differd before, the boys in the experimental groups had a significantly higher mean test quotient (a measure of intelligence) and significantly lower mean qualitative error score than those in the control group. Training
in self-directed verbal commands thus appears to have reduced these children's
impulsive approach to the maze test, thereby improving their performance.

Unfortunately, neither the study just described nor its replication (Palkes,
Stewart, & Freedman, 1971) addressed the question whether the more adaptive
response strategy the boys had been taught in the laboratory experiment generalized to other tasks or had long-term effects on the children's school behavior. This issue was explored in a frequently cited study conducted by Meichenbaum and Goodman (1971) who also used verbal self-instruction as a means
for reducing impulsive responding in learning-disabled, hyperactive children.
These investigators not only taught self-instruction to the children but they
also had an adult model the behavioral strategies appropriate for solving such
tasks as maze tracing and matching familiar figures. This combination served
to reduce impulsive responding and led to improved performance on the MFF
test and on selected subtests of the Wechsler Intelligence Scale for Children
(1949). When these children's appropriate classroom behavior, such as activity
level, self-control, and cooperation was assessed, however, it was revealed that
the training procedures had failed to have an effect.

In view of the fact that training in solving paper-and-pencil tasks bears little similarity to being cooperative in the classroom, it is not surprising that
Meichenbaum and Goodman (1971) failed to find a generalization across time,
situation, and behavior. Clearly, if the desired outcome of an intervention is
that a child be more cooperative in the classroom, then this behavior and not
maze-tracing should be the object of training. Conversely, if one has trained
children to approach paper-and-pencil tests with greater care, it does not seem
reasonable to ask whether such training affects their activity level or cooperation in the classroom. Training must be relevant to the target behavior and
outcome assessment should be on the effect of that training on that target.
When Kendall and Finch (1978) selected children's impulsive behavior as the
target of their intervention and later asked teachers to rate the children's impulsive behavior in the classroom, they were able to show an effect that held
up over a three months period of follow-up. The combination of self-instruction and response cost used by these investigators to reduce impulsive behavior
thus seems to deserve further exploration but the question whether reduced impulsive behavior leads to improved academic performance remains to be answered.

The importance of focusing an intervention on the specific skills one
wishes a child to learn was recognized by Egeland (1974) who also conducted a

study with so-called impulsive children. Out of a total of 260 second-grade children who were all given the MFF test, Egeland (1974) selected 72 whose short response time and high-error scores defined them as impulsive. These children, who ranged in age from 6 years, 10 months to 8 years, 11 months, were assigned at random to one of two training groups or to a control group. The control group received no training while the training groups were given eight 30-minute training sessions spread over 4 weeks. Training consisted of exercises in matching geometric designs or nonsense words, drawing geometric designs from memory, and verbally describing geometric designs. The two training groups differed in that one was instructed to wait 10 to 15 seconds before responding; to "think about your answer and take your time." This is analogous to the usual admonition given impulsive children when they are told, "Take your time; pay attention; think." The other group was, in effect, taught what to do during the time delay, to what to pay attention, what to think about. They were given a set of rules and basic strategies they were to follow while working on the training tasks. The rules were designed to induce the children to focus attention on the relevant features of the stimuli, to examine and compare alternatives, to analyze the component parts of the alternatives by looking for similarities and differences, and to discard alternatives until only the correct one remained. This strategy was intended to counteract the impulsive child's tendency to attend to only one alternative without considering others before making a response. In short, these children received explicit training in the specific skill needed to deal with the tasks that were presented to them, not generalized exhortations of little specific relevance.

At the end of the four-week training period, all children were given an alternate form of the MFF test. Comparison between the pre- and posttest scores revealed that both training groups had increased their response time and decreased their error scores while the score of the control group had remained unchanged. At this point the strategy group did not seem to have an advantage over the exhortation group. When the children were tested once again two months later, however, only the group that had received training in the use of problem-solving strategies had maintained the improved performance. Not only that—this strategy group also achieved significantly higher scores on a test of reading comprehension (the Gates-MacGinitie Reading Test) which was administered to the classes five months after completion of the training. These encouraging results indicate that so-called impulsive children can be taught to change the way in which they process information and solve problems. Egeland's (1974) work strongly suggests that the poor performance so often found with "impulsive" children stems not so much from the precipitous nature of their responses as from their not using adaptive strategies in focusing their attention on the distinctive features of the stimulus material.

This conclusion receives further support from a study reported by Zelniker and Oppenheimer (1976) who worked with 135 kindergarten children, identified as impulsive on the basis of their MFF test performance. The children were given the task of comparing letterlike forms with their rotated transformations. One group was trained in a matching procedure ("Find the one that is the same") while a second group was given differentiation training ("Find the ones that are different"). Zelniker and Oppenheimer (1976) report that the differentiation training procedures were superior to the matching training procedure and that the introduction of novel transformations enhanced the effect of the differentiation training. They attribute this to the fact that the task of finding differences among novel alternatives forces a child to attend to the distinctive features of the stimuli and they conclude that impulsive children are not deficient in problem-solving ability but that they approach tasks requiring information processing with a strategy that is different (less appropriate) than that used by so-called reflective children. From the standpoint of therapeutic–educational intervention with children who persistently give wrong answers in a precipitous manner this means that one should focus on teaching them task-appropriate response strategies, not on having them simply "slow down."

Recapitulation

Attention is a useful construct in that it permits one to conceptualize a mediational link between the presentation of a stimulus and the production of a response. Children who consistently fail to emit an appropriate response when presented with a stimulus may not be attending to the distinctive features of that stimulus. In tracing the development of attention one finds the very young child to be attending to the environment in an overexclusive manner. With increasing age, this gives way to an overinclusive mode of attention that in turn, is replaced by selective attention, the mature and highly adaptive form of coping with the demands children encounter in the academic tasks of school. Individual differences in the development of selective attention and possible fixations at the earlier stages of this development may account for some of the difficulties of learning-disabled, autistic, and retarded children. Treatment of the attentional deficits of such children seems most productive when it is focused on helping them to acquire strategies for responding to complex or multidimensional stimuli. This can be done by modifying the stimuli that are presented to the child, by reinforcing attention to distinctive features, by teaching verbal labeling and rehearsal, or by inducing self-instruction. As in all interventions, the target must be the skill that the child lacks and not some aspect of behavior that, like precipitous responding, is only indirectly related to the tasks with which the child is having difficulty.

6

Hyperactivity

CONCEPTUAL ISSUES

Among the characteristics often attributed to learning-disabled children is that of hyperactivity. Some investigators, in fact, have approached learning disability and hyperactivity as if they were synonymous or at least parts of the same "syndrome" (e.g., Werry, Weiss, & Douglas, 1964). While learning disability and hyperactivity are frequently found to be positively correlated, a study by Lahey, Stempniak, Robinson, and Tyroler (1978) has demonstrated that the two conditions are independent dimensions of children's problem behavior. It is very likely that the high correlation between these conditions is the spurious result of the referral process by which the troublesome, hyperactive child is selected for study and found to be learning-disabled while the equally disabled child who is not hyperactive remains unnoticed, being considered merely a child with low intellectual potential (Ross, 1976). As with other correlated phenomena, it is impossible to ascertain from the correlation whether learning disability leads to hyperactivity; whether hyperactivity causes learning disability; or whether the two derive from a third, common source. In order to treat children who are observed to have trouble learning and who are also excessively active, however, some formulation of the relationship between these phenomena is needed in order to know where to focus the intervention.

If one construed hyperactivity as an excess behavior, treatment would focus on reducing the child's activity level by extinction, punishment, or differential reinforcement procedures. Such an approach should result in an increase of the periods during which the child sits without moving—but that is clearly not the goal of the intervention. Sitting still is, at best, merely a means to an end; a requisite for attending to a task that must be accomplished in a sedentary position. In fact, sitting still might be construed as a by-product of working on a task that has reinforcing consequences. Given this reasoning, might it not be productive to focus intervention on strengthening weak or absent constructive response patterns that are incompatible with excessive movement? In other words, if one were to view hyperactivity not as a behavioral excess but as the indirect result of a behavioral deficit, the treatment approach would take a different direction. In view of the reciprocity between task-oriented behavior and task-disrupting hyperactivity it is logical to proceed on the assumption that if task-oriented behavior were strengthened, the task-disrupting excess motility would perforce have to decrease and hyperactivity would thus cease to be a problem without ever having been the target of intervention. As we shall see in the following, the most successful programs of intervention with hyperactive children have followed this logic, focusing not on reducing hyperactivity but on establishing constructive work or study habits or the attentional skills these require.

It may seem paradoxical to find the chapter on hyperactivity among those dealing with behavior deficits when the very word "hyperactivity" connotes that one is dealing with an excess of activity. The reasoning outlined above should resolve this paradox.

TREATMENT FOR THE HYPERACTIVE CHILD

One of the earliest demonstrations of the systematic application of behavioral principles to the modification of hyperactivity was presented by Patterson, Jones, Whittier, and Wright (1965) who treated a 10-year-old brain-injured, retarded boy whom they identified as Raymond. This child was enrolled in a special school for physically handicapped children and his teacher described him as hyperactive, having a short attention span, and exhibiting a tendency to aggression against younger children. Clearly, this boy was more severely impaired than the children typically classified as hyperactive but if it can be demonstrated that behavioral treatment is effective in such an extreme case, it follows that the principles involved can also be expected to work with less severely impaired children.

Patterson et al. (1965) report that at the beginning of their study Raymond would spend most of his time in the classroom walking about the room, moving his arms or legs, staring into space, and engaging in other behavior typical of hyperactive children. Since such behavior is incompatible with attending to academic tasks, the investigators selected attending behavior as the target of intervention. From behind a one-way screen, observers recorded various "nonattending" behaviors such as swinging arms, fingering objects, looking out the window, and walking about. During the baseline period, Raymond and another child, who served as a control, engaged in a mean of approximately five such behaviors per minute.

After the baseline had been established, Raymond was introduced to the training procedure which was described to him as a way to learn sitting still so that he could study better. He was to wear a small radio receiver and an earphone through which he would be getting a signal to indicate that he had earned a piece of candy. During a series of training trials given away from the classroom the experimenter would activate the earphone and pair the signal with the delivery of a piece of candy for every 10-second period during which Raymond did not display any hyperactive, nonattending behavior.

After he had been thus prepared, Raymond wore the equipment to class. The other children had been told that the receiver and earphone had the purpose of helping Raymond learn better by telling him when he was sitting still. In addition, the children in the class had been informed that Raymond would be earning candy which he would share with them at the end of the period. This strategem led to much peer support and social reinforcement since the other children viewed Raymond's success as benefiting them as well. The actual intervention lasted for three weeks with conditioning periods ranging in length from 5 to 18 minutes. Data collected on eight days revealed that Raymond made approximately 3.3 fewer nonattending responses per minute, significantly fewer than the control child whose rate remained at the baseline level. Observations were continued over a four-week period after the end of the conditioning phase. This revealed that the difference between Raymond and the control child was maintained although the other child also showed a decrease in the frequency of nonattending behavior.

The fact that the untreated child in the study by Patterson et al. (1965) eventually reduced his hyperactive behavior too, reflects a spillover effect that has also been observed by other investigators (Kent & O'Leary, 1976). It is an intriguing phenomenon that reflects the disruptive influence a hyperactive child has on other children in the classroom. In the case of Raymond, the control child had sat near him in the classroom and Raymond's improved behavior may have reduced the number of distracting stimuli to which he had previously reacted with hyperactivity of his own.

The pioneering study just discussed used a DRO (differential reinforcement of other behavior) procedure in that reinforcement was contingent on the nonoccurrence of nonattending behavior which, presumably, represented periods of attending behavior. Given this definition of attending, it is conceivable that Raymond learned no more than to suppress overt movement responses. Whether he was actually "paying attention" to the academic tasks cannot be ascertained from the data presented. The presence or absence of attention can only be inferred by noting whether the child displays evidence of having learned the academic material to which attention was to be directed. Since Patterson et al. (1965) did not present information about Raymond's school achievement it is impossible to know whether Raymond had actually increased attention to his work. It must also be noted that the use of a radio receiver and the need of an observer who signals the delivery of reinforcement is rather cumbersome. More sophisticated instrumentation has since simplified the application of conditioning principles for working with hyperactive children. Thus, Ball and Irwin (1976) describe a portable, automated device that is worn by the child and contains a mercury sensor switch that activates a buzzer at the end of two-minute periods of sitting still. In their work with one hyperactive child, these investigators delivered a tangible reinforcer at the end of a 20-minute period for each instance of buzzer activation. After in-seat behavior had been increased by this method, the automated device was replaced by a kitchen timer which, in turn, was successfully faded out at the end of the study. Still, even here, the focus was on sitting still, not on constructive studying behavior.

Teaching Task-oriented Behavior

For a demonstration of a behavioral approach to working with hyperactive children that did not focus on activity level, did not require electronic instrumentation, and was applied to groups of children in regular classrooms, we turn to a study reported by O'Leary, Pelham, Rosenbaum, and Price (1976). These investigators treated nine hyperactive children whose average age was 10 years. Eight other hyperactive children served as a control group. These children were of average intelligence but seven of the nine in the treatment group scored below average on an achievement test. None of the children displayed definite symptoms of brain damage and none was receiving medication for hyperactivity at the time the study was being conducted.

The behavior of the children was evaluated both before and after treatment by means of an abbreviated version of the teacher rating scale developed by Conners (1969) and by a rating scale of problem behaviors that was individually prepared for each child so as to provide a measure of the severity of four or five problems that this particular child manifested.

The Abbreviated Conners' Teacher Rating Scale (Sleator & von Neumann, 1974) consists of the following ten descriptive statements:

Restless or overactive

Excitable, impulsive

Disturbs other children

Fails to finish things he starts; short attention span

Constantly fidgeting

Inattentive, easily distracted

Demands must be met immediately—easily frustrated

Cries often and easily

Mood changes quickly and drastically

Temper outburst; explosive and unpredictable behavior

Each of these items is rated by the teacher to reflect the degree to which a child displays the behavior. Zero represents "not at all," one "just a little," two "pretty much," and three "very much." The maximum possible score is 30 and in order to be classified as hyperactive, a child must receive a score of at least 15 points. In the O'Leary et al. (1976) study the hyperactive children in the experimental and control groups had an average score of 19.7, while randomly selected same-sex peers in the same classroom as the hyperactives had an average score of 5.1.

The treatment approach employed by O'Leary et al. (1976) called for the cooperation of home and school because it was a teacher-managed, home-based reward program that had the following components: At the beginning of each day the teacher specified the child's classroom goals and throughout the day praised the child for efforts to achieve these goals. At the end of the day the teacher evaluated the child's behavior relevant to the goals that had been set and sent the parents a daily report card on their child's progress. The parents, in turn, had the responsibility of rewarding the child for progress toward his or her goals.

At the beginning of the program the therapist met with the parents of each child to obtain information about the child's behavior at home, and to explain the parents' role in the treatment plan, with particular emphasis on the selection of suitable rewards. The therapist also had a meeting with the child's teacher. This lasted for approximately one hour and was primarily devoted to choosing the behavioral goals for the child. After these initial meetings and throughout the 10-week program, the therapist maintained weekly telephone contact with the parents and visited the teacher once a week.

It is particularly noteworthy that the children's classroom goals and the behaviors for which they received reinforcement did not have activity level as their focus. The children were not reinforced for sitting still, for attending, or for not fidgeting. Instead, the focus of treatment was on academic and pro-social goals such as completing assigned math problems, helping a neighbor with a class project, bringing homework to class, and not fighting. Thus, unlike the studies discussed earlier, the target for behavior change was not the hyperactivity *per se* but the learning-compatible behavior that is usually emitted with low frequency by children who are identified as hyperactive.

O'Leary et al. (1976) point out that the selection of appropriate rewards delivered by the parents was perhaps the most critical element of the program. Selecting maximally effective reinforcers required care and ingenuity since it is a well-established fact that no single type of consequence will serve as a reinforcer for all children. In fact, even a consequence that was reinforcing at one time may lose its reinforcing properties so that new rewards may have to be introduced. In this study the following were frequently used rewards: A half-hour of extra television viewing; a special dessert; spending time with either parent playing a game such as checkers; money with which to buy items of the child's choice. In addition to such daily rewards, the children could earn weekly rewards when four out of five daily report cards sent home by the teacher had reflected improvement. These weekly rewards were such things as a fishing trip with father, a dinner at a favorite aunt's, or a family meal at a drive-in restaurant. In two cases, where the parents failed to reward their children consistently, an in-school reward program had to be instituted. For one of these children the reward consisted of a piece of candy per day; for the other the privilege of spending free time in the school library was found to be reinforcing.

The results of this study attest to the effectiveness of the approach. At the start of the program the treated children and their controls had not differed in mean hyperactivity rating on either the Conners scale or the individualized scale of problem behaviors. When these instruments were administered again after 10 weeks of treatment, the two groups differed significantly on both scales (see Figures 7 and 8). On the individualized problem behavior rating scale only the treated group showed a significant ($p<.005$) improvement from before to after treatment. On the Conners scale both groups showed significant improvement ($p<.005$) but the treatment children had significantly lower posttreatment scores than the controls ($p<.066$). These results are, unfortunately, based on the ratings made by the teachers before and after they themselves had been instrumental in conducting the treatment program. While O'Leary et al. (1976) present fairly robust validity data gathered by independent observers, these are available only for the pretreatment ratings so that the outcome data may be influenced by an unknown rater bias.

A word must also be said about the finding that the untreated control children who had no contact with the therapy team at any time during the study also showed some improvement. On the one hand, this may attest to a lack of rater bias on the part of the teachers whose bias, if any, should have favored the treated children. On the other hand, these results might indicate that hyperactive children become less hyperactive after 10 weeks of the school term have passed, regardless of whether they are subjected to a treatment program. There are no data to support this speculation against spontaneous improvement; in fact, anecdotes from teachers suggest that this does not take place. Conceivably, hyperactive children stimulate each other so that, as one child settles down as a result of a therapeutic intervention, the untreated ones also

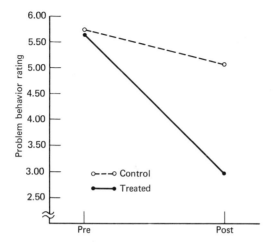

Figure 7. Comparison of the mean problem behavior ratings of nine hyperactive children treated with behavior therapy and of eight similar controls. (O'Leary et al., 1976. Copyright by J. B. Lippincott Co.)

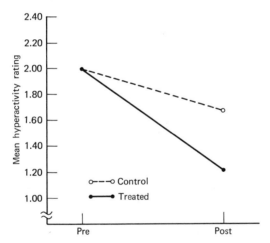

Figure 8. Mean hyperactivity ratings of the same children as in Figure 7, obtained from the Conners scale. The data reflect the mean item ratings (range 0.0 to 3.0) on the 10-item scale. (O'Leary et al., 1976. Copyright by J. B. Lippincott Co.)

settle down. Such a spillover effect had been found by Patterson et al. (1965) in their work with Raymond and while this should be a welcome phenomenon from the standpoint of practical work with hyperactive children it raises the question whether research on treatment outcome should not also include untreated controls in classrooms where none of the children is being treated.

Behavioral versus Chemical Intervention

O'Leary, Pelham, Rosenbaum, and Price (1976) had focused their treatment of hyperactive children not on the hyperactive behavior but on academic and prosocial behaviors. While they present data showing the effect of this approach on the hyperactive and related problem behaviors, they do not report whether the academic performance of the treated children had improved. We thus turn to the work of Ayllon, Layman, and Kandel (1975) who, approaching hyperactivity in a similar manner, report the effect of their treatment on both academic performance and hyperactive behavior. As had others (e.g. Pelham, 1976; Shafto & Sulzbacher, 1977), they addressed their study to comparing the effectiveness of medication and drug-free behavioral intervention in the treatment of hyperactive children. Their research questions were thus twofold in that they asked whether behavioral techniques, when used to decrease the disruptive behavior of hyperactive children, are at least as effective as medication and whether such techniques further the hyperactive child's educational progress.

Ayllon, Layman, and Kandel (1975) worked with three children who were enrolled in a self-contained learning-disability class of 10 children and one teacher. By using a multiple-baseline design, each child could serve as his or her own control. All three children had been clinically diagnosed as chronically hyperactive and all were receiving the drug methylphenidate to control their hyperactivity. One of them, an 8-year-old girl identified as Crystal, had been on the drug for five years, while the two boys, 9-year-old Paul, and 10-year-old Dudley, had been taking the drug for one and four years, respectively. The intelligence test scores of the three children ranged from 94 to 118.

For the purpose of their study, Ayllon et al. (1975) defined academic performance in terms of arithmetic ("math") and reading. They measured math performance as the percentage of correct problems requiring the addition of whole numbers under 10. Reading was quantified by using the percentage of correct workbook responses related to stories previously read in a basal reader. Hyperactivity was defined in terms of gross motor behavior, making disruptive noises with objects, disturbing others, and blurting out answers or screaming. These categories of hyperactive behavior were used by observers who were present in the classroom and who observed each child approximately 50 times during each 45-minute class period. Scores for hyperactivity were expressed in terms of the percentage of observation intervals during which such behavior was present.

The experimental design of the study is reflected in Figure 9. It included four phases. During the first phase, lasting 17 days, the children were observed while they were on medication so as to establish a baseline for hyperactivity and academic performance under that condition. As can be seen in the graphs, the hyperactivity level (solid line) of all three children was fairly low, averaging

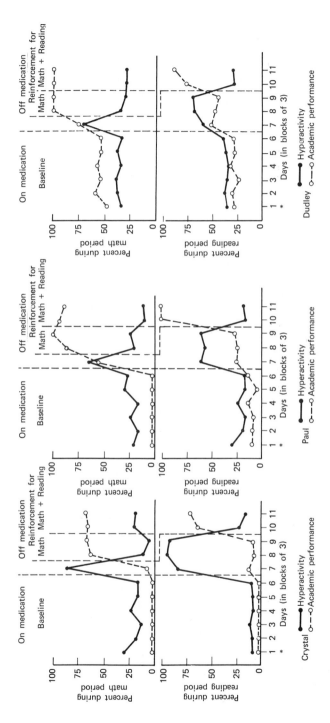

Figure 9. The percentage of intervals in which hyperactivity was observed and the percentage of correct math and reading performance for Crystal, Paul, and Dudley. The asterisks indicate data points averaged over only two rather than three days. (Redrawn from Ayllon, Layman, & Kandel, 1975. Copyright by the Society for the Experimental Analysis of Behavior, Inc.)

about 20 percent, while academic performance (dotted line) was near zero for all but Dudley who managed to get about 50 percent of his math problems and 25 percent of his reading problems correct. On the eighteenth day and with the full cooperation of the children's parents and physicians the medication was discontinued. After a three-day period during which the chemical residues of the medication had a chance to leave the children's system, classroom observations were resumed for the second phase of the study. This phase lasted for three days with respect to the math performance (top half of figures) and continued for an additional six days with respect to the reading performance (bottom half of figures). As shown in the graphs, when medication was discontinued, hyperactivity increased sharply for all three children and for all but Crystal academic performance showed some improvement. This reflects the phenomenon, reported by Sprague and Sleator (1977), that methylphenidate interferes with academic performance when it is administered at a dosage level that is high enough to reduce hyperactive behavior.

In line with the experimental plan that called for a multiple-baseline-across-subject-matter design, different treatments were introduced with the beginning of the third phase. While maintaining the no-medication condition and continuing all observations, math performance was now placed under a reinforcement regimen while reading performance continued as before. The reinforcement system used the token approach. The teacher awarded the children a checkmark on an index card for each correct academic response. These checkmarks could be exchanged later in the day for a choice among a large array of backup reinforcers ranging in price from 1 to 75 checks and consisting of such items as school supplies, candy, or picnics in the park.

Turning again to the graphs in Figure 9, we can see that the introduction of the reinforcement system resulted in a marked increase in the percentage of math problems correctly completed during the 10 minutes of class time available for this task. Crystal now got 65 percent of the problems correct while she had failed them all when she had been on medication, whereas Paul and Dudley turned in nearly perfect performances. At the same time a rather startling effect is found for the hyperactivity ratings. Without medication and with no behavioral intervention other than a reinforcement of academic performance, all three children's activity level falls to or below the level where it had been while they were taking the drug. The multiple baseline design now permits one to see that this change was correlated with the introduction of the reinforcement procedure. Thus, a look at the lower half of the three figures reveals that in reading, where reinforcement is not yet in effect, activity level is still high and academic performance still low. It is only with the beginning of the fourth phase, when both math and reading performance are placed under reinforcement contingencies, that academic performance improves and hyperactivity declines. Given the fact that all three children responded in highly similar fashion, it would seem warranted to conclude that the improved academic performance and control of hyperactive behavior had been the result of the reinforcement procedure.

A multiple baseline design, such as the one employed by Ayllon, Layman, and Kandel (1975) is eminently suited for the kind of applied study as the one they conducted. The limited number of subjects often used in such studies precludes data analysis based on measures of central tendency. Averaged results for the three children in this study, shown in Figure 10, are thus no more than a convenient summary of the information displayed in the three preceding figures. The bar graphs in Figure 10 reflect the fact that when the children were on medication, hyperactivity was held to about 24 percent during math and reading sessions but that the average accuracy of their performance in these academic subjects was only 12 percent. When medication was withdrawn and academic performance was placed under the reinforcement program, the average of correct responses in both academic subjects rose to 85 percent while hyperactivity, at an average of 24 percent, was close to where it had been while the children were under medication. It is difficult to escape the conclusion that behavioral intervention with so-called hyperactive children is far preferable to the pharmacological approach which, while suppressing activity level, apparently also interferes with academic performance. This conclusion is supported by similar findings that have been reported by investigators who studied individual hyperactive children and compared treatment by medication with behavioral management programs (Shafto & Sulzberger, 1977; Wulbert & Dries, 1977).

Group Contingencies. When a reinforcement program is introduced for one child in a regular classroom one must consider the effect on the other children in the class. The classmates of the treated child can presumably help or hinder

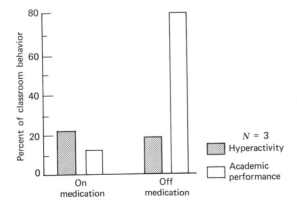

Figure 10. Average percent of hyperactivity and academic performance in math and reading for three children. The first two bars summarize findings from the 17-day baseline under drug therapy. The last two bars show results for the final six-day period without drug therapy but with a reinforcement program for both math and reading performance. (Ayllon, Layman, & Kandel, 1975. Copyright by the Society for the Experimental Analysis of Behavior, Inc.)

the treatment program. One way to assure that help is more likely than hindrance is to involve the entire class in the project. This had been done by Patterson, Jones, Whittier, and Wright (1965) in their work with Raymond and their approach was extended by Rosenbaum, O'Leary, and Jacob (1975) who worked with 10 children, each of whom was attending a different classroom. The primary interest of these investigators was in ascertaining the effect of group consequences when used as a supplement to individual contingencies. The 10 children in this study were boys between the ages of 8 years, 9 months and 12 years, 1 month who had been selected on the basis of their scores on the Abbreviated Conners' Teacher Rating Scale (Sleator & von Neumann, 1974) from among a larger group of children whom their teachers had identified as hyperactive. Five of the boys were assigned to an individual reinforcement condition, while the other five were placed under a group contingency.

Unlike Ayllon, Layman, and Kandel (1975) who had focused reinforcement contingencies on academic performance while ignoring hyperactive behavior, Rosenbaum et al. (1975) targeted more general behaviors for the purpose of intervention. These behaviors included such activities as completing assigned work, staying in one's seat, not fighting, working on one task at a time, and remaining in the room. The appropriate target behaviors were determined individually for each child during a meeting with the teacher in which the principles and procedures of the intervention program were explained and discussed. The teacher was given a package containing an instruction manual with the rules of the program, a stack of reward cards, and a supply of backup reinforcers. The reward cards were colored 3 × 5 index cards with a smiling face on the front and the backup reinforcers consisted of a selection of penny candies.

The individual reward program entailed a private contract between the teacher and the child in that the teacher approached the child privately and explained the program to him. A typical explanation went somewhat as follows:

> Johnny, you know that you have trouble sitting still and concentrating on your work. You are lucky to have been chosen for a special program designed to help you do better. There are certain rules you must follow. There are . . . (list targets) . . . At the end of each hour I will come over to your desk and give you a reward card (show card) if you have been following the rules. After school, you will be allowed to trade in each card for a piece of candy from this box (show selection of candy). No one else in the class has to know about it . . . it will be our secret deal (Rosenbaum, O'Leary, & Jacob, 1975, p. 318).

For the classes where the focus was to be on group rewards, the teachers were instructed to present the program to the entire class, including the target child. Here, some variation of the following statement was to be used:

> Class, we all know that Johnny has trouble sitting still and completing his work. He has been lucky enough to have been chosen for a special program designed to

help him work better. There are certain rules Johnny must follow (list target behaviors). At the end of each hour I will evaluate Johnny on how well he has followed the rules, and if he has been good, I will given him a reward card (show
card). If he has not been following the rules, he does not get a card. At the end of
the day, everyone in the class will get a piece of candy for each card he has earned.
You may get from zero to four pieces each, depending on how well Johnny has
followed the rules. You can all help Johnny earn candy by ignoring him when he
is acting bad and by telling him when he is behaving or working well (Ibid.).

At the start of each day the teachers were to repeat the rules—to the entire
class in the group reward program, to the target child alone, in the individual
reward program. The teachers were asked to rate the child's behavior at the
end of each hour of the four-hour day and to give him a reward card, when appropriate. In giving the ratings, the teachers were supposed to enumerate the
positive and negative behaviors the child had engaged in and to tell why the
boy had or had not earned a reward. In classes where the group contingency
was operating, teachers were to draw on the blackboard a chart showing each
reward card earned so that the class would have a running account of the number of candies they would be receiving at the end of the day.

The token phase of this investigation lasted for four weeks. At the end of
this period the children were told that they had been doing very well, that the
supply of candy was depleted, that they would no longer be receiving reward
cards, but that the teacher would nonetheless expect them to continue to behave well. Four weeks later, the teachers were asked to fill out the Abbreviated
Conners' Teacher Rating Scale once again, having done so three times previously, twice—three months apart—before intervention began, and once at
the end of the token phase. The effect of such repeated administration on the
validity of this instrument is not known. Two other measures used were a specially constructed Problem Behavior Report which the teachers had completed
at the end of each week, and a questionnaire designed to assess the teachers'
satisfaction with the program and its results.

Before presenting the results of this investigation it is well to point to two
flaws in the experimental method that detract from the value of this study.
While the teachers had been carefully instructed in what they were to say to the
children and how they were to conduct the token program, Rosenbaum et al.
(1975) fail to present information about how or whether they ascertained that
the teachers actually implemented the program in the way they had been instructed. Without some form of monitoring teacher behavior it is impossible
to know whether the independent variable under investigation was really in effect. This, unfortunately, relates to the second flaw of the study. It is that the
dependent variables were the ratings and reports provided by the teachers who,
in effect, were being asked to evaluate the effectiveness of their own behavior.
If some of the teachers had carried out the program of intervention less faith-
fully than one might hope, is it not likely that these teachers might have re-

sponded to the rating scales and problem behavior reports in ways that would mask their delinquency? Data gathered by independent observers would have made this study much more convincing.

The results of the study, viewed with some reservations, show that the behavior of the hyperactive children as measured by the Conners' scale improved under both the individual and the group contingencies. After the contingencies had been withdrawn, the children in both treatment conditions showed some increase in problem behaviors but the average ratings remained below the pretreatment level. The data from the Problem Behavior Report essentially parallel the Conners' data although here the children in the group-contingency condition continued to improve slightly between the end of the token phase and the follow-up assessment. Interestingly, the teachers in the group-contingency condition viewed the procedure more positively than did those who had been assigned to the individual condition. Inasmuch as teacher acceptance of an intervention program is crucial to its implementation, the fact that in this study the teachers showed such a positive reaction to the group-contingency condition is quite noteworthy, especially considering that this procedure takes more of a teacher's time than the individual-contingency condition.

The Effect of Self-Instruction

The approaches to intervention with hyperactive children we have discussed thus far focused either on the reinforcement of attending behavior or on the strengthening of academic and prosocial behaviors. If, as in the case of the study by Ayllon, Layman, and Kandel (1975), hyperactivity declines as academic performance improves in the course of being reinforced, one might conclude that the children had learned to focus their attention and were thus able to do better academic work. That is to say that the excess activity level of children who are classified as hyperactive can be construed as the indirect result of a deficit in the child's ability to focus attention on the task at hand. Following that reasoning, it would appear that a program of intervention should focus on developing the weak or absent attentional skills by an explicit training program and that this should lead to improved academic work and reciprocal reduction of hyperactivity.

The above reasoning seems to have formed the basis of a treatment approach reported by Bornstein and Quevillon (1976) who used self-instruction to help overactive preschool boys to control their own behavior. Self-instruction has the considerable advantage over externally managed contingencies that the child, in effect, carries the contingencies around with him, thus enhancing the probability that the learned controls will generalize to a variety of situations and be maintained over time. Self-instruction thus may well be the answer to the ubiquitous problems of the generalization and maintenance of treatment effects. The work of Bornstein and Quevillon (1976) suggests that this is the case, at least with very young children.

The three children with whom Bornstein and Quevillon (1976) worked were four-year olds, enrolled in one classroom of a preschool Head Start program. They had been selected on the basis of teacher and teacher-aide reports of highly disruptive and undesirable classroom behavior. One boy, identified as Scott, was described as unable to follow directions for any length of time, unable to complete standard tasks, and subject to violent outbursts of temper. Another, Rod, was seen as "out of control in the classroom"; as having a short attention span and being generally aggressive and overactive. The third boy, Tim, was reported as highly distractible both at home and in school. He spent most of his classroom time walking around the room or staring into space and he failed to attend to assigned tasks or to listen to instructions.

The target of intervention selected by the investigators was on-task behavior; that is, performing prescribed and accepted classroom activities and being silent and attentive when the teacher was giving instructions. In terms of recording on-task behavior, movement about the room or playing with toys when such behavior was inappropriate with respect to teacher-directed class activity were considered off-task behaviors as were shouting, fighting, kicking, or leaving the classroom without permission. Treatment, however, did not focus on these "hyperactive" behaviors. Data were gathered on four out of five school days per week by two independent and trained observers who recorded behavior as either on-task or off-task during two 30-minute observation periods per day, using a 10-second observe, 1-second record procedure. Interobserver agreement was at the 94 percent level and agreement with a third observer who conducted covert reliability checks during ten sessions was 92 percent. The reliability of the data thus appears encouragingly high.

In order to assess the effect of the self-instruction training on the children's on-task behavior, Bornstein and Quevillon (1976) used a multiple-baseline design across subjects. During the first eight days, all three children were under baseline conditions during which Scott's mean rate of on-task behavior was recorded as 10.4 percent. At this point he was given a two-hour session of self-instruction training (to be described below) whereupon his on-task behavior immediately jumped to near 90 percent and remained at a mean of 82.3 percent until the end of the 40-day posttreatment observation period. Rod, who had remained under baseline conditions for 16 days during which his mean rate of on-task behavior was 14.6 percent, was given self-instruction training on the seventeenth day. His behavior also improved immediately and he maintained a mean on-task behavior of 70.8 percent during the posttreatment period. Tim remained on baseline for 24 days and showed a mean of 10 percent on-task behavior during that time. He too improved dramatically immediately after he received self-instruction training and his posttreatment mean for on-task behavior was 77.8 percent. On the sixtieth and again on the ninetieth observation day of the study the observers returned to the classroom to gather follow-up, postcheck data. These showed that the boys had maintained the high level of on-task behavior they had manifested during the post-treatment observations. Scott was on task 70 and 77 percent of the time (for the first and second postcheck, respectively) while the data for Rod were 64 and 67 percent and for Tim 70 and 68 percent. This is rather remarkable maintenance of an effect of two hours of treatment especially considering the fact that the final day of follow-up occurred 22½ weeks after baseline, there having been only four observation days per week.

The results of the Bornstein and Quevillon (1976) study are shown in graphic form in Figure 11. It reflects in a convincing fashion that the children's behavior changed in direct consequence to the introduction of the self-instruction training. Improvement was clearly not a function of passage of time, nor did the improvement in the behavior of one child affect the behavior of the other children. A multiple baseline design permits one to draw reliable conclusions from a small number of subjects and it facilitates the display of behavior changes of individuals that are invariably obscured when group data are analyzed with measures of central tendencies. Let us now turn to a detailed presentation of the training procedures that produced these remarkable results.

As described by Bornstein and Quevillon (1976), their procedure entailed a massed self-instruction session for each child, lasting two hours and including one 20-minute break. In the words of the investigators:

> The self-instructional training was similar to that described elsewhere (Meichenbaum and Goodman, 1971) and proceeded as follows: (1) the experimenter modelled the task while talking aloud to himself, (2) the subject performed the task while the experimenter instructed aloud, (3) the subject then performed the task talking aloud to himself while the experimenter whispered softly, (4) the subject performed the task whispering softly while the experimenter made lip movements but no sound, (5) the subject performed the task making lip movements without sound while the experimenter self-instructed covertly, and (6) the subject performed the task with covert self-instruction.
>
> The verbalizations modelled were of four types: (a) questions about the task (e.g., "What does the teacher want me to do?)", (b) answers to questions in the form of cognitive rehearsal (e.g., "Oh, that's right, I'm supposed to copy that picture."), (c) self-instructions that guide through the task (e.g., "OK, first I draw a line here. . ."), and (d) self-reinforcement (e.g., "How about that; I really did that one well.").
>
> It should also be noted that, in numerous tasks, the experimenter consciously erred and then corrected his error without hesitation. In addition, since initially the children did not seem motivated to work, the experimenter paired self-praise with material reward (M&M's) as a means of creating incentive. This reward was quickly leaned [thinned] out as the children found they could complete the tasks

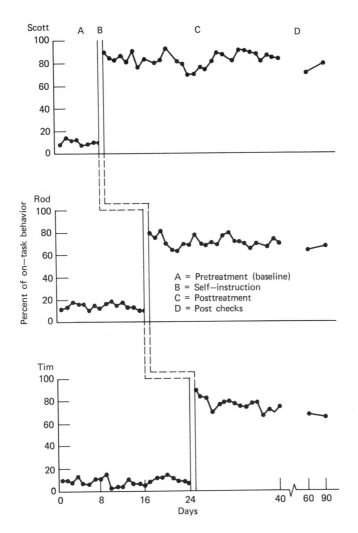

Figure 11. Daily percent on-task behaviors for Scott, Rod, and Tim across experimental conditions. (Bornstein & Quevillon, 1976. Copyright by the Society for the Experimental Analysis of Behavior, Inc.)

successfully. Lastly, the entire training session was presented in a story-like manner. In each situation, the subject was told that the teacher (not the experimenter) had asked him to complete the task in question. When using self-instructions, then, the subject would respond as if he were in the classroom (e.g., "Mrs. B wants me to draw that picture over there. OK, how can I do that?").

More specifically, the self-instructional protocol consisted of the experimenter initially instructing the child "_____(child's name), watch what I do and listen to what I say." Immediately, on gaining his attention, an M&M was placed in the child's mouth. When the first trial was completed, and if the child's attention had not shifted away from the experimental task, he was again given a candy reinforcer. The experimenter then said to the child, "_____(child's name), this time you do it while I say the words." Contingent on correct performance, the experimenter dispensed an M&M to the child paired with self-praise at the conclusion of this second trial. Candy reinforcers were then leaned [thinned] out quite rapidly and given only at the close of a trial. No more than 10 reinforcers were given to any one child during a training session. Later in the training sequence, when the child was asked to verbalize on his own, acceptable responses were those that included correct performance and the four elements outlined above (i.e., questions about the task, answers, self-instructions, and self-reinforcement). If the child did not produce an acceptable response, the experimenter again modelled the task while talking aloud to himself. Following such demonstrations, the child was then returned to that part of the sequence where his error had been committed. If the child refused to comply, the experimenter merely reiterated his instructions and again modelled an appropriate response. When the child successfully completed a trial, he was given instructions for the next step in the training sequence. When all six steps in the sequence had been completed, the experimenter presented a new task and again modelled its performance while talking aloud to himself (i.e., step one).

A wide variety of tasks were employed in the 2-hr training sessions, with difficulty level increasing over time. These tasks varied from situations tapping simple sensorymotor skills (e.g., copying of lines and figures) to more complex problem-solving situations (e.g., block design and conceptual grouping tasks). In all instances, subjects were required to verbalize the nature of the task and their problem-solving strategy. All tasks were modified slightly from those on the Stanford-Binet, Wechsler Intelligence Scale for Children or the McCarthy Scales of Children's Abilities (Bornstein & Quevillon, 1976, pp. 181f. Copyright by the Society for the Experimental Analysis of Behavior, Inc.).

The observers in the classroom would have noticed when a child was absent from class for the two-hour self-instruction training. Even though they were naive as to the design of the study, they might thus have developed expectancies about changes in that child's behavior that could have influenced their observations. For this reason an expectancy control had been included in the design of this investigation. It consisted of having each of the three children leave the classroom for a two-hour session with the investigator on the days when one of them was to be given the self-instruction training. During this time the other two children were individually exposed to the stimulus material used in the training but they were not exposed to the actual self-instruction procedure. Instead, the investigator modeled appropriate responses without verbalization, other than saying to the child, "Watch what I do," and rewarding the child for attending to his demonstration. Following this, the investigator asked the child to perform the same task while he watched, the entire procedure being repeated a second time before another task was presented. In this manner the children who were not receiving self-instruction training on that day experienced what might be termed a placebo condition entailing individual adult attention, removal from the classroom, interaction with the stimulus materials, and receipt of some reinforcers. All of this further increases the robust nature of the results obtained in this significant study which convincingly demonstrates that a self-instructional program for preschoolers can affect their behavior in such a way that the improvement generalizes from the training session to the classroom situation and is maintained for a considerable period of time.

The Bornstein and Quevillon procedure was, of course, a "treatment package" that made use of instruction, self-instruction, verbal modeling, prompts, reinforcement, and fading. Which of these various components or which of their combinations represents the critical independent variable is not known and future research will have to explore whether individual components of the package might be equally effective. Meanwhile, these investigators have clearly presented a readily implemented procedure for increasing the on-task behavior of preschool children who are frequently labeled as hyperactive. Unfortunately, the procedure seems to be less effective when it is used with somewhat older children for when Friedling and O'Leary (1979) attempted to apply it with second- and third- grade hyperactive children they failed to obtain the same results as Bornstein and Quevillon (1976) until they introduced a token program that rewarded on-task behavior.

Recapitulation

The most productive treatment approaches for hyperactive children have focused not on reducing hyperactivity but on strengthening behaviors that are incompatible with the excess motility that leads these children to be called hyperactive. One of the first behavioral treatments of hyperactivity involved the differential reinforcement of attending behavior. Studies since that time have shown that the direct reinforcement of appropriate classroom behavior or of academic performance results in a reduction of hyperactivity. Such programs of intervention, employing either individual or group contingencies, can be instituted in the classroom by the regular teacher and there is evidence that this approach is superior to one that relies on medication to suppress children's activity level. One of the most promising approaches to helping hyperactive, disruptive preschool children is based on a self-instruction procedure in which children are taught in relatively short time to control their own on-task behavior, thereby enhancing both generalization and maintenance of the improvement.

CHAPTER 7

Problems with Elimination

INCONTINENCE: A BEHAVIORAL DEFICIT

In few psychological disorders are the utility and logic of the distinction between behavior deficits and behavior excesses quite as apparent as in the case of problems around the elimination of urine or feces. Although the complaint is usually phrased in terms of the child's wetting or soiling "too often" so that a behavioral excess might come to mind, it is clear that what is involved is the child's deficient ability to control these bodily functions in a socially acceptable manner. Even the word "incontinence," defined in the dictionary as an inability to control eliminative functions, tells us that these problems should be conceptualized as behavioral deficits, as control deficits. The therapeutic task must therefore focus on establishing these missing or deficient controls as a means to reducing the more readily apparent excessive number of wet bedsheets or soiled pants. More specifically, the controls these children must learn entail two related responses. One is to retard elimination through sphincter control and the other is to eliminate in the place society has designated as "proper."

The most frequently encountered problem in the area of sphincter control is nighttime bedwetting (nocturnal enuresis). Daytime wetting (diurnal enuresis) and day or nighttime soiling (encopresis) are reported far less frequently. Azrin and Thienes (1978) cite data showing that about 20 percent of all three-year olds are enuretic, the incidence dropping to 15 percent by age 6, and to about 3 percent by age 14.

DEFICIENT BLADDER CONTROL

The frequency of bedwetting, the relative ease with which it can be treated by methods based on principles of learning, and the objectivity of the criterion for measuring treatment outcome (a bed is either wet or dry), have made the treatment of this problem the object of a number of rather well-controlled investigations (Azrin & Thienes, 1978; Baker, 1969; DeLeon & Mandell, 1966; DeLeon & Sacks, 1972; Finley, Besserman, Bennett, Clapp, & Finley, 1973; Jehu, Morgan, Turner, & Jones, 1977; Lovibond, 1964; Novick, 1966; Young & Morgan, 1972). Most of these studies deal with the use of the bell-and-pad method developed by Mowrer and Mowrer (1938).

The Mowrer Pad

The basic mechanism involved in the bell-and-pad method of treating enuresis is a combination of wire gauze or metal foil sheets that are separated by an insulating pad and wired in such a way that the electrolytic effect of a single drop of urine will close a battery-powered circuit, activating a bell or buzzer that continues to sound until is it manually turned off. This device is placed under the bedsheet of the child who is instructed to get out of bed when the signal sounds and go to the toilet to complete the urination that the alarm will usually have interrupted. To assure complete wakefulness, the child is also asked to wash his or her face as a part of the routine. Afterwards the wet sheet is changed, the signal reset, and the child goes back to sleep. With young children this procedure is supervised by a parent who will also have been awakened by the sound of the alarm (James & Foreman, 1973). The device and its use are described in detail by Turner (1973) and commercially available models come with complete instructions.

Theoretical Issues. As we shall see, there is little doubt that the bell-and-pad method of treating nocturnal enuresis is effective in many cases, some reporting success rates between 80 and 90 percent (Turner, 1973). The principles underlying this effect are, however, less well established. Mowrer and Mowrer (1938) had originally conceptualized their method as an application of the principles of respondent conditioning and these seem, indeed, to be among the central aspects of the process. A carefully controlled study by Collins (1973) "substantiated the view that the effectiveness of the conditioning treatment depends primarily upon the contiguous pairing of bladder cues with the UCS, which induces sphincter contraction and/or awakening" (p. 305). Yet, as Collins (1973) has also observed, certain experimenter and placebo effects seem to contribute to favorable treatment outcome. Even Mowrer and Mowrer (1938) had stressed the importance of a positive parent–child relationship to the success of their conditioning method. In other words, more variables than the CS–UCS contingency of classical conditioning appear to be operating so that the effect of this intervention should be viewed as based on a combination of psychological principles. At the very least, one has to consider the fact that the procedure has some aversive qualities, ranging from the mild discomfort of sleeping on the pad and the startling sound of the alarm, to having to wash one's face in the middle of the night and involving other members of the family who are also awakened by the alarm. Lovibond (1964) pointed out that passive avoidance learning may be the process that plays a major role in this procedure and negative reinforcement is no doubt also one of the contributors to the learning process. Lastly, since contemporary methods stress the importance of keeping a record so that progress can be rewarded by praise and prizes, it seems evident that positive reinforcement also play an important role.

Just as the specifics of the psychological processes that are involved in this form of treatment continue to be a source of debate (see, for example, the exchange between Turner, Young, and Rachman, 1970; Lovibond, 1972; and Turner, Rachman and Young, 1972), so there remains uncertainty about the neurophysiological processes underlying the development of a child's ability to sleep through the night without wetting. The formulation used by Mowrer and Mowrer (1938) speaks of the stimulation produced by bladder distention reflexively leading to sphincter relaxation and onset of urination. When the awakening stimulus is introduced immediately following the onset of urination it will elicit an awakening response and sphincter contraction. On the basis of Pavlovian conditioning principles, the Mowrers then expected that an increasingly strong functional connection would develop "between the stimulation arising from the distention of the bladder and the responses of awakening and contracting the bladder sphincter" (p. 446). Beyond this, the Mowrers' formulation reads as follows:

> Soon this connection should become sufficiently well established to cause the awakening response and the contraction of the bladder sphincter to "come forward" in time and occur actually in advance of the onset of urination, instead of afterwards. The conditioned contraction of the sphincter in response to bladder distention would thus tend to inhibit the occurrence of reflex sphincter relaxation during sleep and to lead to awakening when bladder pressure finally becomes sufficiently great. We thus have a theoretical basis for the expectation that soon the subject would not only cease to urinate reflexly during sleep but would also become capable of retaining his urine longer than had previously been possible, without necessarily awakening (p. 446).

In their pioneering formulation Mowrer and Mowrer (1938) postulated only bladder distention and sphincter contraction as the physiological mediators. Years later, Collins (1973) still speaks of the wake-up signal as inducing contraction of the sphincter muscle. Other writers, such as Young and Morgan (1972), however, focus on the inhibition of the detrusor muscle. The *detrusor urinae* is the muscle that, when activated, pushes down and facilitates the emptying of the bladder. The urinary sphincter, on the other hand, is a ringlike muscle that contracts, thereby closing the urethral canal and retaining the urine in the bladder. The detrusor and the sphincter thus work as antagonists; for urine to be discharged, the detrusor must contract while the sphincter must relax. The ability to hold urine, therefore, calls for detrusor inhibition and sphincter activation. The conditioning process that is involved in the use of the bell-and-pad, therefore, must somehow effect both inhibition and activation but just how this comes about is only vaguely understood by those who write about the use of the Mowrer-type apparatus. They prefer to focus on the outcome, the dry bed, accepting the mediating processes as a given.

Treatment Effects. Outcome studies on the effect of treating bedwetting with a Mowrer-type procedure have generally been highly favorable. DeLeon and Mandell (1966) demonstrated the superiority of this approach over treatments based on psychodynamic formulations and a follow-up of their treated cases by DeLeon and Sacks (1972) conducted four years later showed that 81 percent of the children had not wet the bed during the year prior to the follow-up telephone contact. Baker (1969) had previously demonstrated that successful treatment of bedwetting by conditioning procedures is frequently accompanied by improvements in areas of the child's behavior that had not been targeted for treatment. This may well result from the fact that bedwetting often precludes a child's sleeping over at the house of a friend or having a friend stay overnight, prevents attending sleep-away summer camp, and leads to feeling inadequate and inferior in comparison with siblings and peers. Once a child has learned to stay dry at night the success is likely to change all this, thus improving peer relations, social development, and self-evaluations (Compton, 1968). For this reason it is important to stress for enuretic children that the bell-and-pad is not a magic gadget that will accomplish something they had been unable to do but that it is a tool with which a child can learn to stay dry at night.

In a comprehensive review of the literature on behavioral treatments of bedwetting, Doleys (1977) summarized 12 studies that employed the bell-and-pad procedure in systematic research. On the basis of this summary, covering 628 children, he reports that for 75 percent of these children bedwetting had been successfully arrested with treatments ranging in length from 5 to 12 weeks. The criterion for success used in these studies is a specified number of successive dry nights, that number ranging from a rather lenient 10 (Collins, 1973) to a rigorous 28 (Baker, 1969). With a child who had been wetting the bed every night before treatment began, a criterion of 14 consecutive dry nights is usually considered to be an acceptable criterion of success. In a large number of instances children who have been treated by the urine alarm system will experience a relapse of wetting within six months of treatment. Doleys'

(1977) summary shows this to have occurred in 41 percent of the cases, a figure considerably higher than the 20 to 30 percent usually cited (O'Leary & Wilson, 1975). When children who have thus relapsed are given a second, usually shorter series of nights with the bell-and-pad, they generally relearn quickly and remain dry after that. Because the experience of resumed bedwetting after having ostensibly overcome the problem can be quite devastating to child and family, most therapists who use the urine-alarm method tell clients that relapse may take place and that this is a normal occurrence that a "booster treatment" will easily remedy.

Overlearning. If one construes the effect of the urine-alarm system as the conditioning of a new response, extinction of that response after a period during which reinforcement contingencies were not in effect is clearly a phenomenon that learning theory would lead one to predict. It is also learning theory that permits one to devise methods designed to reduce or eliminate the troublesome relapse problem. One procedure that makes a response more resistant to extinction, and to which we shall return later, is to use intermittent reinforcement during training; another is overlearning, that is, to continue training trials beyond the point where the response has reached a predetermined criterion for learning. In the conditioning treatment of bedwetting a training trial consists of pairing the wetting response with the ringing of the alarm. Once a child no longer wets the bed, further training trials for the purpose of overlearning cannot be given unless one somehow arranged for additional wettings. Mowrer and Mowrer (1938) recognized this dilemma and sought to deal with it by having the child's fluid intake increased by one or two cups of water just before retiring once their training criterion of seven dry nights had been reached. They would then continue this practice until the child had once again gone seven successive nights without wetting. Young and Morgan (1972) conducted a systematic study on the effect of such an overlearning procedure on the resistance to extinction of the ability to sleep through the night without wetting.

From among a group of children who had reached the success criterion of 14 consecutive dry nights Young and Morgan (1972) randomly selected 67 who were instructed to drink two pints of liquid within an hour before bedtime and to continue using the wake-up alarm as before. This overlearning regimen was continued until the child once again reached the criterion of 14 dry nights. It is of practical interest to note that Young and Morgan (1972) had no difficulty getting the families in their overlearning group to cooperate with their procedure. They seem to have expected some resistance to their procedure which places increased demands upon parents and children through the renewal of bedwetting after the child had become dry. As they put it, "Having once known the joys of dry beds, it is possible that patients and their families may become antipathetic towards any procedure destined to produce enuresis once again" (p. 150).

In order to investigate the attitudinal factor, Young and Morgan (1972) compared the dropout rate in the group who participated in overlearning with that of the group of children who had been discharged immediately upon first reaching the criterion of success. Although this fails to control for length of time in treatment, their results show that instead of the requirements for over-learning increasing the rate of premature termination, they had the opposite effect; that is, the overlearning group had a significantly lower rate of termination (6 out of 61) than the group that did not have these requirements imposed on them (37 out of 83). The investigators explain this result by speculating that by the time a child reached the overlearning stage, the efficacy of treatment had already been demonstrated by the experience of 14 dry nights. This demonstration, they suspect, may have disposed the children and their parents so favorably toward the treatment (and toward the therapists?) as to make them willing to implement the instructions required to produce overlearning and to continue in treatment during this period. In only 6 of the 67 cases with whom overlearning was attempted did the required fluid intake result in a relapse of bedwetting of such severity that the procedure had to be discontinued and the child discharged without further recourse to attempts at overlearning once the criterion of success had been regained.

Since the purpose of overlearning is to reduce the relapse rate, the critical information obtained from the Young and Morgan (1972) study lies in the data on relapse. These were gathered by sending follow-up letters to all parents whose child had been treated. The first such letter was sent three months after discharge, another after six months, with further letters every six months thereafter. The reply form enclosed with these letters asked whether the child had continued to have a dry bed and whether the parents wished a further appointment at the clinic. For the purpose of their study, Young and Morgan (1972) defined relapse "as a recurrence of bedwetting, subsequent to discharge sufficient to cause the parent to request a further appointment" (p. 149). By this somewhat subjective criterion, relapse occurred in 22.8 percent of the 101 children who had reached the success criterion at the time they were discharged from the clinic. The 46 children in the total group who had not undergone overlearning training showed a relapse rate of 34.8 percent, while the 55 children who had participated in and completed overlearning had a rate of only 12.7 percent. This is a statistically significant difference leading the investigators to recommend strongly that overlearning be included in the conditioning treatment of enuresis.

It is not clear from the information presented by Young and Morgan (1972) whether all of the children in the overlearning group actually started wetting the bed again once the increase in fluid intake was introduced. In their discussion of the rationale for overlearning they speak of such fluid intake as putting additional stress on the detrusor muscle (to contract) as the kidneys produce more urine. When this additional stress is not tolerated by the detrusor so that the acquired inhibiting response is overwhelmed, wetting would take place, the alarm would go off, and an additional training trial would thus have been achieved. If, on the other hand, the additional stress on the detrusor were tolerated, the learned response (inhibition of urination and/or awakening) "would correspondingly be progressively strengthened" (p. 148), presumably by stimulus generalization to larger bladder content. Since these investigators thus provide a rationale for resistance to relapse when there is no opportunity for overlearning, one must assume that not every child reacted to the increased fluid intake by once again wetting the bed. Unfortunately the report does not reveal how many such children there were in this study and how their relapse rate compared with that of the children who actually experienced a series of additional training trials. This issue is raised here for two reasons. One is that the implications of having a child sleep with the wake-up apparatus in place but inoperative have been investigated in other studies to which we shall now turn. The other is that a treatment method based solely on increasing a child's fluid intake in hopes of raising the threshold is also available (Kimmel & Kimmel, 1970) and will be explored shortly.

Intermittent Reinforcement. It has long been known (e.g., Jenkins & Stanley, 1950) that in respondent conditioning a response that has been acquired under conditions of intermittent UCS–CS pairing (reinforcement) will be more resistant to extinction than one established under conditions of continuous reinforcement in which every presentation of the conditioned stimulus was paired with a presentation of the unconditioned stimulus. As pointed out earlier, the usual method employed in treating enuresis by the bell-and-pad method is to have every instance of wetting followed by the sounding of the alarm and by the sequence of waking up and voiding in the toilet which the alarm presumably initiates. From the stand-point of conditioning theory, this represents a schedule of continuous reinforcement. Once the dry-bed response is established and conditioning, that is, reinforcement is discontinued, one should expect the response to undergo extinction. This, as we stated, may well be what happens in the 41 percent of treated cases who resume wetting after having reached a success criterion (Doleys, 1977). While this formulation begs the question of what maintains the bladder-control response in the other 59 percent of successfully treated children it does suggest a method for reducing the relapse rate. From what is known about conditioning, relapse (i.e., extinction) should be counteracted if one were to place the initial acquisition of the response on a schedule of intermittent reinforcement. The effectiveness of such a procedure has been studied by a number of investigators; among these are Lovibond (1964), Turner, Young, and Rachman (1970), Taylor and Turner (1975), as well as Finley and his associates (Finley, Besserman, Bennett, Clapp, & Finley, 1973; Finley, Wansley, & Blenkarn, 1977).

The usual way of introducing intermittent UCS–CS pairing is to have the alarm apparatus inoperative some of the time so that the child will experience instances where wetting does not result in the activation of the wake-up signal. When the alarm is operational and when it is not must, of course, be randomized so that the child does not know the prevailing condition. In some studies (Turner, Young, & Rachman, 1970; Taylor & Turner, 1975) this was accomplished by having the child's mother switch the alarm system on by following a prearranged schedule. In others (Finley, et al., 1977) an automated, programmed system was used so that no member of the family could know beforehand whether the next trial (wetting) would result in the activation of the alarm.

In all cases it is important that the child's bedsheets are changed and the alarm reset after every wetting because as many as 80 percent of enuretic children wet several times a night (Finley et al., 1977). This being the case, such a child would be on an uncontrolled (and predictable) intermittent schedule if the alarm were to be operational only when the first wetting of the night took place. If such an intermittent schedule were to be operating at the beginning of treatment, it would, in fact, interfere with the acquisition of the dry bed response. This is the case because *acquisition* of a response is enhanced when training is on a continuous schedule while *resistance to extinction* is increased when an intermittent schedule is in effect. The most efficient way of scheduling training trials therefore is to have a continuous schedule operating at the beginning of training and to shift gradually to a schedule that becomes more and more intermittent until reinforcement is completely faded out as training approaches termination.

Pursuing work from an earlier study (Finley, Besserman, Bennett, Clapp, & Finley, 1973) that had demonstrated intermittent reinforcement to reduce the frequency of relapse, Finley, Wansley, and Blenkarn (1977) conducted research with 80 chronically enuretic children using a 70 percent intermittent reinforcement schedule. To maintain a variable interval schedule they employed a specially designed automated alarm apparatus that permitted the programming of any ratio of nonreinforced trials (wettings that do not activate the alarm). The alarm combined the ringing of a loud bell with the illumination of a bright light over the child's bed. Concurrent with these signals, designed to awaken the child, a small beeper alarm was activated in the parent's bedroom so that one of them could monitor the child's using the toilet, change the sheets, and reset the alarm. Because a change of sheets was necessary after every wetting in order to permit the sensors in the pad to function properly, the beeper also alerted the parents after a 20-minute delay when one of the nonreinforced trials had taken place. In addition to these responsibilities, the parents were instructed to keep accurate records containing data on the child's bedtime, time of each wetting, number of wettings per night, the diameter of the wet spot, and whether the alarm activated in the child's room or only in the parent's room.

For the first seven wettings all children were on a schedule of continuous reinforcement. After that the intermittent, 70 percent, variable interval schedule was initiated and continued until the child had reached the criterion of 14 consecutive dry nights. All cases were then followed for a median time of 10 months and relapse was defined as three or more wet nights per week during that follow-up period.

The results of the treatment conducted by Finley, Wansley and Blenkarn (1977) are quite impressive in that 94 percent of the children reached the dryness criterion after a mean of 21.5 wettings during a mean of 46.8 treatment nights. The child's age (the range had been from 5 to 14 years with a median of 8 years) was unrelated to these outcome data but when the relapse data were examined it was clear that they were a function of age. With children of all ages combined, the relapse rate was 25 percent but this low rate was due particularly to the extremely low rates in age groups 5 to 6 (15 percent) and 7 to 8 (5.25 percent). For children between the ages of 9 and 10 years, the rate was a disappointing 50 percent while those 11 years of age and over had a relapse rate of 22 percent. Finley et al. (1977) compared their data with a relapse rate of 47 percent, calculated from studies published over the past 10 years where schedules of continuous reinforcement had been applied. From this comparison they concluded that their variable 70 percent schedule was significantly more effective despite the fact that it did not seem to improve the relapse rate for the 9 to 10 year age group. Whether a different ratio of reinforcement would work better with that age group remains to be investigated.

Before leaving the study by Finley et al. (1977) note should be taken of the information they provide about the frequency of multiple wettings per night. It seems that in the beginning stages of treatment, enuretic children wet the bed more than once per night and that this shows a linear decrease until just before the dryness criterion is reached. In the first week of treatment, approximately 80 percent of the chidren in this study had at least one night of multiple wettings. This information is important to keep in mind when planning a variable interval schedule since it means that one must count each instance of wetting as a trial and not merely record whether a given night was wet or dry. By viewing the whole night as one trial and having the apparatus connected or disconnected for the entire night, one may inadvertently lose control over the ratio of reinforcement one wishes to employ.

On the whole, it appears that both overlearning and intermittent reinforcement are procedures that effectively reduce the rate of relapse in treated children. Morgan (1978) reviewed the available literature concerning this problem and concluded that of the two procedures, published results generally tend to favor overlearning as the more effective for preventing relapse after treatment.

Retention Control Training

The ultimate aim of any intervention with enuretic children is to have them acquire the ability to sleep through the night without wetting the bed. In order for this end result to come about, urine that accumulates in the bladder during the night must be retained in the bladder. The fact that enuretic children seem unable to do this, combined with reports that these children have a high frequency of urination during the daytime, has led to the suggestion (Muellner, 1960) that their problem might be that they have an unusually small bladder so that treatment ought to focus on increasing bladder capacity and/or raising the amount of pressure the detrusor muscle can tolerate before it initiates voiding of bladder content. While the hypothesis about bladder capacity might apply in the case of the chronic enuretic who has never been dry at night, it does not seem to fit the large number of regressed enuretics who, once having been dry, revert to wetting at a later age (Doleys, 1977). On the other hand, the speculation about the threshold of the detrusor muscle might well apply to both types of enuretics.

In discussions of "bladder capacity," measurement is always indirect. Since the actual amount of urine the bladder is capable of holding is very difficult to ascertain, investigators usually resort to measuring the amount of urine being discharged when the child has been asked to delay urination for as long as possible. It is then assumed that this represents the maximum amount the bladder is capable of holding. It was on the basis of such an indirect measure that Starfield and Mellits (1968) had reported a positive correlation between bladder capacity and improvement in remaining dry at night. As is usual with correlations, this does not tell us whether increased bladder capacity caused the decreased bedwetting or whether decreased bedwetting increased bladder capacity. Early suggestions for retention control training (Muellner, 1960), however, were based on the assumption that a child should be able to remain dry at night if one were able to increase the capacity of his or her bladder.

Retention control training, as introduced by Kimmel and Kimmel (1970), avoids speculations about the physiological mediators and focuses instead on teaching the child to delay urination for longer and longer periods. This is done during the day, while the child is awake, by increasing fluid intake and asking the child to withhold voiding for two or three minutes longer than the day before. Success in doing this is then followed by reinforcement and the procedure is continued until the child is able to delay urination for as much as 45 minutes after the need to urinate was first reported. When Kimmel and

Kimmel (1970) first used this operant approach with three enuretic children the retention interval was only 30 minutes, yet they reported that two of the three children ceased bedwetting within seven days while the third child became dry within two weeks. All three remained dry during a 12-month follow-up period. It seems that the ability to delay urination for a relatively brief period, when learned during the day, generalizes to nighttime retention when it must be practiced for a considerably longer time. As is often the case in behavior therapy, practice has outpaced theory as the mechanisms by which such generalization takes place are not known.

Following the apparent success in the exploratory study by Kimmel and Kimmel (1970), Paschalis, Kimmel, and Kimmel (1972) conducted a controlled investigation of retention control training. The parents of 35 children who had never been dry at night and the parents of a nonenuretic control group (number not reported) were instructed to record the number of times per day their child used the toilet for urination during waking hours. During this 15-day baseline period the number of urinations per day ranged from 4 to 12 for the enuretic group, while the range for the control group was only from 3 to 5. On the basis of this information, the authors speculated that bedwetting is associated with a lower threshold of bladder-distension cues needed to evoke urination.

Following the baseline period, Paschalis et al. (1972) held a two-hour meeting with the parents during which they were taught the reinforcement procedures they were to use. Each child was to decide on the initial duration of withholding urination following his first reporting a need to urinate. The withholding time was then to be increased by two to three minutes each day until the child could wait 45 minutes before urinating. A reinforcing token and praise were to be delivered at the end of the withholding period just before the child went to the toilet. The child was to chart the withholding times and at the end of each day tokens were to be exchanged for a choice of trinkets. Once the child had been dry for one complete week, a gift, chosen at the beginning of the shaping period, was to be delivered to reward this accomplishment.

Paschalis, Kimmel, and Kimmel (1972) report that 15 children attained a minimum of one continuous week without bedwetting, while eight children had improved to between two and six dry nights a week. Since the parents of four children failed to apply the procedure, this leaves ten children who were unimproved. Ninety days after the end of the reinforcement period, which had lasted for 20 days in all but two cases, the parents were asked whether any further bedwetting had occurred and the authors state that "no relapses were reported," presumably for the fifteen cases where complete dryness had been achieved. Although Paschalis et al. (1972) conclude that their method "has great promise" (p. 255) for the treatment of chronic enuresis, one must agree with Doleys (1977) that available data "do not provide strong support for retention control training as a treatment procedure for enuresis" (p. 46). Studies with the bell-and-pad method report an initial arrest rate of 75 percent with criteria considerably higher than 7 days, while Paschalis et al. (1972) show an arrest rate for the treated children of only 48 percent. Since the eight children they consider as significantly improved are not usually counted in the success column by other investigators, one must view this study to have had a failure rate of 52 percent. Hardly an "especially impressive" result as the summary of the report by Paschalis, Kimmel, and Kimmel (1972) would lead one to believe. In fact, when Doleys, Ciminero, Tollison, Williams, and Wells (1977) applied retention control training to nine children over a period of six weeks, they found no changes at all in the number of wet nights per week. For that matter, they found no consistent changes in bladder capacity (amount of urine voided) which, unlike Paschalis et al. (1972), they had measured both before and after treatment. On the other hand, when Harris and Purohit (1977) applied a retention control procedure for 35 days to nine enuretic children they did find an increase in bladder capacity but, they too, reported no reduction in bedwetting.

On the whole, the results of retention control training may well be "suggestive of further research" as Doleys (1977) concludes but they hardly provide support for considering this form of intervention "a viable alternative" to the bell-and-pad method, as O'Leary and Wilson (1975) would have one believe.

Dry Bed Training

A method of treating enuretic children that combines aspects of a variety of techniques was introduced by Azrin, Sneed, and Foxx (1974). It is an extension of a rapid method of toilet training that Foxx and Azrin (1973a) had successfully used with children whose difficulty was that they had not yet learned to maintain urinary continence during the day. That method, which is also described in a book written for the general public (Azrin & Foxx, 1974), entails one day's intensive practice of going to the toilet from various parts of the house while a high rate of urination is maintained by frequent fluid intake. Appropriate urination is strongly reinforced and "accidents" have the consequence of *positive practice overcorrection*, consisting of ten rapidly conducted trials during which all responses involved in using the toilet (short of actual urination) are rehearsed.

In modifying this method for the treatment of bedwetting, Azrin, Sneed, and Foxx (1974) referred to it as dry bed training, a term that places the emphasis on the positive goal to be learned and not on the negative behavior that is to be eliminated. In the dry bed method an outside trainer joins the family for one intensive day's training during which the child is taught the series of re-

[""]

sponses needed for remaining dry at night. In later work (Azrin, Hontos, & Besalel-Azrin, 1979) the outside trainer was dispensed with and the parents and their child were instead given their instructions during a single office visit of about 1½ hour duration.

The dry bed program begins while the child is awake. One hour before bedtime he or she is informed of all phases of the training procedure. A bell-and-pad alarm is then placed on the bed and the child proceeds to engage in 20 trials of *positive practice* in toileting. This entails having the child lie down in the bed, counting to 50, getting up and going to the toilet where an attempt is made to urinate, returning to bed and starting the sequence anew. At bedtime the child drinks a large amount of liquid so as to increase the number of practice urinations. Every hour thereafter the child is awakened and walked to the toilet. At the bathroom door the child is asked to delay urination for one hour and if the child indicates being able to do so, the trainer (or parent) delivers praise statements and returns the child to bed. On the other hand, if the child feels unable to tolerate the delay, he or she urinates in the toilet, is praised for correct toileting, and returned to bed. In either case, the child is to feel the bed-sheets after returning from the toilet and to comment on their dryness. The adult praises the child for having a dry bed and has him or her drink some more fluid before returning to sleep.

If the child wets the bed during the night of intensive training, the adult disconnects the alarm, awakens the child, and delivers a reprimand for wetting. After the child has been directed to the bathroom to finish urinating, cleanliness training is provided. Azrin, Sneed, and Foxx (1974) view this as a form of *overcorrection*. It consists of having the child change to dry night-clothes, to remove the wet sheets and place them with the dirty laundry, to obtain clean sheets, and to remake the bed. This natural negative consequence of bedwetting is followed by 20 trials of positive practice in correct toileting, identical to the procedure that had been followed earlier that evening. Such positive practice is also to be performed on the evening following this, or subsequent to any later wettings.

A period of posttraining supervision by the child's parents begins the following day. At bedtime, the alarm apparatus is placed on the bed and the child is reminded that it is important to remain dry and that cleanliness training and positive practice would be required were wetting to take place. The parents then awaken the child and send him or her to the toilet just before they retire for the night. After each dry night these awakenings take place 30 minutes earlier than the night before until they occur within one hour of the child's bed-time at which point they are discontinued. When the child wets the bed during the night, cleanliness training and positive practice are instituted immediately upon wetting and again at bedtime the following night. On the other hand, if the child remains dry through the night both parents give praise and repeat such praise at least five times during the following day. Significant relatives are also encouraged to praise the child and the success is entered on a conspicuous progress chart. This chart is part of a behavioral contract between the parents and the child who have previously agreed on a reinforcer to be obtained once dryness is achieved.

After seven consecutive dry nights the bell-and-pad device is removed from the bed and a normal routine instituted, except that the parents continue to inspect the child's bed each morning. If the bed is wet, the child receives cleanliness training immediately and positive practice the following evening but if two wettings occur within one week, the posttraining supervision regimen is reinstated.

As this detailed outline of dry bed training reveals, it includes aspects of retention control training, nighttime awakening approaches, positive reinforcement for having a dry bed, the urine-alarm procedure, scolding and other negative consequences for wetting, especially the bothersome positive practice which, regardless of its euphemistic label, must be viewed as a form of punishment. With so many different aspects a part of the procedure, it is impossible to know which of them or which combination of them is to be credited for the rather remarkable success Azrin, Sneed, and Foxx (1974) reported for the 26 children with whom dry bed training had been used. As Doleys (1977) has observed, it is possible that some aspects of the procedure account for the improvement of some children while for some other children other aspects supply the crucial elements. Enuretic children are not likely to be a homogeneous group who all respond to a specific treatment in the same way so that a comprehensive approach may have the best chance of being successful. At any rate, Azrin et al. (1974) found that the median child in their sample had only two wettings before reaching the criterion of two consecutive weeks of dryness. All 24 of the 24 children treated (2 had become dry during the baseline period) became dry within four weeks and only 7 (29 percent) suffered a relapse during a six-month follow-up and had to undergo a second treatment sequence.

A replication of the dry bed training procedure for enuretic children was carried out by Doleys, Ciminero, Tollison, Williams, and Wells (1977) who compared that procedure with the retention control training originated by Kimmel and Kimmel (1972). While dry bed training proved superior to retention control training, the results were not quite as remarkable as those reported by Azrin et al. (1974). Of the 13 children who had received dry bed training, 8 reached the success criterion of 14 consecutive dry nights in a mean of 10.4 weeks of treatment while 5 discontinued treatment at various stages of therapy. A follow-up three months after termination showed 4 children to have had from zero to 2 wettings per month, while the rest had wet 3 or more times per month or could not be contacted. Williams, Doleys, and Ciminero (1978) published a further follow-up study of these children two years later. By then, of the 8 who had successfully completed the dry bed training, 5 were wetting less than once a month, while 2 were wetting four times per month and 1 six times. Four of the five families who had terminated treatment prematurely could be contacted and these parents reported a mean frequency of 14.5 wettings per month. If one considers three or more wet nights per month to be a criterion of relapse, approximately 38 percent of the treated group must be considered to have relapsed within the two-year follow-up period. Interestingly, none of the parents sought renewed treatment when it was made available to them.

Further research with dry bed training was conducted by Bollard and Woodroffe (1977) who, like Azrin, Hontos, and Besalel-Azrin (1979), had the child's parents conduct the entire procedure, thus eliminating the outside trainer who had spent the first night with the child in the original method. The 14 children treated in this manner were all dry within a median of 12 days and only 2 (14 percent) required retraining during a six-month follow-up period. With a closely matched group of 10 children these investigators used parent-administered dry bed training with one important modification—omitting the bell-and-pad alarm. They were thus able to shed some light on the question regarding which of the various aspects of the Azrin et al. (1974) procedure contributes an element that is critical to the success. The results showed that the urine-alarm may be one of these crucial variables inasmuch as none of these children reached the success criterion of 14 consecutive dry nights during the 13-week treatment period although there was a drop in the number of wet nights per week after the first week of training. While the median number of wet nights per week had dropped to zero by the third week of training for the children who had used the bell-and-pad, the group in which this device had been deleted from the training procedure still had a median of three wet nights during that week and remained at that level for the remaining 10 weeks of treatment.

Bollard and Woodroffe (1977) suggest that the urine-alarm is an important, perhaps essential component of the dry bed training procedure but they stress that its function may not be limited to the postulated conditioning effect. When the bell-and-pad is used in dry bed training, the ringing of the alarm not only wakes up the child but it also serves as a signal to the parents who then immediately institute the cleanliness training and positive practice. When the alarm is omitted, as in the Bollard and Woodroffe (1977) modification, the parents are unable to know exactly when a wetting takes place since they find out about it only at the scheduled awakening or the following morning unless the child happens to wake up on his own during the night. Under these circumstances, the cleanliness training–positive practice contingency may be temporally removed from the actual bedwetting by as much as 9 or 10 hours thereby reducing the effectiveness of this consequence. In addition, where multiple wettings occur, the absence of an alarm limits the number of detected wettings to one per night thereby reducing the number of possible training trials and further weakening the potency of the procedure.

In order to test the relative contribution of the direct conditioning effect and the signal effect of the bell-and-pad alarm, Azrin, Sneed, and Foxx (1974) had one group of children in their study sleep on a pad that activated an alarm only in the parents' room. Upon hearing the buzzer, one of the parents would wake the child and institute the cleanliness training and positive practice consequences of the dry bed training procedure. Since this group of children became dry just as quickly and effectively as the group for whom the alarm was also activated next to their own bed, Azrin et al. (1974) concluded that respondent (Pavlovian) conditioning did not contribute to the effectiveness of their procedure.

Whatever the basis of the urine alarm's contribution to the success of the dry bed training approach, it does seem that without it the procedure is less effective. When Azrin and Thienes (1978) attempted to conduct that procedure without the conditioning apparatus they had also found that the original Azrin, Sneed, & Foxx (1974) approach had been superior. In what they call their "new training method" for the rapid elimination of enuresis, Azrin and Thienes (1978) have introduced additional modifications, designed to make the procedure more convenient for the parents. One of these modifications was to hold the intensive training on the first day during the afternoon and early evening rather than during the night; another was to have the child rehearse during the day the toileting action to be taken at night. Those children who voided only small amounts of urine during any one toileting were instructed to inhibit urination until a large volume had accumulated so as to increase the threshold of bladder sensations at which the need to urinate would become urgent. Lastly, a "strain-and-hold" procedure was added to the method in order to teach voluntary control over urination. This entailed asking the child every half hour during the afternoon of the first training day to strain at the toilet until feeling the need to urinate and then to try to hold it back. When the child was successful at this, the trainer praised the performance but when the child indicated that longer delay was becoming impossible he or she was asked to lie on the bed in the darkened bedroom pretending to be asleep while concentrating on the feeling of the full bladder and describing it aloud. Only then was the child to go to the toilet to urinate, thereby re-creating the conditions that would prevail at night when the child was asleep.

In order to compare the effect of their new method with a traditional urine-alarm procedure, Azrin and Thienes (1978) randomly assigned half (27) of the 55 children who participated in their study to a control group which used only the bell-and-pad but under the supervision of an outside trainer who spent the first day and part of the night in the home. The results showed that during the first two weeks of training the children using the bell-and-pad wet their beds 76 percent of the nights while those who received the modified dry bed training wet their beds only 15 percent of the nights.

The parents in both groups had been told that they could transfer their child to the other condition after two weeks if they were dissatisfied with the progress. None of the parents in the dry bed group requested such transfer. Of the 27 in the bell-and-pad condition 23 requested such transfer and their children too reduced their wetting to 14 percent of the nights during the first two weeks under the new procedure. Combining the data for all the children who had been given the new method of the dry bed training, Azrin and Thienes (1978) report that all but four of these 51 children eventually reached the criterion of 14 consecutive dry nights. The four children who did not were those whose parents dropped out of the program by failing to perform the required posttraining activities. During a 12-month follow-up period 10 children (20 percent) experienced a relapse following an illness or a traumatic event involving their family but all of them regained control when the maintenance procedures were reinstated.

The above are highly impressive results yet they fail to equal those of the original dry bed training method of Azrin et al. (1974) in that there the average child had only two wettings before reaching the dryness criterion while with the new method this number was four. On the other hand, the relapse rate in the earlier study had been 7 out of 24 children (30 percent). A close examination of the difference in results between the two approaches shows that the use of the alarm system in the context of the Azrin training method does bring an important advantage, which Azrin and Thienes (1978) for some reason fail to mention in their report. It is that the old Azrin method which employed the urine-alarm as part of the dry bed training procedure resulted in a median number of zero wet nights per week by the fourth week following the institution of training (Azrin, Sneed, & Foxx, 1974). For the "new method," on the other hand, Azrin and Thienes (1978) report that there was still an average of 9 percent wet nights during the second month, 6 percent during the third month, 4 percent during the fifth month, and one year later accidents still took place, though at a rate of less than 2 percent of the nights. Similar results were reported by Azrin, Hontos, and Besalel-Azrin (1979) when they eliminated both urine-alarm and outside trainer and instructed the parents and their child in the dry bed procedure during an office visit. There they found bedwetting to occur during 13 percent of the nights in the second month, 11 percent during the third month, 9 percent during the fourth, and 4 percent during both the fifth month and one year later.

On the whole, it appears that the dry bed training method is both more efficient and effective when it includes a urine alarm that alerts the parents as soon as a wetting has taken place so that the consequences can be instituted immediately. Available research also leaves little doubt that in terms of the speed with which bedwetting can be stopped, this combination is significantly more effective than the standard urine-alarm procedure by itself (Azrin, Sneed, & Foxx, 1974).

The Role of Parents

In reviewing research reports on the use of behavioral methods to treat enuresis, one is repeatedly reminded of the important role that parents play in the success or failure of the intervention. Whether it be their implementing the bell-and-pad or dry bed procedures or following through with the post training supervision when the dry bed method is first initiated by an outside trainer, unless the parents are able and willing to cooperate, the treatment has little chance of success.

When the bell-and-pad method is used to treat enuresis, the mother's attitudes and interests are factors that contribute to the variance of treatment outcome. This was found by James and Foreman (1973) who measured maternal attitudes and interest with the so-called A–B therapist scale that Dublin, Elton, and Berzins (1969) had described. Mothers whose responses on that scale show them to have a high interest in, and aptitude for natural science and engineering, to be willing to take risks, and to be socially affiliative, field independent, and "masculine" tend to be more successful in implementing the bell-and-pad method with their enuretic childen than mothers whose responses show them to fall at the low end of these attributes. Many of these A–B characteristics would seem to be related to mothers' attitudes toward a technological approach to treating their child's problem, but it is not only in the implementation of the mechanics of treatment that the parents' role is important. Also to be considered are parents' relationship to the child, their attitude toward bedwetting, and the function the bedwetting serves in the parent–child relationship. As with any other form of behavior therapy, a careful and thorough assessment is an essential first step in the treatment of enuresis.

Mowrer and Mowrer (1938) are often thought of as having introduced the use of a mechanical conditioning device that can simply be placed in the child's bed so that the laws of learning will bring about the desired improvement. It is therefore of interest to recall that in the second paragraph of the Mowrers' classical paper they observed, using the language of their day, "that in order for child training of any kind to proceed smoothly and effectively and to be enduring, the love of the child for the adult in the situation must be strong enough to counteract, or at least hold in bounds, the negative impulses which are certain to be engendered by the educative process" (Mowrer & Mowrer, 1938, p. 444). They went on to say that the first requirement for the establishment of satisfactory toilet habits "is the existence of thorough confidence in, and respect and affection for the adults who are commissioned to carry out the requisite training.'' (Ibid.) They also observed that in two of the thirty children in their study the enuresis had "a conspicuously aggressive connotation" and that for various other children an element of hostility seemed also to be involved. For such cases, they wrote, "it is obviously essential that the child's attitude toward parents or parent substitutes be changed from one of ambivalence in which negative feelings predominate to one in which positive feelings are stronger" (Ibid.).

In somewhat different words, it should seem clear that one must investigate whether bedwetting is being maintained by such reinforcing consequences as parental indulgence or parental exasperation. In either case, these contingencies would have to be modified before the treatment of enuresis could be expected to succeed. Similarly, where parental praise is to be used to reinforce desired toileting behavior and dry nights, it is essential to know whether praise statements are indeed positive reinforcers for the child. Such relationship and attitudinal factors have been investigated by Nordquist (1971), James and Foreman (1973), and Morgan and Young (1975) all of whom demonstrate their importance. These factors are just as important as, they may in fact enter into, the parental cooperation with the therapist that Lovibond (1972) and Doleys (1977) point to as the single most common reason for treatment failure.

DEFICIENT BOWEL CONTROL

Compared with the extensive research literature on the behavioral treatment of enuresis there is a dearth of studies dealing with the less frequent but in many respects more dismaying problem of encopretic children, those who fail to maintain bowel control. In almost all of the cases reported, encopresis occurs during the day rather than at night. Hence, while a child's problem with bedwetting may be known only to the immediate family, fecal soiling very quickly comes to the attention of outsiders and the child's peers are often quick to coin an uncomplimentary sobriquet and to avoid their malodorous classmate. The fact that these negative social consequences do not lead to a cessation of the soiling behavior reflects that the problem results not from an excess response that must be suppressed but from a deficit in a skill (sphincter control) that must be acquired.

As with other responses that must be acquired before they can be performed, punishment alone is incapable of establishing the deficient skill. The only thing punishment can do in these and similar situations is to teach the child to avoid the punishing agents or to find ways of keeping these agents ignorant of the transgression. In the case of encopretic children, avoidance of peers is not unusual and where the parents are the punishing agents, such children have been known to find ingenious ways of hiding the evidence of soiling by secreting dirty underwear in various parts of the house. All of this points to the need to establish the required bowel control and toileting skills through the use of positive reinforcement combined, where necessary, with the delivery of negative consequences for instances of inappropriate defecation. This is the approach that has been used by therapists who have reported cases involving the successful treatment of encopresis by behavioral methods (Ayllon, Simon, & Wildman, 1975; Bach & Moylan, 1975; Gelber & Meyer, 1965; Edelman, 1971; Plachetta, 1976; Tomlinson, 1970; Wright & Walker, 1978).

In almost all reported case studies the management of the reinforcement contingencies was the responsibility of the child's parents to whom the therapist had given appropriate instructions. Here, as was true in the case of bedwetting, a careful assessment of the parent–child relationship in the context of a functional analysis of the soiling is an important first step before intervention can be instituted. There is another question that should be raised during assessment although it is rarely mentioned in the published reports. This question has to do with the exact nature of the problem. To know that a child has feces in his or her underwear is important but not sufficient information. There are several ways by which that end result may have come about. Some children retain their stools (having very good control over their anal sphincter) until colonic pressure reaches a point where it overwhelms the sphincter so that involuntary bowel evacuation takes place. These children often stain their underwear between the actual soilings that take place after fairly lengthy intervals. In extreme cases, stools may be retained so long that they harden and become impacted, requiring medical intervention for their removal. It would seem that these children avoid bowel movements and assessment must establish the basis of this avoidance response which may be related to fear and should be approached like any other excessive avoidance behavior. From the standpoint of classification it is probably best not to include such stool retention problems under the rubric of encopresis.

Another group of children who soil also seem to have good sphincter control but the reinforcement contingencies operating for them make defecation in their pants more potent than the use of the toilet. It has been speculated that the consequences of maintaining such behavior are related to the reaction of one or both parents whose sympathy, concern, or even anger may be serving as a positive reinforcer for the so-called accidents. It is not unlikely that cases of this nature are found among the discontinuous or regressed encopretics who had at one time acquired appropriate toileting habits but resumed soiling at some later point. For them a change in reinforcement contingencies would obviously be the first step in any attempt at intervention.

In addition to the groups just mentioned, there are the chronic or continuous encopretics, children who have never been toilet trained with respect to bowel functions and for whom a program aimed at helping them to acquire such control has to be instituted. Young (1973) has reported that the encopretic children he treated lacked the ability to recognize when they had to move their bowels and could therefore not exercise control over their eliminatory functions. For this reason he treated them with a mild laxative and had them sit on the toilet for 10 minutes following food intake 20 to 30 minutes earlier. When a bowel movement then took place, the parents would reinforce the child with praise and Young reports that this approach was successful within a mean of seven months for 22 of the 24 children in his sample. Young (1973) unfortunately fails to report whether the children thus treated had attained perception of their gastroilial or gastrocolic reflexes on the absence of which he had based his approach. That it is possible to conduct such treatment without making assumptions about the physiological or sensory mechanisms that might underlie the problem was demonstrated by Wright and Walker (1978) whose intervention was based on positive reinforcement for continence and appropriate toilet use, combined with response-cost, time-out, and other negative consequences for soiling. A parent-implemented training program of this kind is clearly preferable to such drastic measures as hospitalization, as was the case in the report by Gelber and Meyer (1965), or the insertion of a fluid-filled balloon in a boy's rectum so as to provide him with feedback on internal pressure changes, a procedure employed by Kohlenberg (1973).

Details of an operant treatment program were described by Crowley and Armstrong (1977) who treated three encopretic boys in a community clinic where client-therapist contacts were limited to one hour per week. This, of course, is the typical milieu where most child behavior therapy is conducted and any approach that lends itself to such a setting has much to recommend it. Professional trainers who can spend time in the child's home or trained observers who can be sent out to gather objective observations are often luxuries the usual clinic or independent practitioner can ill afford. These considerations led Crowley and Armstrong (1977) to opt for a home-based, parent-delivered treatment that consisted of positive practice combined with overcorrection.

The three boys in the Crowley and Armstrong (1977) study were 12, 7, and 5 years old, respectively. All had once been toilet trained for both bladder and bowel control but they had lost consistent bowel control when they were between 3 and 4 years of age. They were therefore so-called regressed, discontinuous encopretics. As is usual in such cases, parental reactions had run the gamut from anger and spanking to sympathy and empathic discussions. Attempts at treatment had included ignoring, reminders, laxatives, enemas, psychiatric consultation, and having the child wash out his soiled pants.

During the first week after initial contact with the clinic, the 12-year-old had 10 recorded "accidents" and the other two children each had five but these data do not represent a true baseline. While the therapist had instructed the parents to continue their previous regimen and to help their child keep a record of his defecations, the children had been told to try using the toilet as much as possible and to sit on the commode for 15 minutes after each meal and "try to go." This procedure had been introduced in order to determine whether instructions alone would result in improvement, but even with these instructions, the children had less than one appropriate bowel movement per day during that week.

Initial assessment had revealed that the parents were inconsistent in the consequences they provided for soiling and that they did not have a repertoire for verbally reinforcing appropriate toilet behavior. The children, on the other hand, were inconsistent in carrying out appropriate toilet behavior. Occasionally they failed to exercise sphincter control when in the company of others because they did not seem to know how to go about excusing themselves when they felt the urge to move their bowels. It was on these behavioral deficits that Crowley and Armstrong (1977) decided to focus their intervention.

During the first of the weekly sessions at the clinic the parents were instructed to emit positive praise statements whenever the child used the toilet appropriately. They rehearsed these statements with the therapist during this and subsequent sessions. Concurrently, the therapist spoke to the child about appropriate toilet behavior and had him practice contraction and relaxation of the anal sphincter. In addition, the child was taught what to say in social situations when he felt the need to use the toilet. It seemed that all three boys could "feel it coming" but would not interrupt activities or request to be excused from the classroom in order to go to the toilet. Here too, behavior rehearsal was used to help the children practice appropriate responses. Motivational strategies included parent–child contracts for weekly treats contingent on a reduction in weekly accidents by one-half of those during the previous week. When accidents did occur, two consequences were to be used; overcorrection and positive practice. The former consisted of a 30-minute period during which the child was to wash himself and the soiled clothes as well as additional laundry items supplied by the parents. These were to be hung up to dry and later folded and put away. Positive practice entailed sitting alone in a quiet room for 10 minutes, followed by spending 10 minutes on the toilet "trying to go," and repeating this sequence three times. The timing and recording of this activity was made the child's responsibility while the parents merely monitored the procedure in a calm and matter-of-fact way.

With this combination of procedures Crowley and Armstrong (1977) achieved quick and lasting success. During the first week after baseline, the number of soilings for the 12-year-old dropped from 10 to 6; during the second week of treatment it was 1, after which it never again reached a higher level. Beginning in the sixth week this boy had only one more accident in the eighth week after which he reached the treatment goal of four consecutive weeks without soilings. Follow-up over an 18-month period revealed that this boy had remained free of toileting problems. The treatment of the other two children progressed fairly similarly. Having had 5 accidents during the week before treatment began, they reduced this to 4 during the first and second weeks of treatment. By the fifth week the 7-year-old was problem free and remained that way throughout the 18 months of follow-up. The 5-year-old had 4 accidents during the first two weeks of treatment, 2 for each of the following 3 weeks, none in the sixth and 1 in the seventh, after which he too reached the treatment criterion and remained continent.

As Crowley and Armstrong (1977) recognize, it is of course impossible to tell which of their treatment procedures or which combination of these had been responsible for this favorable outcome. The answer to this awaits future research. As we said in connection with the discussion of enuresis, it is conceivable that different children will show a favorable response to different treatment approaches so that a combination of many approaches has a better chance of success with an unselected group of clinic cases than would any one procedure alone.

Most of the case studies reporting successful behavioral approaches to the treatment of encopresis have used a combination of methods. Thus, overcorrection, positive practice, and contingent use of positive reinforcement was successful with three children treated by Butler (1977), while Plachetta (1976) who used scheduling, contingency contracting, and self-charting with a 6-year-old boy, reports him to have become continent after eight weeks of treatment and to have remained so over a two-year follow-up. On the other hand, procedures limited to the straightforward use of positive reinforcement for appropriate toilet use have also resulted in the successful treatment of encopresis (Ayllon, Simon & Wildman, 1975; Edelman, 1971; Tomlinson, 1970).

From the standpoint of clinical application it might be a desirable strategy to institute a regime of positive reinforcement and self-recording as a first phase of treatment. Not only is this the simplest procedure which even parents with impaired competence can follow (Bach & Moyland, 1975), but it also lacks the negative component that overcorrection and positive practice invariably introduce into treatment. Only when the record shows that the simpler intervention has no effect should one add these more involved procedures so that the problem would then be attacked both by strengthening the desired toileting responses through positive reinforcement and by weakening the undesirable soiling responses through the punishment entailed in the negative consequences of positive practice and overcorrection.

Recapitulation

Incontinence involving bladder and bowel functions is best construed as a skill deficit so that treatment must take the form of teaching the child how to maintain the necessary sphincter control. By far the more frequent of the two problems is difficulties with bladder control, particularly while the child is asleep. Much research has been done on various behavorial approaches to the treatment of bedwetting among which the bell-and-pad method is both the oldest and the most frequently employed. This method has been shown to be effective in a large number of cases although the psychological processes through which it works remain in the realm of speculation. A phenomenon that is frequently encountered when the bell-and-pad are used to treat bedwetting is that the child has a relapse some weeks after having reached the criterion of treatment success. Such relapse can be construed as the extinction of an acquired response and procedures involving overlearning or intermittent reinforcement have been demonstrated to reduce the relapse rate. Some investigators have combined the signaling function of the bell-and-pad with other training methods, among which the so-called dry bed training, a procedure that teaches the child appropriate toileting behavior during the day while he or she is awake has proved to be singularly effective. Whatever the method used for treatment, the child's parents play a crucial role as auxiliary therapists since the intervention invariably takes place at home. While few large-scale studies have been conducted on the less frequently encountered problems associated with bowel control, there too, methods based on behavioral principles are reported to have been successful.

CHAPTER 8

Norm-violating Behavior

GENERAL CONSIDERATIONS

A child or adolescent who violates the norms of society that have been codified into laws comes to be labeled a juvenile delinquent if he or she is apprehended and processed through our system of juvenile justice. Many forms of behavior enaged in under a great variety of circumstances represent violations of laws so that juvenile delinquency is not a unitary phenomenon and juvenile delinquents are not a homogenous group. It could, in fact, be said that the only thing all juvenile delinquents have in common is that they got caught.

At the risk of making an unwarranted generalization, we here construe juvenile delinquency as reflecting a behavior deficit, as stemming from a failure to have learned the ability to postpone immediate and often unlawful gratification and from a lack of socially endorsed skills for finding alternate, legal forms of gratification. When the focus is thus placed on the deficit, it follows that intervention must be aimed at teaching needed controls and missing skills. If one postulates furthermore that the norm-violator may not have acquired the ability to discriminate between acceptable and unacceptable behavior, the logical treatment is the teaching of this discrimination. Since controls, skills, and discriminations are best learned under contingencies of positive reinforcement, it follows that mere punishment for disapproved behavior would be ineffective in reducing the frequency of delinquent behavior.

A formulation of juvenile delinquency in terms of a behavioral deficit not only shifts intervention with norm-violating youth who have been apprehended from a punitive to a constructive base, but also opens the way for a preventive approach with children who are at risk of becoming delinquent. Such preventive work would be aimed at teaching constructive social skills as alternatives to such unacceptable behavior as aggression, noncompliance, and stealing. This can be done within the child's own family or in treatment-oriented, family-style community settings and we shall cite several examples of such approaches in the following pages.

A discussion of norm-violating behavior must take cognizance of several issues that complicate work in this area. One of these issues has to do with the relationship between magnitude (severity) and frequency of the target behavior. The ultimate definition of a psychological disorder, no matter what form it may take, is a function of the judgment of society regarding what is acceptable behavior and this judgment involves either the frequency or the magnitude of the behavior (Ross, 1980). When a behavior occurs too frequently or if it occurs at too high a magnitude it is deemed changeworthy. Only in the case of the most profoundly disturbed (and that may be why they are so defined) will the unacceptable behavior be found to be high in both frequency *and* magnitude. Generally, frequency and magnitude stand in an inverse relationship. In the case of bedwetting, for example, any individual instance of wetting is a relatively minor event (it is of low magnitude) and parents do not deem it a problem that calls for professional help unless it occurs at a high frequency, such as every night. It thus is the high frequency of this low magnitude event that brings it to the clinician's attention. Conversely, setting fire to the house is a behavior of such high magnitude that even a single instance will make it seem as abnormal and an occasion for intervention.

The inverse relationship between magnitude and frequency poses a problem for the behavior therapist. It is far easier to work with a frequent response than with one that occurs rarely because with the former many learning trials can take place in a relatively short time. When a response, such as fire-setting, takes place only rarely, the learning trials in whatever intervention might be chosen are widely spaced and small in number. There are three conceptualizations that may facilitate the treatment of high-magnitude–low-frequency behaviors. One of these is to consider the behavior a member of a response class and to use that response class as the target of treatment. In the case of fire-setting, for example, the lighting of matches might be viewed as a member of that response class. A second, and related conceptualization is to postulate the high magnitude behavior to be at the end of an escalating sequence of responses so that treatment might focus on interrupting that sequence at an early stage, thus aborting the high magnitude response before it is emitted. This was the procedure Burchard and Tyler (1965) employed in the case of "Donny," to be discussed shortly. The third possibility is to conceive of high magnitude behavior as a reflection of a lack of alternative, constructive skills on the part of the person who engages in such behavior. Treatment would thus aim at teaching these alternative skills on the assumption that once they are in the person's repertoire, the unacceptable, high magnitude behavior will no longer be emitted. An example of this approach will be found in the work of Cohen and Filipczak (1971) that will be presented in this chapter.

Yet another difficulty one faces when working with high-magnitude–low-frequency behavior is that the effect of treatment is much more difficult to monitor here than in the case of high-frequency responses. With a child who has been wetting the bed every night, for example, one can tell that treatment is having an effect when wetting begins to occur only three times a week and the criterion of treatment success can be set with considerable confidence at two weeks of consecutive dry nights. A follow-up of 18 months is readily acceptable proof that the problem has been fully alleviated. What about the occasional fire-setter, on the other hand? If the frequency of this high-magnitude behavior has been on the average of one fire every 10 months, how will a therapist know whether the treatment has an effect? How many months without fire-setting must elapse before treatment is terminated? How many years of follow-up before one can consider the treatment to have been effective?

Much of the behavior that results in a youth's being classified as a juvenile delinquent is of the high-magnitude–low-frequency variety. Car theft, for example, may be committed only once in several years yet its magnitude ("grand" larceny) leads to serious sanctions. Even shoplifting is rarely a behavior a youngster will engage in every day even though a parent might report that "he steals all the time." In fact, such distorted reporting is often the result of the observer's mistaking magnitude for frequency and it can only be guarded against by insisting on a quantitative record of the behavior in question. It may well be that the difficulties encountered in many attempts at therapeutic intervention with juvenile delinquents are at least in part due to the low frequency of their high-magnitude behavior.

Another source of difficulty in treating norm-violating behavior lies in the fact that much that society deems delinquent are actions that carry their own inherent and immediate reinforcement. Stealing is the most obvious example. The moment the stolen item is appropriated the reinforcer is delivered. Against such immediate, regular (FR-1) reinforcement, therapeutic attempts to teach a youngster to respond under conditions of delayed gratification operate under considerable disadvantage. It is probably for this reason that the more promising programs of intervention have been those conducted in institutional settings where access to reinforcers can be reasonably well controlled. Unfortunately, behavorial improvements achieved inside the institution often fail to generalize to the community setting to which the youngster is returned upon discharge. This is the case largely because the same contingencies of reinforcement in which the delinquent behavior had been originally emitted are then once again in effect. It is for this reason that thoughtful observers of the issues involved in juvenile delinquency have repeatedly pointed to the social environment as a principal contributor to the problem and thus as the crucial focus of any attempt to deal with it in a lasting and constructive fashion (Davidson & Seidman, 1974).

Before we turn to a review of some of the treatment approaches that have been employed with youngsters defined as juvenile delinquents, another dilemma must be pointed out. It is that any measures of treatment outcome, hence of the effectiveness of intervention, depend on the detection of norm-violating behavior. When a youngster has been apprehended for delinquent behavior and given therapeutic help intended to keep him or her from engaging in such behavior in the future, the only way one can tell whether this goal has been reached is by noting the absence of further delinquencies. Like attempting to prove the null hypothesis, this is an impossible task since one can never be sure than an event has not taken place; it may have taken place when nobody was there to notice it. To deal with this dilemma, data on the effectiveness of work with delinquents are customarily presented in terms of recidivism rates. That is, one reports not how many treated youngsters have desisted from further norm violations but how many of them have once again been apprehended in a delinquent act. A low recidivism rate may thus as readily reflect a high number of norm violators who have succeeded in not getting caught as it may document a successful treatment program. Given this state of affairs, a program of intervention that manages to teach youngsters how not to get caught could report a highly successful outcome!

TREATMENT PROGRAMS IN INSTITUTIONAL SETTINGS

While detention homes, training schools, youth farms, or whatever they might be called almost always profess the purpose of rehabilitation, fiscal constraints and inadequate staffing patterns usually force them to function primarily as places of confinement. As such, the immediate aim of those operating such facilities becomes two-fold; to assure that the inmates behave in an orderly, nondisruptive fashion and to keep them engaged in more or less constructive activity. These interrelated aims, designed primarily for maintaining smoothly running institutions, are then rationalized as providing their charges with a preparation for a norm-abiding life after discharge where they are expected to use the social and academic–vocational skills they were presumably taught.

The emptiness of this rationalization is reflected in recidivism rates of the magnitude of 76 percent during the first year after discharge (Cohen & Filipczak, 1971).

When behavioral approaches are introduced into institutions of this type they are often employed for similar aims, to improve the personal–social behavior of the inmates while they are in the institution and to teach them academic–vocational skills that they might use after discharge. Davidson and Seidman (1974) are among those who have raised the question whether behavior therapists should lend their efforts to the aims of traditional institutions but, as Burchard and Harig (1976) have recognized, as long as society continues to maintain and use such institutions, something needs to be done for the young people who are sent there and that "something" might as well be effective. What then is some of the evidence for the effectiveness of behavioral intervention with institutionalized delinquents?

Most of the early reports on the systematic use of behavioral principles with institutionalized delinquents were no more than demonstrations of the not-too-surprising fact that these principles are also effective with that population. Tyler and Brown (1968), for example, showed that contingent reinforcement is superior to noncontingent reinforcement in raising the number of correct answers to quizzes about the day's news given to 15 institutionalized boys. The same investigators (Tyler & Brown, 1967) had previously shown that rule violations while playing pool during recreation periods could be more effectively reduced by brief contingent isolation than by the usual verbal reprimand delivered by the staff. While such demonstrations may be valuable in that they might convince the institutional staff to employ contingency management in their daily work, they leave the question of their impact in terms of lasting effects largely unanswered.

Contingency Management

Since the inevitable, ultimate recourse for the control of unacceptable behavior used by institutional staff (as by the rest of society) is to employ some aversive consequence, it is instructive to review an early case study by Burchard and Tyler (1965) which showed that these aversive consequences often fail to serve as punishment if punishment is defined in its technical sense as a response-contingent consequence that reduces the frequency of that response. The case presented by Burchard and Tyler (1965) is that of "Donny," a 13-year-old institutionalized delinquent boy whose antisocial, aggressive–disruptive behavior in group situations had led to his having spent a total of 200 days in an individual isolation room during the year preceding the investigators' intervention. During that year Donny's behavior had become increasingly unmanageable, a clear indication that the presumed punishment did not have the desired effect. Observations of the events surrounding the use of isolation to control the boy's behavior showed why it was so ineffective.

As described by Burchard and Tyler (1965) the steps taken by the institutional staff tended to follow a fairly regular sequence. When Donny first began "acting up," staff members would try to ignore this behavior as long as possible. During that time, peer encouragement and peer attention seemed to serve as reinforcers since the boy's behavior continued and increased in magnitude. At this point, the attendant would resort to attempts at supportive persuasion along the lines of, "Come on, Donny; cut it out." This seemed to serve as further reinforcement with the magnitude of the boy's disruptive behavior continuing to increase until the staff member finally became angry and, in desperation, ordered Donny into the isolation room. Now, however, the staff members apparently felt guilty for they would visit the boy in the isolation room, bring him food, and talk to him in sympathetic fashion, hoping to reason him into behaving better next time. As reflected in the staff's report that the boy's behavior had become more and more unmanageable during the year these contingencies were in effect, it would seem that they had been using reinforcing rather than punishing consequences.

Burchard and Tyler (1965) now proceeded to introduce a systematic time-out regimen that entailed removing Donny from the group immediately upon the first signs of his disruptive behavior and placing him in the isolation room for three hours or overnight. The staff was instructed to do this in a matter-of-fact, perfunctory manner immediately upon the onset of any behavior that would normally require a sanction. Time-out was to be used on an all-or-none basis, never as a threat. This procedure was combined with the delivery of positive reinforcement in the form of a token for each hour that Donny did not have to spend in the time-out room. The tokens could later be used to purchase various canteen items or privileges. The approach was thus a combination of time-out for unacceptable behavior with differential reinforcement of other behavior (DRO). The investigators report that their approach resulted in marked improvement of Donny's behavior within the institution during a period of five months. In contrast, a year's use of the prior management technique had been not only ineffective but, in fact, counterproductive. It must be pointed out however, that making a youngster's behavior within the institution more manageable is not really what institutionalization is supposed to be all about. The crucial question is how Donny behaved after he was discharged and on that point the record is silent.

In the case of Donny, Burchard and Tyler (1965) had no reliable baseline or objective observations on the boy's behavior, the report being based solely on the institutional record and the recollections of the staff. This shortcoming was remedied in a study conducted by Burchard and Barrera (1972) that is one of the few investigations on the systematic modification of institutional behavior that employed both a baseline and controlled variation of treatment methods.

Through the vagaries that determine the labeling and hence the disposition of young people who engage in norm-violating behavior, the adolescents in the Burchard and Barrera (1972) study were confined in an institution for the mentally retarded. Their intelligence test performance was in the mildly retarded range, not an unusual status for delinquents who have often spent little constructive time in school. All had committed various types of delinquent and antisocial behavior, including theft, arson, and assault. The study here under discussion was conducted in the Intensive Training Unit at Murdoch Center in North Carolina where a programmed environment based on the principles of a token economy was in operation. All residents of this Unit could earn tokens through achievement in the workshop and these tokens were spent for such things as meals, store items, privileges, clothes, recreation trips, and transportation. Time-out or response cost were used as consequences for specified categories of unacceptable behavior. These were swearing, personal assault, property damage, and such miscellany as being too noisy, taking things from others, disobedience, and trying to escape. Again we see a set of goals that seems to focus more on the smooth running of the institution than on helping the participants learn to function adaptively in outside society.

The time-out contingency entailed social isolation in that the offender had to sit on a bench behind a partition for a predetermined period of time. Anyone refusing to go immediately to time-out or who created a disturbance while there, was fined 15 tokens and taken to an empty seclusion room where he had to remain until he had been silent for 30 consecutive minutes. The latter condition is usual in this procedure because if time-out were for a fixed period of time so that it might terminate just as the youngster is behaving in an unacceptable fashion, being released at that moment would serve as a negative reinforcement, thus strengthening that unacceptable behavior.

The response-cost condition in this study consisted of the removal of a specified number of tokens from the offender's possession. Since the tokens served as the sole medium of exchange in the economy, it constituted the equivalent of a monetary fine. If the offender did not have enough tokens to pay the fine or did not want to pay right away, he could do so later but this entailed the payment of "interest" in the form of five extra tokens for the delay. Some of the issues surrounding the use of response cost have been discussed by Kazdin (1977). Of particular concern in the use of response cost is the potential devaluation of the token in cases where a person owes so many tokens that it becomes pointless to earn any more since they would have to be given up immediately in order to pay off the debt. Analogous dilemmas are, of course, well known in the monetary economy of the "real world" where a person can be so hopelessly in debt or have to pay so much of his income in alimony that he might as well stop trying to earn money by working.

What Burchard and Barrera (1972) sought to investigate in their study was the relative effectiveness of time-out and response cost and the conditions under which these consequences are effective in reducing the frequency of undesirable behavior. Two quantities of response cost (5 and 30 tokens) and two lengths of time-out (5 and 30 minutes) were analyzed for six residents who were exposed to each of the four contingencies at different times and in different combinations. The dependent variable in this study was the total frequency of the imposition of a response consequence (time-out or response cost). This is an indirect measure of the frequency of unacceptable behavior and rests on the unverified assumption that the cottage staff imposed a consequence every time a resident emitted such behavior.

The baseline condition consisted of the contingencies under which the Unit had been operating during the previous two years; a combination of 5-minutes time-out and a 5-token response cost. During 12 consecutive days when a baseline record was kept of the frequency with which these consequences were imposed, the total mean frequency for the six residents was approximately 64 (see Figure 12). During the experimental condition which lasted for 48 days the combination of time-out and response cost was broken up and each of these two consequences was used alone at each of its two levels of magnitude. During this experimental period, each resident was exposed to each of the four conditions three times following a prearranged, counterbalanced schedule. Each exposure to a condition lasted for four days and the results were analyzed in terms of cumulative 12-day blocks per condition. Combining the data for their six subjects and comparing the frequency with which the two magnitudes of the response consequences had been imposed, Burchard and Barrera (1972) found that the higher response cost and the longer time-out periods were more effective than the lower response cost and shorter time-out. Under the high-magnitude conditions of the consequences, their use (and presumably the unacceptable behavior for which they were imposed) fell to a frequency of about 50 for cumulative 12-day blocks. The two lower magnitudes of the response consequences (5 tokens or 5 minutes) unexpectedly resulted in an increase of the need to impose these consequences. The total frequency of consequence imposition under the 5-token condition was approximately 92 and under the 5-minute condition it was approximately 75 (see Figure 12).

Inasmuch as the data presented by these authors are based on the frequency with which the various response consequences had been imposed and not on the frequency of the unacceptable behavior that occasioned the consequences, the obvious question arises whether the consequence-imposing behavior of the institutional staff was a function of the magnitude of the consequence in effect for a particular group of residents at any given time. Conceivably, the lower frequency with which the high-magnitude consequences were employed was not so much a function of the residents' reduced inappropriate behavior as of the staff members' hesitancy to impose high-magnitude consequences, thus

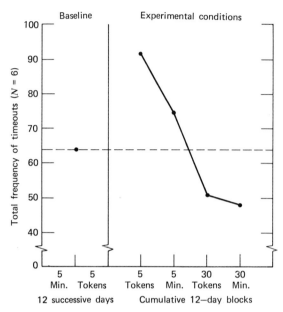

Figure 12. Total frequency of consequences (time-out plus response cost) for all subjects during baseline and each of the experimental conditions. (Burchard & Barrera, 1972. Copyright by the Society for the Experimental Analysis of Behavior, Inc.)

tolerating more unacceptable (but unrecorded) behavior. Burchard and Barrera (1972) seek to allay this concern by showing that when they analyzed only the data based on the very first consequence imposed on each day (when the staff members were presumably less apt to know which contingency was in effect for a particular youngster) the relationship of the frequencies of high-to low-magnitude consequences was similar to that found for the study as a whole. This information also militates to some extent against the possibility that the reduced number of instances of unacceptable behavior on days when the longer time-out condition was in effect might have been the result of the fact that while a resident was in the 30-minute time-out he had less opportunity to engage in unacceptable behavior than on days when he was under the shorter, 5-minute time-out condition.

The ambiguities just mentioned, and to which Burchard and Barrera (1972) were fully sensitive, place some limit on the persuasiveness of their data. There is also the point that the group data obscure important individual differences in the manner the six residents reacted to the imposition of the various contingencies. While the results, when combined for all six subjects, suggest that more response suppression can be effected by using the higher magnitude of either tokens or time-out, the analysis these authors present of the records of each of the six boys reveals an interesting paradoxical effect. It is that the generalization about the greater effectiveness of the higher magnitude holds true for only five of the six boys while for the sixth the very opposite is true. This boy engaged in more disruptive behavior under the 30-minute or 30-token conditions than under the 5-token or 5-minute conditions. As Burchard and Harig (1976) have pointed out, this finding has the important implication that any consequence that is imposed on unacceptable behavior on the assumption that it is a punishment may, for a given individual, not function as a punishment at all. As is true of reinforcement, the definition of punishment is based on the observed function of a consequence with respect to the behavior on which it is contingent. Only when the frequency of that behavior decreases subsequent to the imposition of a given consequence, can that consequence be called a punishment. If the frequency of the behavior increases or remains the same, the consequence serves a reinforcing function and must be called a reinforcer, no matter what the people administering the consequence might think they are doing. To refer to response cost or time-out as punishment, regardless of their actual effect, is confusing and interferes with the discovery of ways for bringing unacceptable behavior under optimal control (Burchard & Harig, 1976).

What can one conclude from the study by Burchard and Barrera (1972)? Provided that the effect of whatever consequences are imposed is carefully monitored so as to detect such individual differences as those just discussed, it would seem that response cost might be preferable to social isolation (timeout). Inasmuch as the higher magnitudes of these two methods seem equally effective in suppressing undesirable behavior, response cost has the advantage of not removing the offender from the opportunity to engage in desirable, hence reinforceable behavior. What is more, removing the offender from the stimulus situation in which the undesirable response was emitted does not provide an opportunity to practice response suppression under the conditions of that situation. By the time an individual returns to the group from the time-out room, the provocative aspects of the situation will usually have diminished and a valuable learning opportunity for acquiring internal controls over one's behavior has been lost.

While response cost provides the advantage just mentioned, Burchard and Barrera (1972) remind us that its effectiveness may be a function of the economic conditions within which it is implemented. It could be that having to forfeit a certain number of tokens is not a potent consequence to a youngster who has accumulated a large number of these tokens or who will soon have the opportunity to earn new tokens. To one who is marginal with respect to his or her token resources, on the other hand, such forfeiture may be a powerful penalty. Yet again, one who already owes a large amount of tokens as the result of earlier fines may shrug off the loss of additional tokens as of no consequence. The Burchard and Barrera (1972) study fails to provide conclusive data on this issue. Lastly, it is well to be reminded that their finding of the greater potency of the higher response cost and longer time-out may have been a function of a contrast effect such as the one reported by White, Nielsen, and Johnson (1972) who had studied various sequences of time-out lengths with a group of retarded children. A contrast effect would be operating when, in a comparison of the effectiveness of a higher and a lower magnitude of a response consequence, the higher magnitude proves superior but owes that superiority to its juxtaposition with the lower magnitude. When used alone, so that a comparison with the lower magnitude is precluded, the relatively higher magnitude might lose its advantage. In the Burchard and Barrera (1972) study, a juxtaposition of the higher and lower magnitudes was present since the two levels of magnitude alternated during the experimental condition. Furthermore, the lower magnitude had been in effect during the baseline period and the prior two years of institutional routine before the higher magnitude was introduced. Whether the higher magnitude consequences would have retained their potency had they alone remained in effect over an extended period of time is a question that remains for future research.

It will be recalled that the Burchard and Barrera (1972) study had been conducted in the context of a behaviorally oriented intensive training program for so-called retarded delinquents. This program was in operation for approximately six years. While it facilitated such studies as the one just presented, the more important question of its overall effectiveness in the habilitation of its residents for the purpose of which the program had been established remained unanswered, largely because administrative and funding arrangements precluded the conducting of meaningful follow-up research. For even a tentative answer to the question of what happens to delinquent youngsters who have been exposed to a behaviorally oriented rehabilitation program we have to look elsewhere.

An Academic-Vocational Program

The behavioral approaches to work with juvenile delinquents that we have discussed thus far had as their principal aim the maintenance of a certain decorum within the institution. While it is probably desirable to reduce the amount of fighting, cursing, vandalizing, and disobedience on the part of institutional inmates, it is doubtful that their learning to control these behaviors while in the institution will either generalize to the outside community upon their discharge or, even if they were to generalize, whether this particular skill will greatly enhance their chances of social survival in that community. On the assumption that these chances will be enhanced if the juvenile's academic and/or vocational skills are strengthened before he or she is returned to the community, some habilitation programs have focused on that goal.

The assumption that acquired academic–vocational skills will be adaptive in the community to which the juvenile is returned has not been directly tested.

If the schools to which such young people are returned are incapable of maintaining their academic achievement or if there are no jobs where their vocational skills can be utilized, it is doubtful that their institutional experience will stand them in good stead. What is needed, as Burchard and Harig (1976) have observed, is for those undertaking a rehabilitation program to conduct a careful analysis of the characteristics of the families and communities to which their charges will be returning in order to ascertain just what behaviors will be adaptive in terms of the reinforcement contingencies operating in those environments. Unless one can change these contingencies, it is folly to assume that teaching a delinquent boy to use grammatically correct language that is free of profanities, and strengthening such middle-class virtues as proper grooming will earn him many positive reinforcements in the low-income community from which many delinquents come and to which most of them are inevitably returned.

An oft-cited, comprehensive behavioral program primarily aimed at strengthening the academic skills of juvenile delinquents so as to permit them to reenter the public school system where they had previously failed and from which most of them had dropped out was established and operated for one year at the National Training School for Boys in Washington, D. C. (Cohen & Filipczak, 1971). This project operated under the acronym CASE II-MODEL, standing for "Contingencies Applicable to Special Education—Motivationally Oriented Designs for an Ecology of Learning," the Roman numeral II indicating that it had been preceded by a pilot study which had been labeled CASE I. The CASE II program, as we shall call it for short, entailed an around-the-clock token economy, facilitated by the fact that the participants who were enrolled in it lived together in a converted dormitory building which had been set aside for this purpose on the grounds of the training school. The adolescents who participated ranged in age from 14 to 18 and had been committed to the institution for such offenses as homicide, assault, armed robbery, auto theft, and burglary.

Upon entry into CASE II the boys were considered to have been hired to work for the project and given the title, Student Educational Researcher. Their work consisted of activities related to the academic objective of the program: studying, reading books, taking and passing tests. Payment was in the form of points that were the equivalent of money and could be used to purchase any of a wide range of privileges and treats. These included the renting of a private room, ordering clothing and other items from a mail order catalog, or gaining access to a recreational lounge. The only way of obtaining these back-up reinforcers was by the payment of points the student himself had earned. Since the academic program was voluntary and individualized, it was possible for a boy not to work and, having no points, to "go on relief." This meant that he would be entitled to no more than the standard institutional food and regular group sleeping facilities.

During the year CASE II was in operation a total of 41 students passed through the project, the census at any one time being held at 25. This meant that the results reported by Cohen and Filipczak (1971) are based on a shifting sample for as one participant left the project, either because the period of his commitment ended or because he escaped (as happened in at least two instances), he was replaced with a new boy selected by the training school administration. This selection was designed to make the CASE II students representative of the entire population of National Training School inmates, an aim that seemed to have been met rather successfully for in terms of the nature of their offenses, race, and type of commitment the two groups are quite similar.

In conducting field research of this nature it is almost impossible to introduce and maintain strict experimental controls. The investigators should therefore not be faulted for the absence of a control group, for the fact that participants did not spend a uniform length of time in the project, or for having had to introduce changes in the operation of the project while it was under way. These changes involved modifications in the price structure (inflation), providing additional back-up reinforcers, and modifying the educational method. It should also be noted that while the CASE II participants had not volunteered for the project, assignment had not been on a random basis. Possible generalizations to the institutional population at large are therefore highly circumscribed. Mindful of these, probably unavoidable, methodological limitations, what were the results of this ambitious project and what conclusions can be drawn from it?

Cohen and Filipczak (1971) present descriptive–anectodal material that reflects improvements in their participants' behavior in such cultural–interpersonal areas as eating behavior, health-care practices, socialization, and maintenance of one's living quarters. Yet while their case for the success of the project is convincingly stated, it is only in the data on achievement and intelligence tests and in recidivism rate that one finds quantitative information about its outcome.

Two forms of the Stanford Achievement Test (SAT) had been used to assess the students' academic progress, changes in scores having been adjusted for the length of time a student had actually been in the program. For students on whom test scores for the 1953 series of the SAT were available the rate of gain in grade level per year was 2.0 while for students who had been given the 1963 series of the test the mean gain for all students was only 1.5 grade levels. The use of two different editions of the achievement test with different students during overlapping periods of time contributes to the difficulty in evaluating the results. The investigators state that the 1953 norms were particularly appropriate to their instructional objectives and that the differences in the results from the two editions might have been due to the fact that the 1963 version tended to be administered to the students who were in the project longest or latest so that "increasingly more rigorous standards were interacting with the increasing stabilization of the project" (Cohen & Filipczak, 1971, p. 126). Be that as it may, it does appear that the CASE II students who, according to the investigators, had spent close to 90 percent of their available study time on academic-related activities, did indeed improve in their achievement test performance. In the absence of appropriate controls, however, it is impossible to tell whether this change was due to their exposure to the programmed teaching material and individualized study, to the fact that they were able to earn points for taking the tests, or to their repeated exposure to the tests and resulting familiarity with the material and the testing situation.

Another measure that presumably reflects improved academic ability and learning was an IQ score based on the Revised Army Beta test. Here the investigators report data on 24 students who had been tested at entry into the National Training School and again an average of approximately seven months later while they were in (but not at the end of) CASE II. For these students the mean gain was 12.5 IQ points, a statistically significant increase. Only one student failed to show an increase, while another gained as many as 27 IQ points. Nineteen of these 24 students were tested again three months later and for them the mean gain since their admission was 16.2 IQ points. Unfortunately, the interpretation of these impressive results is again handicapped by the fact that on the second and third testing "high scores were rewarded by a generous point payoff in proportion to the score" (Ibid., p. 132).

The explicit goals of the CASE II project, as stated by Cohen and Filipczak (1971), had been to increase the academic behaviors of all of its students and to prepare as many of them as possible "for return to the public school system" (p. 7). Achievement test scores suggest that the boys' academic behavior had indeed been increased; whether they returned to the public school system and how they fared there is not reported. Since the investigators had made no other assumptions regarding the potential effect of their project on the students' adjustment after discharge, this discussion of CASE II could end here. The effect of programs in the field of penology, however, is usually evaluated by asking the question how discharged inmates fare in the community and the customary measure for this is to count how many of them are later again institutionalized. This so-called recidivism rate is a poor substitute for careful follow-up of individuals since all it shows is whether ex-inmates were able to avoid apprehension by law enforcement agencies and renewed commitment to an institution (Repucci & Clingempeel, 1978). Whether they avoid this development by desisting from norm violation, by escaping detections, or by moving to a different community remains unknown. Nonetheless, to provide some basis for comparing CASE II with other forms of dealing with juvenile delinquents, a study was undertaken some two and one-half years after that project had terminated to ascertain what had happened to the students.

Attempts were made to contact or at least locate each of the 41 students who had passed through CASE II. For ten of these no information could be obtained. Of the remaining 31, 26 were interviewed and given reading and achievement tests that showed that they had retained and in some cases increased the skills they had learned in the project. Again, the absence of a control group does not permit one to draw a meaningful conclusion from these data. In the case of the crucial recidivism rate, Cohen and Filipczak (1971) offer a comparison with the average for the National Training School for prior years; this had been 76 percent within one year of discharge. In other words, 76 percent of the boys discharged from that Federal institution had been returned there within one year because they had committed new offenses; a rather dismal record that is considerably higher than the national average of about 50 to 60 percent (Burchard & Harig, 1976). In order to compare the CASE II record with that 76 percent figure, Cohen and Filipczak (1971) made a post hoc decision; it was to consider only those students who had participated in their program for at least 90 days. This reduced the number of those on whom follow-up data were available to 27 (the 26 who had been interviewed plus one who, being overseas with the Army, was assumed not to be in trouble). These 27 were further divided into 11 who had been released directly from CASE and 16 who had been moved from CASE to other programs or institutions before their final release.

Of the eleven students who had been released directly from CASE, three (27.3 percent) were recidivists within the first year after discharge. By the end of the third year after discharge, one additional youth was reinstitutionalized, raising the total recidivism rate to 36.4 percent. For the 16 students who had other institutional experiences after leaving CASE and for whom a different set of contingencies had thus been in effect, the recidivism rate is considerably higher. Within the first year after final discharge, ten (62.5 percent) had been returned to an institution. With an additional student who had become a recidivist during the following year, the total rate for that group of former CASE students is 68.8 percent. The combined recidivism rate for all CASE II students, both those discharged directly from the program and those who had spent further time elsewhere is thus 55.6 percent, a record considerably better than that of the Training School as a whole, but not much different from the national average, especially not if two students who had warrants pending for their arrest on violations of parole and who, because they could not be located, are not included in the CASE follow-up data are added to the record at which point the overall rate rises to 63 percent.

When one looks at the recidivism rate for only those students who had been discharged directly from CASE, the record of the project is impressive but there are some troubling ambiguities in the information provided in the mere ten pages Cohen and Filipczak (1971) devote to these follow-up data. We are not told, for example, about the nature of the difference, if any, between students who had been assigned to CASE II and who dropped out in less than 90 days and those who remained longer and on whom the assessment is based. Nor do we know what determined whether a student was discharged directly from the project or had to spend more time in other parts of the institution. Were the latter, per chance, those with longer sentences or those who for some reason were not eligible for parole in which case their higher recidivism rate would have to be viewed in a somewhat different light. The fact that 27 percent of the CASE population could not be located for follow-up is another source of ambiguity. Who were they and how had they fared since discharge? Lastly, there are the questions that plague any such study conducted in a natural setting. These are perceptively discussed by Repucci and Saunders (1974) and include administrative interference and pressure, personnel changes, and subtle sabotage based on misunderstandings and rivalries among the staff. Such problems can result in the introduction into a program of variables that the research investigators cannot identify so that the assumption that the independent variables in the study are those the investigators wish to evaluate may or may not be tenable.

Despite these misgivings, the work of Cohen and Filipczak (1971) stands as a landmark demonstration of constructive changes that can be introduced in the rehabilitation of institutionalized juvenile delinquents when established principles of learning are systematically applied. Studies with more circumscribed goals where tighter experimental controls are generally possible have repeatedly attested to the effectiveness of behaviorally oriented programs for juvenile deliquents in improving their behavior within the institution (e.g., Barkley, Hasting, Tousel, & Tousel, 1976; Hobbs & Holt, 1976; Tyler & Brown, 1968). But, as we said before, the ultimate test of effective intervention is not whether institutional inmates show greater obedience to often irrational institutional rules but whether they can function adaptively once they are returned to their community. Let us therefore examine one more such institutional program where the focus was on a combination of personal–social *and* academic–vocational behavior, covering, as it were, the inmates' entire institutional experience.

A Comprehensive Program

As part of a wider investigation that sought to compare two approaches based on different theoretical orientations (behavioral and transactional), Jesness, DeRisi, McCormick, and Wedge (1972) organized one of the institutions of the California Youth Authority along behavioral lines. The setting was the Karl Holton School for Boys near Stockton, California which is designed to house approximately 390 boys in eight 50-bed living halls. During the time this study was being conducted, the average age of the residents was 18, ranging from 15 to 21 (Jesness & DeRisi, 1973). The behavioral treatment program that was established at the school covered all aspects of the boys' life in the institution, including personal, social, and academic behavior. While the most basic approach entailed a comprehensive token economy and behavior contracting, use was also made of systematic desensitization, assertiveness training, extinction, and avoidance conditioning. As the program evolved over the years of its existence, changes were introduced in order to make it more effective or more practical and this, together with the mixing of procedures makes it impossible to conclude which aspect or combination of aspects of the "treatment package" led to the reported outcome.

Three categories of behavior were covered by token programs. The first, entitled "convenience behavior," had as its focus the efficient and orderly functioning of the institution. It covered such daily routines as getting up on time, dressing appropriately, maintaining the living area, following rules, and being courteous to and cooperative with peers and members of the staff. As Jesness and DeRisi (1973) observed, such behavior may not be crucial to the institution's goal of turning the residents into law-abiding citizens but it is necessary in order to run an institution. Probably more functional from the point of view of the boys' later adaptation in the community, was the category "academ ic behavior." The classroom-based token system centering around academic behavior was separated from that covering behavior in the living units because of several problems that had arisen there, such as inflation, excessive debts, and poor bookkeeping on the part of the staff. The third category of behaviors under the token/contract system was entitled "critical behavior deficiencies" and focused on the kind of conduct most immediately related to a boy's succeeding or failing on parole. Identified by a behavior checklist, these included such characteristics as friendliness, responsibility, and other forms of socialized behavior.

As in other token economy programs, back-up reinforcers for which the tokens could be exchanged consisted of privileges, personal items, and special services that were listed on a reinforcement menu. In addition to this short-term reinforcement system, an important long-term incentive was built around the number of points a boy had to accumulate in order to become eligible for referral to a parole board hearing. The minimum number of points (7,875) needed for this was calculated to allow a resident to reach parole in approximately 30 weeks but the acquisition of these points had to be distributed over the three categories of behavior so that 45 percent had to be earned for convenience behaviors, 28 percent for academic behaviors, and 27 percent for correction of critical behavior deficiencies. It is not clear why this particular distribution had been decided upon but it is likely that it was related to the relative ease or difficulty with which points could be earned in the different program areas. On the other hand, the heavy emphasis on "convenience behavior" probably reflected the attitude of staff and administrators that values a clean and orderly institution (and thus their own convenience) almost as highly as preparing the residents for life in the community.

The outcome of the program at Karl Holton School was compared with the record of that school in prior years and with that of other institutions operated by the California Youth Authority but the comparison of greatest interest was with the transactional analysis program that had been implemented in the adjacent O. H. Close School and which also entailed the negotiation of treatment contracts but without explicit reinforcement contingencies. Both institutions involved in the overall study reported a reduction in the amount of misconduct and rule violations. Detention, the ultimate sanction to which staff was able to resort, dropped more than 60 percent at both schools. The two schools were also similar in the 12-month follow-up data of parole violations which were 31.4 percent for the transactional and 31.9 percent for the behavioral program, significantly lower than during the two previous years. In the same follow-up year, two other facilities of the California Youth Authority reported 46 percent parole violations, a level not signifcantly different from that of previous years.

While the short-term outcome of the two programs is encouraging, the fact that two approaches based on rather different theoretical premises led to almost identical results raises the question whether the improvement was at least in part a function of a Hawthorne effect whereby any change from an established routine has some gratifying consequences. Data on long-term maintenance of the effect both within the institutions and for the discharged program participants are needed in order to throw light on this issue.

Meanwhile, it is worth noting that from the point of view of the participants in the two programs, as reflected in the ratings of satisfaction that the investigators collected from the boys, the transactional analysis program with its small group therapy sessions was clearly favored. The boys who had been in the O. H. Close program gave their staff higher ratings in competence and likability and rated their living units higher than did those who had been at Holton. Furthermore, the average length of stay in the Close transactional analysis program was significantly shorter than that in the Holton behavioral program. Given these outcomes, it would seem that a program established along transactional lines might be preferred to one following behavioral principles but before a firm conclusion can be drawn about this, questions such as differential background and training of staff, specifics of student characteristics, and— most of all—long-term follow-up on the adjustment of the discharged residents would have to be available.

TREATMENT PROGRAMS IN COMMUNITY SETTINGS

In parallel with the development in the area of care for psychotic and mentally retarded individuals, there has developed a forceful movement aimed at moving the care of the delinquent from large and isolated institutions to small, community-based treatment facilities. Probably the most widely publicized

and extensively adopted model of this type is the home-style rehabilitation setting, based on operant principles and directed by a trained staff of house-par-
ents, which was pioneered by Phillips (1968) and has come to be known as
Achievement Place.

Achievement Place

Programs based on this model operate on the premise that delinquent behavior
is the product of inadequate social learning experiences and have as their goal
the development of appropriate behavior patterns. In other words, delinquency is viewed as a skill deficit. Accordingly, those who follow the Achievement Place or Teaching-Family model of intervention establish a structured,
systematic program, aimed at teaching social skills such as how to make an introduction, academic skills such as how to study and do homework, self-care
skills in areas such as meal preparation and personal hygiene, and prevocation-
al skills that are designed to enable a young person to find work in the community. All of this takes place in and around a group home, located in the youngster's own community in which he or she remains from nine to twelve months.
Typical residents in such a setting are of junior high school age, about three to
four years below grade level on academic achievement tests, whose norm-violating behavior had led to their being adjudicated delinquent. A group home
houses from six to eight such adolescents and is operated under the direction
of professionally trained teaching-parents.

The details of an Achievement Place program have been presented by
Phillips, Phillips, Fixsen, and Wolf (1971) who describe it as a token economy.
The boys or girls in one of these family-style group homes earn points as reinforcers for specified desired behaviors that their past environments had presumably failed to teach them. The points that are earned can be converted into
a great variety of privileges such as the use of tools, telephoning, snacks, or an
allowance. While clearly defined, desirable behavior thus receives positive reinforcement, similarly defined undesirable behavior or rule violations, such as
aggressive speech or not being punctual, has the consequence of losing points
so that a response-cost system is also in operation.

In the beginning, behavior is heavily reinforced through a daily point system. This is later faded to a weekly point system and, ultimately, the resident
progresses to a merit system in which all privileges are free and reinforcement
for desirable behavior takes the form of praise, approval, and affection on the
rationale that these are the contingencies that operate in the youth's natural
environment to which he or she is soon to be returned. All behavior is carefully
monitored either by the staff or by peer monitors and after four successful
weeks on the merit system, the resident advances to the homeward bound sys-

tem. Here, the adolescent returns to his or her own home, spending occasional nights at Achievement Place for discussions of problems that were encountered while at home. This return to the youth's own home is coordinated through regular meetings between the parents or guardians and the program staff. These meetings are discontinued when the problems have abated.

The original Achievement Place program in Lawrence, Kansas has been the site of numerous studies, designed to assess specific aspects of the endeavor and to evaluate its outcome. Most of this work has been devoted to rigorous functional analyses of specific behaviors such as room cleaning, interview skills, and doing homework (Phillips, 1968), or to evaluating the efficacy of such methods as self-reporting (Fixsen, Phillips, & Wolf, 1972) or self-government (Fixsen, Phillips, & Wolf, 1973). Such process research is very important for it permits an investigator to demonstrate that the manipulations that have been introduced are indeed the effective independent variables that control the target behavior. At the same time, the question whether the program is effective in its principal aim, the prevention or reduction of delinquent behavior, that is outcome research, must be considered to be at least as important. Here the efforts of the Kansas research team are somewhat disappointing, largely because the experimental rigor they were able to bring to their process research is difficult to apply when conducting outcome studies. Random assignment of large numbers of cases to experimental and control groups, equation of length of stay, and counterbalancing of staff assignments are simply not possible when one conducts research in the natural environment, nor are the available criterion measures there as objective and quantifiable as are those that can be applied to specific behaviors taking place within the controlled group home. Yet given these considerations, the outcome results presented by Fixsen, Phillips, Phillips, and Wolf (1972) are very impressive.

In a comparison of 16 boys whom the juvenile court had committed to Achievement Place with 15 boys who had been sent to a state institution for delinquents, and 13 boys who had been placed on probation, Fixsen, Phillips, Phillips, and Wolf (1972) found that the Achievement Place boys excelled the other groups on such measures as school attendance, police or court contacts, and academic performance. In terms of recidivism rate, Achievement Place was far superior to the other two dispositions. Within the first 12 months after discharge, 6 percent of the Achievement Place boys, 13 percent of the state school boys, and 31 percent of the boys on probation had committed a delinquent act that led to their being readjudicated by the court and placed in an institution. By the end of 24 months following discharge, the cumulative totals of readjudicated youths was 19 percent for Achie ement Place, 53 percent for the state institution, and 54 percent for the probationary status. Similar results were later reported by Kirigin, Braukmann, Fixsen, Phillips, and Wolf (1975) who found that within two years after treatment participants in the Achievement Place program had an institutionalization rate of 22 percent while those who had been committed to the state reformatory for boys had a rate of 47 percent. These investigators also report that Achievement Place youths were more likely to remain in school following treatment than comparison cases who had been sent to the state institution; the former remaining at a rate of 56 percent, while of the latter only 33 percent continued to attend school. While these data are preliminary and must be qualified in terms of the unavoidable constraints that reality places on almost all such outcome research, there can be little doubt that the Teaching-Family model is a viable alternative to the institutionalization of delinquent youths.

INTERVENTION IN FAMILIES OF DELINQUENTS

Behavioral Contracting

When a treatment program is based on a token economy, the participants are informed that they can earn a specified number of tokens for behaving in a specified manner. Such a bilateral agreement is essentially a contract, similar to a commercial transaction where one party undertakes to deliver a specified item or service for which the other party is obligated to pay a previously agreed upon sum of money. The contract, in other words, spells out a contingency that will arise *if and only if* one party does a certain thing in which case the other party will respond in a certain way. This, of course, is the principle behind any contingent reinforcement procedure but in a laboratory experiment the contingency is usually not announced in advance; the subject comes to be exposed to the reinforcement contingency only after the operant has been emitted. In clinical practice with verbal clients, reinforcement contingencies are generally announced ahead of time. This, however, does not usually take the form of a contract that the parties have developed in the course of explicit negotiations. It is such negotiation of contingencies that sets a behavioral contract apart from other, less formal programs of reinforcement. In behavioral contracting the parties agree on the response that must be emitted before a specified consequence will be forthcoming. This consequence is usually not a token or other tangible reinforcer but a behavior that the other party to the contract has agreed to perform. In some respects then, a behavioral contract is similar to a bartering agreement.

Behavioral contracting can be used in any relationship where two or more people seek to interact in a mutually agreeable fashion, whether this be in a work setting, in a marriage, in parent–child relations, or in an institution. As is true of any therapeutic intervention, a behavioral contract is needed only when an identified problem is to be resolved or when an imminent problem is to be avoided. When a marriage or a parent–child relationship is functioning smoothly there is little point in formalizing the interaction by an explicit understanding of who is to do what for which consequence. In fact, it is likely that a good marriage or a constructive parent–child relationship is characterized by various implicit understandings about the functions of the respective partners. In situations where such smooth functioning has broken down a behavioral contract can be very helpful because once such a contract has been agreed upon it precludes arguments, misunderstandings, cajoling and pleading, thereby reducing conflicts and emotionally charged, hostile interactions.

In the family of a delinquent child, interactions frequently revolve around the child's undesirable behavior and are marked by hostile exchanges and coercion while, as Stuart (1971) has observed, the rate of positive exchanges is usually quite low. By the time such a family comes to seek help, matters have often reached a stage where members refuse to talk to each other and where mutual anger colors all interactions. In such circumstances Tharp and Wetzel (1969) found that formalizing the relationships by means of a behavioral contract can improve the situation and the delinquent member's behavior.

Underlying Assumptions. When used in a family, a behavioral contract can be viewed as a structured basis for the scheduled exchange of positive reinforcements when the reciprocal pattern of reinforcement between parents and child has broken down (Stuart, 1971). Four assumptions that underlie a behavioral contract have been stated by Stuart (1971) who made extensive use of this vehicle in the Family and School Consultation Project, a community-based family intervention project for school-referred, predelinquent children (Stuart, Jayaratne, & Tripodi, 1976; Stuart, Tripodi, Jayaratne, & Camburn, 1976).

The first of Stuart's (1971) assumptions is that the receipt of positive reinforcements in an interpersonal relationship is a privilege and not a right. This assumption, so diametrically opposed to the notion of unconditional (that is, noncontingent) positive regard, makes the point that the privilege of receiving positive reinforcement is a special prerogative that one may expect from another person only upon having engaged in some qualifying behavior. Under this assumption, it is therefore the responsibility of one member of a family to grant the privileges sought by another on the basis of reciprocity. An adolescent wishing to have the privilege of time to himself, for example, may have to agree to undertake the responsibility of attending school; the privilege will not be forthcoming unless the responsibility has been fulfilled.

The second assumption is related to the first in that it states that effective interpersonal agreements are governed by the norm of reciprocity. As Stuart (1971) points out, it is inherent in the use of behavioral contracts that the partners to the contract accept the notion that everyone must be fairly compensated for all that is received; no gifts are to be expected within a contractual relationship.

The third assumption underlying a system of behavioral contracting expresses the principle of interpersonal attraction. It is that two persons' attraction to each other is a function of the positive reinforcements each is able to receive within that relationship. In Stuart's (1971) words, "The value of an interpersonal exchange is a direct function of the range, rate, and magnitude of the positive reinforcements mediated by that exchange" (p.4). In negotiating a behavioral contract, each party to the contract seeks to extend to the others the maximum rate of positive reinforcement because the more positive reinforcements he or she delivers, the more will be received in return. A good intrafamilial contract thus encourages the highest possible rate of mutual reinforcement for every member of the family and thereby improves the relationship between and among the members of that family.

Positive reinforcement, it should be recalled, is not limited to the receipt of tangible objects or services since, by definition, positive reinforcement is any consequence that accrues to an individual following a given action that makes it likely for that action to be repeated at a future time. In a smoothly functioning interpersonal relationship it is often difficult to ascertain just what reinforcers the various partners obtain that makes them continue to emit positive behaviors. One would obviously not wish to introduce a behavioral contract when interpersonal relationships are operating smoothly and to the satisfaction of all concerned. It is when a relationship has broken down, where people do things for each other grudgingly or not at all, that a formalization of the relationship through a contract may help and where the assumption about positive reinforcers increasing mutual attraction finds its implementation.

Stuart's (1971) fourth assumption about behavioral contracts is that rules create freedom in interpersonal transactions. A contract specifies contingencies in terms of "if you do this, you will receive that." All parties to the contract therefore know exactly what to expect, leaving room for neither argument nor disappointment. Stuart (1971) uses the example of an adolescent girl whose contract provides that she can visit friends after school (a privilege) provided that she returns home by six o'clock (a responsibility). This rule governs an exchange of reinforcers between the girl and her parents; though it sets limits to the scope of her privilege, it grants the girl the choice of when or whether to take advantage of the privilege. Making the exchange explicit in the contract also frees the girl from arbitrary sanctions or unspecified consequences that she encountered in the past. Before the contract had been arranged, the girl would ask whether she could visit her friend and often receive an arbitrary refusal. Further, without a rule regarding her clear-cut responsibility as to when she was to return home, she would one day return at seven o'clock and be greeted warmly, return at six o'clock the next day and be ignored, yet arrive home at half past five the following day only to be reprimanded. Stuart (1971) points out that only through the explicit agreement regarding an acceptable hour for returning home, "can the girl insure her freedom, as freedom depends upon the opportunity to make behavioral choices with knowledge of the probable outcome of each alternative" (p. 5). One need not necessarily endorse Stuart's somewhat idiosyncratic use of the word "freedom" to agree that an explicit spelling out of contingencies and consequences will reduce frictions in a relationship and pave the way for more positive interactions.

Elements and Requirements of Good Contracts. In addition to stating the assumptions that underlie a behavioral contract, Stuart (1971) discusses the elements that are required for making such a contract accomplish its goal of establishing an effective parent–child interaction. These elements deal with the need for the contract to specify the privileges (reinforcers) each member of the family expects to gain after carrying out his or her responsibilities (responses) which, in turn, must be clearly detailed and defined. Typical privileges are free time with friends, choice of hair and dress styles, spending money, and the use of the family car. Privileges must be restricted to norm-abiding behavior; a boy cannot be granted the privilege of driving a car if he is legally not allowed to do so. Typical responsibilities include school attendance and minimally adequate academic performance, adherence to specified curfew hours, completion of explicit household chores, and keeping parents informed of one's whereabouts. Stuart also stresses that in order to have a workable and effective contract, the responsibilities expected from an adolescent must be kept to a minimum. In negotiating contracts, parents of somewhat rebellious, predelinquent adolescents readily generate long lists of requirements to which they want their offspring to conform but when they are asked to list the privileges they are willing to grant as consequences for this behavior, they usually find that they control comparatively few salient reinforcers. For this reason, the few available reinforcers must be apportioned with care if desired behavior is to be established and maintained.

Further requirements of an effective contract are that its provisions be such that the parents can monitor them and that clear sanctions be available for contract violations. There is no point in having unenforceable provisions in a contract. If enforcement is to be consistently carried out, parents must be able to know whether the adolescent adheres to his or her end of the bargain, for otherwise the contract becomes meaningless. As soon as a term of the contract has been violated by the adolescent's failure to meet an agreed-upon responsibility, the direct consequence must be that the contingent privilege is forfeited. Where this alone is not sufficient to assure compliance with the terms of the contract, Stuart (1971) advocates contractual provisions for additional sanctions, similar to a response-cost system in a token economy. These sanctions, however, must be carefully managed lest a point of diminishing returns be reached where it is no longer worth the adolescent's while to adhere to any portion of the contract.

Another requirement of a good behavioral contract, as advocated by Stuart (1971), is that it includes a bonus provision so that compliance with the contract is itself a behavior that earns specified positive reinforcement. Extended periods of nearly flawless compliance with the contractual responsibilities would thus earn extraordinary privileges or extra money. In order for such a bonus provision to work, it is of course necessary that the family keep some sort of record so that everyone's compliance with the contract can be reviewed. The availability of such a record also serves as a feedback system around which members of the family can exchange positive comments that enhance constructive interaction and strengthen prosocial behavior.

Factors Contributing to a Successful Contract. A behavioral contract provides a vehicle around which the mutuality of parent–child interaction can be organized and made explicit. A good contract must meet the assumptions and requirements just outlined but the specific content of a contract will vary from family to family. The question whether behavioral contracts are an effective treatment method is therefore as difficult to answer as similar questions about other complex treatment approaches. The answer to this question is further complicated by the fact that the Family and School Consultation Project conducted by Stuart and his associates (Stuart, Tripodi, Jayaratne, & Camburn, 1976) was a large-scale experiment in social engineering of which the behavioral contract was only one, albeit important, part.

While the use of behavioral contracts in that project resulted in small but statistically significant improvements of treated youths relative to an untreated control group, the most meaningful outcome of this project is the list of suggestions it engendered regarding the factors that seem to contribute to the effectiveness of the behavioral contract as a tool of intervention. These factors involve the type of family, the nature of their problem, and the qualities of the therapist who helps them establish their contract. The specific nature of the contract itself appears to contribute relatively little to the success or failure of the intervention. As Stuart and Lott (1972) speculated in discussing their study, families with strong histories of constructive social facilitation seem more likely to be able to use a behavioral contract constructively than those whose transactions have long been chaotic. In addition, contracts seem to work best in families where conflict is most acute. More important than these factors, however, seems to be "the therapist's skill in structuring a climate of compromise in which no one loses face" (p. 169). The therapist serves a mediating role that calls for considerable skill and this skill may be more important than the structure or content of the contract. It thus appears that in the hands of a skilled therapist a behavioral contract can be a useful tool but whether such a therapist might be able to reach the same goal by other means remains a question for further research.

Short-term Intervention

A relatively short-term family intervention program lasting four weeks and built around the principle of contingency contracting was conducted and evaluated by Alexander and Parsons (1973). More focused than Stuart's (1971) "social engineering" approach, this project also included better controls and more objective outcome measures, thus presenting a more conclusive test of the effectiveness of behavioral contracting than the earlier work.

Like Stuart (1971), and Snyder (1977), Alexander and Parsons (1973) see the interactions in problem families as characterized by low rates of mutual positive reinforcement, by what Patterson and Reid (1970) had identified as a lack of reciprocity in family interaction. Their therapeutic intervention was designed to replace these maladaptive interaction patterns by patterns of reciprocity. Therapists therefore modeled, prompted, and reinforced for all family members such interpersonal skills as clear communication of messages and feelings, as well as the clear presentation of demands and alternative solutions. The aim was to enable the family members to enter into negotiations with each other so that each could receive a privilege for every responsibility undertaken, even where this required a compromise.

In describing their intervention technique, Alexander and Parsons (1973) point out that when introducing contingency contracting in a family it is important to begin with relatively minor issues around which the members of the family may be willing to compromise rather than opening negotiations around a topic of major conflict where positions may have hardened and strong feeling become involved. Once members of a family can recognize the reduction in conflict that results from having developed a working contract around one issue, they are often willing to extend the system to more adamant problem areas. This is a principle well worth generalizing to other areas of child therapy. By starting an intervention with a relatively minor problem that has a high probability of showing quick improvement a therapist can demonstrate to clients the benefits they can derive from accepting therapeutic recommendations and following required procedures, thereby increasing the likelihood of their cooperating in more extensive and more difficult tasks.

Two major procedures were applied with all of the families in the short-term behavioral intervention used by Alexander and Parsons (1973). One entailed introducing greater structure into the family interaction pattern by making explicit the difference between rules and requests. Rules were defined as established limits that regulate and control the behavior of all members of the family. Everyone was to adhere to these rules and infractions led to clearly stated and enforceable consequences. Requests, on the other hand, were defined as ad hoc statements addressed by one person to another and as not possessing the demand characteristics of a rule. A person being requested to perform an act thus had the privilege of complying or refusing without having to fear negative consequences for a refusal.

The other major intervention procedure that was applied with all families in the treatment group was the therapist's systematic use of social reinforcement to improve the family's communication pattern while they were negotiating the contingency contract. The specific communication patterns that were reinforced by the therapist's praise entailed interrupting another person in order to (a) seek clarification; (b) offer clarifying information; and (c) provide informative feedback to other family members. By increasing the rate of such interruptions, the therapist sought to raise the level of clarity and precision of the family members' communications since, as Alexander and Parsons (1973) point out, families of delinquents, when compared with those of nondelinquents, tend to be more silent, talk less equally, have fewer positive interruptions, and are, in general, less active.

Therapists trained in these procedures applied them with 46 families referred by the Juvenile Court of Salt Lake County, Utah because an adolescent member (between 13 and 16 years of age) had been arrested or detained for such offenses as running away, being habitually truant or ungovernable, shoplifting, or possession of alcohol, soft drugs, or tobacco. The authors report their results in terms of two kinds of data, process measures and outcome measures. Process measures were designed to evaluate whether the families' communication patterns had an effect on the norm-violating behavior of the delinquent member of the family. The use of both of these measures represents a most laudable aspect of the research by Alexander and Parsons (1973). As O'Leary and Turkewitz (1978) pointed out in their discussion of methodological errors in marital and child treatment research, investigators all too often neglect to provide data to show that the manipulation of the independent variable (treatment process) that was expected to effect changes in the dependent variable (treatment outcome) had indeed been implemented. Particularly when the actual treatment is in the hands of someone other than the investigators, such as parents, teachers, or other auxiliary therapists, the question whether they actually carried out the procedures for which they had been made responsible must be answered in the affirmative if the results of the investigation are to be correctly interpreted. In the absence of reliable process measures it is impossible to state unequivocally that the treatment under study had actually been the effective independent variable even if outcome data show a change in the target behavior. Conversely, when outcome data fail to reveal such change it is impossible to know whether the negative results were due to a failure of the treatment or to a failure of the therapists to implement the treatment.

In the case of the study by Alexander and Parsons (1973) process measures were gathered on the first 20 families who completed the treatment program by observing their interactions in a series of tasks and scoring the reciprocity and clarity of their communication. This revealed that the families who had received the short-term intervention designed to increase these aspects of family interaction had indeed significantly more equality in talk time, fewer silences, and more interruptions than ten families who had been exposed to a comparison condition consisting of client-centered family group therapy, and six families who had received no formal treatment.

In a different study, in which the same intervention method was used with another group of 21 families of delinquents, Alexander, Barton, Schiavo, & Parsons (1976) demonstrated a direct relationship between process measures and treatment effectiveness. There the process measures were ratings of the families' defensive and supportive communications. Defensive communications were defined as behavior that is threatening or punishing to others and elicits defensive behaviors in turn. Supportive communications, on the other hand, were those involving genuine information seeking and giving, spontaneous problem solving, empathic understanding, and equality. The frequency with which each family member used such communications was rated by trained judges who listened to tape-recorded samples of therapy sessions at the beginning and just before the end of the four-week treatment program. A supportiveness/defensiveness ratio was then derived for each family and these were shown to be significantly related to whether a family terminated treatment contact against their therapist's advice and without having changed their communication pattern or whether they continued in treatment until termination was mutually agreed upon because they had achieved an effective communication pattern. It is important to note that the supportiveness/defensiveness ratios did not differentiate among the outcome groups at either the beginning or the end of the first treatment session but that a significant difference was found for the ratios based on the next-to-the-last session in the direction of the more supportive families having the better outcome. This suggest that differences in outcome were not a function of differences in communication patterns at the beginning of treatment but that the intervention was responsible for changing the communication pattern and thus affecting the outcome.

While these are important data, the most crucial outcome measure for a program of intervention with families of juvenile delinquents is obviously one that gauges the effect of the intervention on the behavior of the delinquent. Here, Alexander and Parsons (1973) turn to the criterion of recidivism. After an interval ranging from 6 to 18 months following termination of treatment the records of the juvenile court were examined in order to ascertain how many of the adolescents in the treated families and in several control or comparison groups had once again come to the court's attention. The adolescents in the ten control families who had received no formal treatment of any kind had a recidivism rate of 50 percent; a rate almost identical with the 51 percent rate recorded county-wide for 2,800 cases during the year in which this study took place. In the 46 families who had participated in the short-term behavioral family treatment (including the 12 cases who had dropped out of the program before completion) the recidivism rate was a significantly lower 26 percent. This was strikingly better than the record of two comparison groups one of which, consisting of 19 families who had received client-centered family group therapy, had a 47 percent recidivism rate and another, who had been given an eclectic, psychodynamically oriented family treatment, where the recidivism rate was 73 percent; significantly *higher* than the 50 percent rate of the no-treatment controls! (The client-centered and psychodynamic comparison treatments had been conducted in agencies and by therapists who subscribed to and routinely practiced these approaches.)

Having demonstrated that their program modified the communication patterns of the treated families and that the adolescents in the treated families had significantly lower recidivism rates than either a group of untreated families or families treated by different methods, there remained for Alexander and Parsons (1973) to show a relationship between improved communication patterns and reduced recidivism rate. They do this by dividing all cases, regardless of treatment, into recidivism and nonrecidivism groups and presenting the communication pattern measures for this dichotomy. It turns out that there is indeed a statistically significant difference between these groups on all of the process measures. That is, the nonrecidivism group showed greater equality in talk time, fewer silences, and more interruptions than the recidivism group, just as the investigators had predicted on the basis of their theoretical formulations about family interaction patterns. This lends a good deal of support to their conclusion "that family intervention programs may profitably be focused on changing family interaction patterns in the direction of increased clarity and precision of communication, increased reciprocity of communication and social reinforcement, and contingency contracting emphasizing equivalence of rights and responsibilities for all family members" (p. 224).

The Role of the Therapist. It will be recalled that in a discussion of the effectiveness of behavioral contracting, Stuart and Lott (1972) speculated to what extent the skill of the therapist is an important variable in the outcome of treatment that employs this method. Research conducted by Alexander, Barton, Schiavo, and Parsons (1976) throws light on this issue and underscores the importance of the therapist's relationship skills in implementing an effective behavioral program.

Using the short-term behavioral intervention that had been found to be successful in their previous study (Alexander & Parsons, 1973), Alexander et al. (1976) assigned 21 families of delinquent adolescents at random to one of 21 different therapists who, in terms of background, ranged from second-year graduate students to doctoral level therapists with extensive experience. All of these therapists had been given 10 weeks of training in the use of the family intervention program and they continued to receive direct supervision while they worked with their family. At the end of the therapists' 10-week training program and before they began work with the family assigned to them, the training supervisor rated each therapist on eight characteristics, basing their ratings on direct observations they had made during training.

Treatment outcome was expressed in terms of how long and with what results the families remained in therapy. This outcome measure was categorized in four levels; families who unilaterally terminated treatment contact after a first, nonproductive session; families who attended several nonproductive sessions before terminating against the therapist's advice; families who continued in treatment until the end of the project and who had made some progress in their communication patterns but were still unable to solve problems without help; and families whose termination was agreed upon jointly with the therapist because their complaints had ceased and they had achieved spontaneous problem-solving ability and effective communication. The number of families at these four outcome levels were 4, 5, 5, and 7, respectively. When this subjectively judged therapy outcome was compared to recidivism it was found that there had been no recidivism within 12 to 15 months following intervention for families at the last two outcome levels, while three families at the first and two families at the second outcome level had further court or clinic referrals. The outcome measures used were thus supported by nonreactive data.

Of the therapist characteristics that had been rated by their supervisors five were found to be positively related to treatment outcome. Three of these fell into a relationship dimension (affect–behavior integration, warmth, and humor) and two into a structuring dimension (directiveness and self-confidence). Alexander et al. (1976), describe these characteristics as follows:

Affect–behavior integration: The degree to which the trainee related a family's expression of affect to behavioral sequences and vice versa.

Warmth: The frequency with which the trainee used smiling, active listening, and forward-lean during sessions, and social small talk before and after sessions.

Humor: The degree to which the trainee would characteristically use humor to reduce tension and relabel sequences.

Directiveness: The frequency of verbal and nonverbal commands, instructions, physical rearrangement of chairs, and interruptions of family interaction sequences.

Self-confidence: Use of eye contact and forward-lean when giving directions; voice level, references to the program, and/or personal effectiveness.

The analysis of the relationship between these therapist characteristics and the treatment results revealed that the scores on the relationship and structuring dimensions jointly accounted for 59.65 percent of the variance in outcome, relationship skills contributing a greater portion. Since each therapist in the sample had worked with only one family it was possible to designate them as poor-outcome therapists and good-outcome therapists on the basis of the result they had achieved in terms of the outcome criteria used with the families. A comparison of these two kinds of therapists and their therapist characteristics showed significant differences; families whose therapist had low scores on the relationship dimension tended to be those who terminated unsuccessful treatment, while those whose therapists had high scores tended to continue treatment until the end of the project or mutually agreed-upon termination. The same significant relationship held for therapists' scores on the structuring dimension.

The results of this study strongly suggest that the behavior of the therapist makes an important contribution to the outcome of a program of behavioral intervention with families of delinquents. The therapist's ability to relate the family's expression of affect to their behavior, to use humor in reducing tensions, and to be directive appear to be among the most critical characteristics. With therapists who possess (or are taught) these characteristics, the structured treatment approach developed by Alexander and Parsons (1973) would seem to be the most effective form of short-term intervention in delinquency currently available for the type of family with which it has been used.

Recapitulation

The norm-violating behavior of young people who—when apprehended—come to be designated as juvenile delinquents is often low in frequency but high in magnitude. This poses difficulties for treatment and for the assessment of treatment outcome. Norm-violating behavior is best construed as reflecting deficits in socially acceptable, alternative behavior, in the skill to discriminate between acceptable and unacceptable behavior, or in the ability to postpone immediate gratification. Behaviorally oriented treatment approaches have focused on the development of these missing or inadequately learned skills and abilities. In settings where juvenile delinquents are institutionalized the aim of interventions has often been to improve the youth's social behavior within the institution while, with rare but ambitious exceptions, the development of the academic and occupational skills that are needed to function adaptively outside the institution has been relatively neglected. Treatment programs conducted in community settings, such as those following the teaching-family model, have shown much promise but the complications involved in conducting rigorous outcome and follow-up studies under relatively uncontrolled field conditions make it difficult to know whether such approaches do indeed prevent or reduce norm-violating behavior. With young people who are viewed as prone to delinquency, intervention within their families has received considerable attention in recent years. Contingency contracts drawn between the various members of these families with the aid of a skilled therapist appear capable of improving family interaction and to reduce the frequency of norm-violating offenses.

The Treatment of
Behavior Excesses

CHAPTER 9

Aggressive Behavior

As pointed out earlier, the separation of problems into those of deficient and excess behavior, which is used as an organizing framework for this book, does not represent a true dichotomy when psychological disorders are considered in terms of the labels that are customarily used to classify disturbed children. When the norm-violating behavior of the juvenile delinquent is discussed in that part of this book which is devoted to behavior deficits while agressive behavior is found under the rubric of behavior excesses, the blurred boundaries of this convenient but artificial framework become especially apparent. The description of the Achievement Place model, for example, made mention of aggressive speech which was reduced by invoking a response-cost system. While it seems logical to view norm-violating behavior as a reflection of behavior deficits that treatment had to try to counteract, it must be recognized that some behavior, such as aggression, that is emitted by a juvenile delinquent represents an excess that treatment must seek to reduce. Nonetheless, an examination of aggression, per se, seems best placed under the rubric of excess behavior for reasons that should soon become apparent. Meanwhile, it is hoped that the reader will not struggle excessively with this problem, created, as it is, by the deficiencies of the classificatory system in the field of children's psychological disorders.

THE REDUCTION OF AGGRESSIVE BEHAVIOR

Aggressive behavior takes a variety of forms. It may involve a physical attack on another person, the destruction or theft of someone else's property, verbal abuse, or the infliction of injury to an animal. In each instance the behavior will be a noxious, aversive stimulus for the victim who will protest, emit avoidance or escape responses, or engage in defensive counteraggression. Partly because it interferes with the smooth functioning of society in that it disrupts interpersonal relations, thus representing a social problem, and partly because its definition poses complicated conceptual issues, aggression has been the subject of extensive analyses (e.g., Bandura, 1973). We need not here concern ourselves with the nature of aggression. Suffice it to assert that aggression is best viewed as an overt response that is maintained by its consequences and can thus be strengthened or weakened by the manipulation of these consequences (Horton, 1970). Support for this assertion comes from an extensive study of the behavior of nursery school children conducted by Patterson, Littman, and Bricker (1967) who demonstrated that aggressive behavior increases in frequency when the victim of the aggression yields to the aggressor, thereby providing a positive consequence for the aggressive act. When, on the other hand, the victim retaliates or otherwise provides a negative consequence, the aggressive acts toward that victim decrease in frequency. The peer group is thus an important source of reinforcement for aggressive behavior and one of the directions that attempts at the modification of aggressive behavior must therefore take is the removal of this form of reinforcement.

Time-Out Procedures

When a child emits aggressive behavior in the presence of other children as is the case in the classroom or a family group, it usually is difficult for the teacher or parent to prevent the peers or siblings from responding and thereby providing reinforcement. The most feasible method for preventing these reinforcing consequences from becoming available to the offending child is the response-contingent removal of that child from the situation and thus from the opportunity to obtain the reinforcement. This entails the method of time-out from positive reinforcement, known as *time-out* for short. Depending on the nature of the identified reinforcing stimulus, time-out can take the form of isolating the child for a brief period in a corner of the room or it can require that the child be physically removed from the room, again for a brief period of time.

When time-out has the effect of reducing the frequency of the response that it follows, it is technically and by definition a form of punishment by removal and children generally perceive it as an aversive event (Clark, Rowbury, Baer, & Baer, 1973; Kanfer & Phillips, 1970; Leitenberg, 1965). Brief removal of a child from the opportunity to obtain positive reinforcement from his or her peers however, must not be confused with extended periods of punitive social isolation. Solitary confinement is not made more acceptable by renaming it time-out!

While some of the parameters of time-out procedures remain to be investigated (Hobbs & Forehand, 1977; MacDonough & Forehand, 1973) there exists fairly convincing evidence that brief periods of time-out are more effective than long periods of punitive confinement (Burchard & Tyler, 1965). It also appears that some schedules of intermittent use of time-out may be as effective as its application on a continuous schedule in which every instance of undesirable behavior is followed by this consequence (Clark, et al., 1973). As in any intervention designed to reduce the frequency of an undesirable response, it is vital that explicit efforts are concurrently made to establish and strengthen alternative, desirable behaviors. To accomplish this, time-out can be embedded in the method of differential reinforcement of other behavior (DRO). Repp and Deitz (1974) used this approach in reducing the aggressive and self-injurious behavior of institutionalized retarded children for whom they linked a 30-second time-out contingency to the positive reinforcement of periods of time when such behavior was not emitted.

Recalling that time-out means the removal of the opportunity to receive positive reinforcement should make it obvious that in order to employ this form of intervention one must first find out what the positive reinforcers are that maintain the undesirable behavior (Solnick, Rincover, & Peterson, 1977). One cannot remove the availability of something one has not identifed. Having this information is, in fact, what differentiates true time-out from undifferentiated, response-contingent social isolation (Drabman & Spitalnik, 1973a). It has been repeatedly demonstrated that contingent teacher attention can serve as a reinforcer for children's aggression (Brown and Elliot, 1965; Pinkston, Reese, LeBlanc, & Baer, 1973). When such attention is withdrawn from a child contingent on an aggressive response, the teacher is using a time-out procedure. Pinkston et al. (1973) instructed a nursery school teacher to introduce such a contingency; ignoring a child's aggressive behavior as much as possible and attending instead to the child who had been attacked. They report that the child's aggressive behavior declined and socially desirable behavior increased, especially when the teacher attended to him when he engaged in non-aggressive interaction with other children. Slaby and Crowly (1977) demonstrated that when teachers attended to speech having aggressive content, the frequency of such speech increased yet when they shifted their attention to children's spontaneous cooperative speech and behavior, cooperative behavior increased while both verbal and physical aggression decreased.

The relationship between aggressive content of speech and physical aggression, reported by Slaby and Crowley (1977), has also been observed by

Firestone (1976) in a study of the behavior of a 4½-year-old boy who had been expelled from nursery school the previous year for his aggressive behavior and who was about to be expelled again for the same reason. In addition to trying to help this child, Firestone (1976) was interested in studying whether a time-out procedure had any undesirable side effects as had been suggested by Pendergrass (1972) who had found the social responses of two retarded children to decrease when their aggressive behavior was treated by a time-out approach. For this reason Firestone (1976) gathered direct observations not only of verbal and physical aggression but also of cooperative behavior, interaction with teachers, and isolate play. After three days of baseline observations the time-out procedure was instituted contingent on acts of physical aggression, which had been defined as striking, hitting, kicking, pulling, and the destruction of others' property. Time-out consisted of requiring the boy to sit in a chair, placed in a corner of the classroom, until he had been quiet for two minutes. The rationale for this procedure had been explained to the child at the time the first aggressive act was followed by time-out and he seemed to accept it, creating very little fuss when he had to sit in that chair.

During baseline, the child's physical aggression took up about 20 percent of the daily observation periods which lasted approximately 2 hours. When the time-out procedure was instituted on the fourth day, during which the boy had to be placed in the time-out chair six times, the rate of aggressive acts dropped precipitously to a 4 percent level (see Figure 13). This rate then continued to decline over the next 9 days, reaching an average of 1.9 percent. Concurrently, incidents of verbal aggression, which had not been placed on the time-out contingency and had been at a 3.7 percent level during baseline, dropped to 0.53 percent of the observed time by the fifth day of the time-out phase. Physical and verbal aggression thus appears to belong to a response class since an induced change in the rate of one so readily generalized to the other. Furthermore, such generalization seems restricted to this response class since Firestone (1976) found that neither the boy's general activity level nor his cooperative play were adversely affected by the time-out procedure; in fact, his cooperative play showed a marked increase from a baseline rate of 42.2 percent to an average of 68.2 percent during the 10 days of the treatment phase. Concurrently, his rate of isolate play decreased from 28.2 percent to 8.2 percent. It seems that as this boy's aggressive behavior decreased, socially acceptable behavior that had already been in his repertoire underwent an increase, possibly because greater acceptance by his peers reinforced such activity.

A somewhat ambiguous result of Firestone's (1976) study is that the child's rate of interaction with the teachers (question-asking, story-telling, helping with chores, and attention-seeking) which had occurred at a rate of 6.1 percent fell to 3.4 percent during the time-out phase. Firestone (1976) was unable to interpret this result because his data had not differentiated between de-

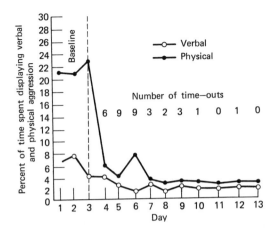

Figure 13. Incidence of verbal and physical aggression during baseline and treatment phase when verbal, but not physical aggression was followed by time-out. (Firestone, 1976. Copyright by Pergamon Press, Ltd.)

sirable interactions with teachers, such as helping with chores, and essentially undesirable "attention-seeking behavior." If the reduction in the category of teacher interactions had been the result of less nonconstructive, "attention-seeking" behavior it could be viewed as a positive side effect of the time-out procedure. On the other hand, it might also be that the teachers, as agents of the time-out procedure, had acquired negative stimulus characteristics so that the boy avoided contact with them. This would obviously have been an unfortunate consequence of the intervention. Lastly, it is conceivable that the child's increased interaction with his peers simply left less time for interaction with adults. In the absence of relevant data it is impossible to tell to what the effect should be attributed. In addition to this defect in the design of this study, the fact that it employed a simple AB format, without reversal, leaves unresolved the question whether the time-out procedure was really the critical independent variable. Admittedly, reversal is undesirable when the dependent variable is something as noxious as aggression but other designs, such as multiple baselines, are available that would permit one to draw firmer conclusions.

Considerations in the Use of Time-out. Because time-out procedures are frequently recommended for use in the reduction of aggressive and disruptive behavior, it is worth noting that, like any other technique, these procedures can be ineffective or even counterproductive when they are applied without the circumspection that only a thorough assessment can provide. Reviews by Mac-Donough and Forehand (1973) and by Hobbs and Forehand (1977) have highlighted some of the parameters that are involved in the use of time-out and that have been investigated.

One of the aspects of time-out that must be taken into account when considering its use is that its onset functions as a punishment by the removal of the opportunity to receive positive reinforcement; it thus has aversive aspects. Like any other aversive stimulus, the *onset* of time-out functions as a punisher while its *offset* functions as a negative reinforcer. Therefore, the termination of time-out, representing the removal of an aversive condition can serve as negative reinforcement of whatever response might be emitted at that moment. If the implementation of time-out takes the form of isolating a child from potentially reinforcing peer contacts it is well to consider what that child is doing at the moment isolation is terminated and return to the peers is permitted. If the child were to be cursing and yelling or kicking the door of the time-out room at that moment, it is these responses that would be reinforced. On the other hand, if the child were quiet at that moment, quiet behavior is likely to be strengthened. This consideration has led to the recommendation that release from time-out should be contingent on the then ongoing behavior and not on some predetermined, fixed period of time. A study by Hobbs, Forehand and Murray (1978) showed that such response-contingent release from time-out is more effective than fixed-period time-out in suppressing noncompliant behavior in young children.

Time-out presumably derives its effectiveness in reducing the behavior on which it is contingent from the fact that the child is temporarily deprived of positive reinforcement. Yet, as is true of any other response consequence, it is important to ascertain the functional relationship of time-out to the behavior in question. If what is supposed to be a time-out procedure increases rather than decreases the target behavior it is obviously not functioning as punishment by removal. Careful studies by Plummer, Baer, and LeBlanc (1977) demonstrated the difference between a time-out *procedure* and a time-out *function*. In one of these experiments the target was a 5-year-old autistic girl's disruptive behavior during individualized lessons. On the assumption that an adult's attention served as a positive reinforcer for this child, the teacher interrupted the lesson and turned away from the girl each time she engaged in disruptive behavior, a procedural time-out. Observer records revealed, however, that this procedure increased the frequency of the disruptive responses. What had been meant to be time-out from positive reinforcement (teacher attention) apparently served the function of a negative reinforcer in that the presumably aversive instruction was terminated contingent on the disruptive responses. The investigators dealt with this problem by substituting paced instruction for time-out. In paced instruction the teacher delivers instructions to the child at a set pace, regardless of the child's behavior. When disruptive behavior no longer resulted in discontinuance of the lessons, that behavior extinguished in the tutoring situation. This finding led Plummer et al. (1977) to conclude that procedural time-out should be used only when its effect is carefully monitored.

The crucial question to be asked is from what a time-out procedure is time out.

A similar analysis of the effect of time-out was presented by Solnick, Rincover, and Peterson (1977) in a study that dealt with the tantrum behavior of a 6-year-old autistic girl who occasionally engaged in this high-magnitude behavior during sessions of color-discrimination training. In an attempt to eliminate these tantrums, the investigators instituted a time-out procedure in that the teacher would leave the room for 10 seconds, taking along the candy which she was using to reinforce correct responses. Contrary to expectations, this procedure increased the frequency of tantrums to as many as 33 per session while they had ranged from zero to three per session before time-out was instituted. Clearly, something in the time-out procedure served as a reinforcer.

Observation revealed that the girl spent virtually every time-out period engaging in self-stimulatory behavior. In terms of the formulation advanced by Premack (1959), the opportunity to engage in high-probability behavior (self-stimulation) served as reinforcement for lower-probability behavior (tantrums). Solnick et al. (1977) tested this assumption by a functional analysis of the self-stimulatory behavior. They used a design in which baseline conditions alternated with three different phases. One was a time-out contingency, another was a phase where 1-second opportunities to engage in self-stimulatory behavior were provided contingent on a tantrum, and in a third phase self-stimulatory behavior was physically prevented for 10 seconds immediately following a tantrum. The data showed that the frequency of tantrums increased when self-stimulation was possible and that it declined to zero when self-stimulation was prevented, suggesting that the opportunity to engage in self-stimulation during the time-out periods had indeed been reinforcing the tantrums. Based on this analysis and on work with a 16-year-old retarded male for whom "time-in" was experimentally enriched or impoverished, Solnick, Rincover, and Peterson (1977) drew the same conclusion at which Plummer et al. (1977) had also arrived: The effect of time-out must be carefully monitored to assure that it does indeed serve the function of reducing the behavior on which it is contingent. They point out that this effect may well depend on the relationship between the conditions existing before, during, and after the time-out period. If time-out provides relief from a boring, demanding, or otherwise aversive situation it can serve as a negative reinforcer, strengthening the behavior on which it is contingent.

A similar contrast effect was commented upon by MacDonough and Forehand (1973) in concluding their review of existing research on the duration of time-out. It seems that very brief periods of time-out can be effective, provided that a given duration is used consistently. If longer periods of time-out are mixed with shorter periods, the shorter periods will lose their effectiveness probably because in contrast to the longer periods they are perceived as negligible consequences. When instituting contingent time-out in order to reduce the frequency of an undesirable behavior it seems best to begin with very brief periods, increasing the time only when these periods prove to be ineffective. Once longer periods have been instituted, it does not seem feasible to revert to shorter periods.

While the punishment by removal that is entailed in the time-out procedure is an attractive alternative to punishment by application, particularly when this involves the infliction of pain, it is not simple to use and must be employed with considerable circumspection. Clinicians, faced with parents who routinely resort to pain-infliction in trying to correct their child's objectionable behavior, are often inclined to induce the parents to substitute time-out procedures for the spankings. Doing this without first ascertaining the reinforcers for the unacceptable behavior and without carefully monitoring the procedure and its effect may be counterproductive. The parents, seeing time-out as failing to work, often resume their old ways of dealing with their child's behavior. Since this behavior, as a result of having been reinforced, may have become more frequent or intense, the parents may now inflict even more pain on their child than they did before the unsuccessful intervention by the hapless (and careless) clinician.

Family Intervention

The most extensive work with the problem of aggressive children has been conducted by Patterson and his colleagues (Patterson, Cobb, & Ray, 1973; Patterson & Reid, 1973). This group of investigators view aggressive behavior in the light of Patterson's coercion hypothesis (Patterson & Reid, 1970) according to which such behavior is a link in a chain of interpersonal events consisting of antecedents and consequences. The coercion process may be initiated by a parent who issues a command that represents an aversive stimulus for the child. The child may respond to this stimulus with any of a number of behaviors that, in turn represent aversive stimuli to the parent; for example, noncompliance accompanied by footstomping and "no." If the parent, in order to terminate these aversive stimuli, withdraws the command or emits some other compliant behavior this reinforces the child's noncompliance while the parent is, in turn, reinforced for giving in by the fact that the child's aversive behavior ceases. The process, as Patterson, Cobb, and Ray (1973) pointed out, provides reinforcement for both the child and the parent because the coercer is reinforced by the removal of the initial aversive stimulus, while the initiator is reinforced for compliance by the termination of the coercive behavior (p. 142). They view such aggressive behaviors as yelling, teasing, hitting, temper tantrums, and noncompliance as elements in the coercion chain that are learned, strengthened, and maintained by their characteristic of eliciting reinforcing responses from others.

Parental Characteristics. Patterson, Cobb and Ray (1973) suggest that parents of children who display a large amount of coercive (aggressive) behavior have identifiable characteristics that must be considered when contemplating a program of intervention. For, as Patterson and Fleischman (1979) pointed out in their review of family intervention programs, the maintenance of treatment effects is, in part, a function of the parents' ability to modify their habitual pattern of responding to their child's coercive behavior. Three distinctive parental characteristics have been described by Patterson, Cobb, and Ray (1973), as follows.

The Diffusion Parent. This is the parent who:

> is inattentive to the antecedents in coercive chains that lead to high amplitude responses. When a terminal behavior such as *hitting* does occur, the parents react with yelling or nagging, behaviors which are more likely to increase rather than reduce rates of coercive behavior unless they are followed frequently with intense punishment. If the parent consistently paired yelling and severe punishment, this might become a decelerating consequence. However, most parents of aggressive children do not react *consistently* enough or early enough in the coercive chain of behavior to produce any effective decelerating consequences.
>
> In addition to inattention and ineffective use of punishment, diffusion parents do not systematically train the child in adaptive responses to aversive situations. In effect, sloppy management techniques permit coercive behaviors to occur and to be reinforced on rich schedules among *all* family members.
>
> The diffusion parents fail to attend to and reinforce the child when he does behave appropriately; in fact, they are likely to describe him as *always bad*. Even when prosocial behaviors are pointed out to them, they are unlikely to reinforce because, as they say, "That's what he is *supposed* to do. Why reward that?"
>
> As the rates of coercive child behavior accelerate, the parents will be trained to yell, nag, and hit at ever-increasing rates. As their own aversive behaviors increase in rate in conjunction with similar increases among other family members, the amount of reinforcement the parents receive for effective parenting will drop and may result in further reducing the overall level of positive reinforcers they dispense to other family members (p. 146).

Patterson et al. (1973) report that in their experience, the diffusion parents who rarely provide positive reinforcement for their children's prosocial behavior have difficulty benefiting from an intervention program aimed at changing the reinforcement contingencies used in the home. While some of these parents respond to a reduction in the rate of coercive behavior by increasing the reinforcement of prosocial behavior, they seem less likely than other parents to find such changes reinforcing. Such parents, these authors say, "forget" to reinforce the competing prosocial behavior consistently and tend to return to the use of sporadic punishment to control the coercive behavior when it occasionally occurs. They thus re-create the very problems that brought the family to seek help in the first place.

The Selective Diffusion Parent. In the words of Patterson et al. (1973), this pattern takes the following form.

> The selective diffusion parents *are* involved, and they *do* track child behaviors; in fact, they may do a creditable job in rearing several children. They may also train the problem child for prosocial skills, but they do not apply effective contingencies in dealing with coercive behaviors. This omission may occur in a number of family situations. One example is the working mother who feels that she deprives the child of *mothering*, and as a result feels that she should permit his coercive behavior. As the behaviors increase in rate, this is seen as proof that the child had *needs* which are not being met, and leads to even greater indulgence. For other parents, serious illness or hospitalization may lead the parent to allow the coercive behaviors to be reinforced because the child is, or was, *sickly*. The diagnostic label of *brain damage* or *retardation* seems to have a particularly iatrogenic effect upon parents' child management approaches (p. 146f).

The Complementary Couple. In the third pattern of child rearing the inconsistent handling of the child stems from the fact that the two parents behave in diametrically opposing, reciprocating fashion. Patterson et al. (1973) gave this pattern a fanciful label, the Sado-masochistic Arabesque, which as they say:

> requires the mutually supportive interactions of both parents. In the minuet, the reactions of each parent to the child are delicately balanced in such a way that only one parent is able to control the child effectively, and the control only occurs when the parent is physically present. Interestingly enough, each parent seems to track the behaviors of both the child and the other parent. One parent elects to play the harsh punitive role. When this parent is present, the behavior of the child is controlled. The permissive member attempts to balance the severity of the other by being noncontingently warm. As a result, when the despot is not present, the behavior is out of control. Aggressive behaviors occuring in the despot's presence are brutally punished.
>
> In our own experience the fathers most frequently function in the role of despot, many of whom summarize the situation, "But, he acts okay when I'm home. She is just too easy on him, that's all." . . . While home observations may show the boys to be reasonably well-behaved, they tend to display high rates of aggressive behaviors in the neighborhood or in the classroom. In the latter situations the stimuli associated with intense punishment are missing, but stimuli for coercion without intense punishment are in plentiful supply. It is also our impression that acceleration in rates of out-of-control behaviors seem to occur shortly after a separation or divorce, when the father is unlikely to be in the home. Among our cases the highest rates of out-of-control behavior seem to be found in such homes (p. 148f).

The Insular Family. The extent to which a parent can learn to modify his or her mode of interaction with a child and be able to maintain the new interaction after the therapeutic intervention has ceased appears to be a function not only of that parent's personal characteristic but also of the social support system in which the parent–child relationship is embedded. The so-called insular family, described by Wahler, Leske, and Rogers (1979), appears especially prone to derive little permanent benefit from presently available modes of family intervention. Insularity, according to these authors, is a characteristic that often accompanies certain demographic features, such as low income, crowded living conditions, limited education, and single-parent households. These families become "insulated" from their interactions with people outside the home who thus have little or no impact on their behavior. Because the children of such families are at high risk for developing psychological and behavioral difficulties, the insular family represents a critical challenge to those seeking to develop effective modes of therapeutic intervention.

Parent Training. The critical role of the parent in perpetuating coercive interactions led Patterson and his colleagues to develop a program of intervention in the families of aggressive boys that has parent training as one of its most important components. The details of such training are outlined in a lengthy report by Patterson, Cobb, and Ray (1973). It begins with a number of home visits during which the family is observed for the purpose of establishing baselines of the child's deviant and prosocial behaviors and the rates and consistencies of the parents' delivery of reinforcement. To this end a coding system consisting of 29 response and consequence categories had been devised and observers trained in its use. Following these baseline observations, the parent training program itself is instituted. This consists of distinct steps or stages, each of which the parent has to master before moving on to the next one.

On the assumption, shared by most child behavior therapists, that parents are in a better position to implement a treatment program if they understand the underlying concepts and that they will later be able to apply these in their everyday child-rearing practices, thus maintaining the progress begun during treatment, parent training begins with a study of basic social learning principles and their application. In the work of Patterson et al. (1973) this was accomplished by requiring the parents to study a programmed text on child management techniques based on these principles. Depending on the parents' educational level, the text used was either Patterson and Gullion (1968) or Patterson (1971). Among other books that may be suitable for this purpose are those prepared by Krumboltz and Krumboltz (1972) and by Morris (1976). Manuals of this type usually focus on such principles of operant learning as reinforcement, shaping, generalization, extinction, time-out, and punishment, providing concrete examples of their application to typical situations in parent–child interaction.

After both parents had completed the assigned programmed text, Patterson et al. (1973) conducted another series of home visits. During these the parents were tested on their knowledge of the basic concepts covered in the text and trained in the basic skills of defining, tracking, and recording a series of targeted child behaviors of both the deviant and the prosocial variety. Between and following these visits, telephone contact with the parents was maintained in order to monitor their adherence to the provisions of the intervention program.

The parents also participated in a parent training group that was used to provide further instruction in child management skills. The focus of these sessions was on strengthening socially adaptive behaviors by a contracted point program and on reducing the frequency of coercive behaviors. For the latter, time-out procedures were emphasized so as to provide the parents with a negative contingency that could replace their frequent resort to physical punishment. Modeling and role-playing were the principal methods used in these groups which consisted of three to four sets of parents who met once a week for eight to twelve weeks. When necessary, training sessions were also conducted in the home where the desired parenting skills could be modeled in the natural environment.

The point of terminating the program was usually determined on the basis of mutual agreement between the family and the clinician. Following termination, home observations were made once again in order to gather data for ascertaining what change, if any, had been made. If at any time during the ensuing follow-up period either the clinicians or the parents felt the need for additional help, arrangements for so-called booster-shot training could be made but Patterson's (1974) review of this work does not reveal of what this consisted or for how many families it was implemented.

Extension to the Classroom. Following the principle that intervention is most effective if it takes place in the setting where the problem behavior is emitted, the investigators working with Patterson (Patterson, Cobb, & Ray, 1972) also implemented procedures for classroom intervention for those cases where the child's aggressive behavior was found not only in the home but also at school. During the first stage of such classroom intervention, one of the investigators served as behavior manager, bringing the disruptive behavior under control by a method that had been used by Patterson, Jones, Whittier, and Wright (1965) with a child described as hyperactive. This consisted of placing a "work box" on the child's desk through which the observer who sat at the back of the class could signal the child when he was displaying nondisruptive behavior and other work-oriented "survival skills." These response-contingent signals were counted and their sum could be exchanged for backup reinforcers consisting of such consequences as extra recess time, movies, or story reading sessions that the target child shared with his classmates. As the child made progress, the work box was faded into a work card for recording the points earned by appropriate behavior. When the program was running smoothly so that only a few moments of bookkeeping were required each day, the contingency management was turned over to the classroom teacher.

With the families treated in the latter phases of his project, Patterson (1974) also instituted contracts negotiated between family and school personnel under which the child would bring his work card home every day so that the parents could provide positive consequences for desired behavior and aversive consequences for disruptive behavior. Such a procedure has the advantage of removing the delivery of consequencs from the classroom although it still requires the cooperation of the teacher who must provide the parents with the needed information on the daily work card.

Another modification introduced later in the project was to train and supervise parents in the administration of remedial teaching methods for those children whose behavior problems were accompanied by inadequate academic skills. Patterson, Cobb, and Ray (1973) point out that the close involvement of the parents in the various parts of the intervention program required that they had to modify their expectations early in the contact with the project. Parents of children who manifest psychological disorders often come to a clinic expecting the professional staff to undertake the treatment of the child while the parents sit by as passive spectators, waiting for treatment to run its course. When the clinic expects the parents to participate actively in the treatment process, to be, in effect, the staff members' colleagues as auxiliary therapists, many are surprised, sometimes hesitant and initially uncooperative. This is particularly true of fathers who often view the details of child rearing to be the mother's responsibility and who try to use their occupational duties as a rationale for noninvolvement. Only firm insistence on the part of the clinic staff, occasionally aided by subtle pressures from the referring agencies, can convince some parents that their full cooperation is a requisite for the treatment of their child.

Outcome of Family Intervention. Patterson (1974) summarizes the results of the intervention program he and his treatment team had conducted for 4½ years during which they had gathered data on 35 consecutive referrals of boys with conduct problems. Of these families, 27 had remained in treatment for longer than four weeks and the reported outcome data are based on that group. Two criteria were used to evaluate the treatment, one based on observers' data, the other on the parents' daily report on the occurrence of specified problem behaviors ("symptoms"). Observers' data had been gathered during the previously mentioned home visits, which were conducted around dinner time and consisted of two five-minute observations on each family member. This produced a sequential account of each family member's behavior and the reaction of others to it, recorded by means of the 29-item observational code. Such observations were made prior to the beginning of actual intervention, immediately following the parents completion of the programmed text, after four and again after eight weeks of intervention, and at termination. To gather follow-up data, two monthly visits were conducted for the first six months, with additional visits in the eighth, tenth, and twelfth months after termination. Complete data, representing observations at every one of these points, were available for only 12 of the 27 families due to the usual vagaries of conducting research in the natural setting. Some families moved away, some refused to participate in the follow-up study, and others withdrew from participation before the entire follow-up could be completed.

For purposes of the data analysis, a criterion score was used that expressed the child's total deviant behavior and represented the average rate of occurrence for 14 noxious responses such as teasing, whining, noncompliance, and other coercive responses. Observations on a carefully matched group of presumably normal families had permitted the determination of a cut-off score of .45 for total deviant behavior and scores falling at or below this level were viewed as "within the normal range" (Patterson, 1974). The mean baseline score for the 27 clinic families was .749. At termination, this score had fallen to .402 and at one-year follow-up (for 17 families) this score was .403. Statistical comparison of the total deviant scores from the observations during baseline, with the three during intervention, and the one at termination showed that these differences are significant. With 14 families for whom the parents' daily report scores were available the comparison between baseline and termination data revealed comparable results as did the classroom observations on the 14 boys with whom classroom intervention had been carried out. Inasmuch as the amount of professional time spent on the family intervention was calculated to have been, on the average, only 31½ hours, the approach would seem to be both efficient and effective. In view of these results, Patterson's (1974) conclusion that the procedures "were moderately successful in producing reductions in noxious behaviors in the settings for which they were designed" (p. 479) would seem excessively modest, especially since a study using a placebo control (Walter & Gilmore, 1973) had shown that similar changes do not take place merely with the passage of time during which parents believe that they are in treatment.

Why then Patterson's (1974) modesty? One basis of this diffidence is found when, instead of looking at expressions of statistical significance for differences between measures of central tendency, one examines what happened to the deviant behavior of individual cases. "At termination," Patterson reports, "approximately two out of three boys exhibited reductions of 30% or more from the baseline level; six showed increases" (p. 476). This means that some 66 percent improved, while 22 percent (6 of 27) got worse, leaving approximately 12 percent who showed no change. Such an outcome would not be overwhelmingly impressive, except for the fact that, as Patterson recognizes, the procedure used in accepting cases into the intervention program militated against such data being particularly meaningful. Although all cases who had been referred as severe conduct problems had been accepted into the program, observational data showed that some of the boys had been mislabeled or that the observational code was inappropriate for them. This can be seen in the fact that 12 of the 27 boys had average baseline "total deviant" scores that were at or below the cut-off point for the "normal range," making it unreasonable to expect a 30 percent reduction as a result of treatment. When outcome data are calculated only for those boys whom baseline observations had identified as socially aggressive, both observation and parent-report criteria showed a success rate of 88 percent.

Another reason for Patterson's (1974) belief that he had been only moderately successful may lie in the fact that during the month immediately following termination, half of the families evidenced an increase in noxious behavior. Many of these families were then offered additional intervention sessions, so-called "booster shots," on which the treatment staff expended an average of 1.9 hours. After this, the behavior returned to the level that had been achieved at termination and which had presumably led to the mutual decision to terminate the intervention.

Yet another reason for Patterson being less than enthusiastic about the results of his "preliminary exploration of the problem of devising effective treatment for younger conduct problem boys" (1974, p. 480) may lie in the fact that response generalization of the treatment effect was quite limited. This was revealed in an analysis of eleven of the later referrals to the project, reported by Patterson and Reid (1973). The noxious behaviors pinpointed by the parents as changeworthy had been made the targets of the intervention but since the observation code provides a record not only of this targeted behavior but also of other deviant behavior that had not been the specific focus of intervention, it was possible to compare the treatment effect on both the targeted and the nontargeted behavior. The observations having been conducted on all family members, they also provide information on the behavior of the referred child's sibling. If one assumes that parents who have learned the principles of contingency management will apply these not only on the most noxious (targeted) behavior of one child but also on other behavior of that child and on the objectionable behavior of his siblings, one would expect that all of these behaviors should reveal concurrent changes. This, however, was not the case. The nontargeted behavior of the deviant child showed proportionately less improvement than the targeted behavior while the siblings' noxious, coercive behavior which had improved during treatment was back to its pre-treatment level at termination. It thus appears that parents do not automatically apply what they have learned to situations that had not been a focus of training so that they may have to be helped to generalize or given specific training in the application of reinforcement principles to a wide variety of responses of different members of their family. As Stokes and Baer (1977) have stressed, the generalization and maintenance of treatment-produced improvement must be planned and programmed by the therapist; they cannot be expected to occur spontaneously.

Intervention in Families of Boys Who Steal

Stealing, in that it delivers a noxious experience to the person whose property has been misappropriated, represents a form of aggressive behavior that is particularly difficult to bring under control. Unlike other aggressive behavior that can be readily observed, stealing takes place in a furtive fashion and is often not discovered and attributed to its perpetrator until considerable time has elapsed, if at all. As a result, the act of stealing receives immediate positive reinforcement by providing the thief with possession of the stolen object while any sanctions that might be applied as a consequence to the behavior occur only intermittently and almost invariably after a delay so that their effectiveness is considerably reduced. Another difficulty stealing poses to therapeutic intervention is that it is a behavior that usually occurs at a relatively low rate. Thus, even if negative consequences could be brought to bear immediately after the transgression, such training trials would be few and far between so that the effectiveness of treatment would still be compromised.

The extensive data gathered in the course of Patterson's program of intervention with families of aggressive boys made it possible to undertake a separate scrutiny of those families where the child's antisocial behavior included stealing (Reid & Hendriks, 1973). Of the 25 families participating in the program and on whom complete data were available at the point this analysis was undertaken, 14 included a child who stole. Compared with the other 11 families, these had far less favorable treatment outcomes. In terms of the success-of-treatment criterion of a 33 percent reduction in the rate of deviant behavior from baseline, 9 of the 11 nonstealers but only 6 of the 14 stealers were categorized as successes. The difference is also reflected when the reduction in rate of deviant behavior from baseline to termination is compared for the two groups. For the nonstealers the average reduction in the rate of observed deviant behavior per minute was .461, while the decline for the stealers was only .171, a statistically highly significant difference. It will be recalled that the behavior observations on which these data are based had been conducted in the families' homes around dinner time and that the observational categories focused on interpersonal behaviors. The act of stealing was therefore neither observed nor counted in the deviant behavior score.

The reduced effectiveness of the family intervention approach when applied to families of boys who steal led Reid and Hendriks (1973) to analyze their data so as to ascertain in what manner these families differed from those where the boy displayed aggressive behaviors other than stealing. In conducting this analysis they also looked at data obtained from a matched control group of 27 normal families who had been paid some money in return for their permission to have observational data gathered on their interactions. From among the 29 observational code items used in the overall project, Reid and Hendriks (1973) selected a subset of 19 items with sufficiently high reliability to warrant further analysis. These items were, in turn, grouped into six that made up the category of positive-friendly behaviors and 13 that combined into a category of negative-coercive behaviors. Items such as attention to other family members, compliance to requests from other family members, and friendly laughing were in the former category, while such items as disapproval of others, destruction of property, noncompliance to requests, and teasing were in the latter.

As one would expect, the normal boys produced the lowest rates of negative-coercive behaviors and the highest rates of positive-friendly behaviors. On both the negative-coercive and the positive-friendly behaviors, the nonstealers had a higher rate than the stealers. While only some of these differences reached the customarily accepted level of statistical significance, it appears that while the stealers are in less negative-coercive conflict with their families than the nonstealers, they also experience fewer positive-friendly interactions. Neither of the categories revealed differences in the behaviors of the fathers of the three groups of boys but significant differences were found for some of the behaviors of the mothers. These differences were similar to those found for the sons in that the mothers of normals showed the highest positive-friendly and the lowest negative-coercive rates, the mothers of the nonstealers showed the highest rates of negative-coercive and intermediate rates of positive-friendly behaviors, while the mothers of the stealers were lowest in the positive-friendly category and intermediate in negative-coercive behavior rates.

For the purpose of what they called a preliminary analysis, Reid and Hendriks (1973) draw the following tentative conclusions from their data, attempting to explain the relatively poor success rate of the intervention procedures with families of boys who steal. It appears, they reason, that the aggressive behavior that forms the basis of the clinic referral is manifested in the home in the case of boys who do not steal, while stealers engage in their antisocial behavior outside the home. When observations are then conducted in the home, focused, as they are, on the interactions of family members, the boys who steal and their mothers are not significantly different from normals in the rate of observable negative-coercive behaviors. This being the case, there will be few deviant behaviors that a family-based intervention program can hope to modify by a response-contingent manipulation of consequences. At the same time, having only the complaints from the community and not direct interpersonal conflict with their boys to motivate them, parents of stealers may not be very highly motivated to implement the treatment procedures recommended by the clinicians.

Reid and Hendriks (1973) interpret the findings that the positive-friendly behaviors occur at the lowest rate of the three groups in the families of the stealers by postulating that the families of these boys are rather distant and have only loose social ties with each other. From this it might be speculated that these parents lack the powerful social reinforcers that could be effectively employed to control the child's behavior. One cannot withdraw positive-friendly responses in consequence of a stealing incident if such responses occur at a low rate in the first place. The low rate of positive social interaction, combined with the moderate rate of negative interactions is viewed by Reid and Hendriks (1973) as reflecting a rather boring family climate and they speculate that this may lead the child to seek out developmental experiences and positive reinforcers in unsupervised, extrafamily settings. It is conceivable that stealing has a great likelihood under such circumstances, particularly since it creates excitement and thus reduces the child's boredom.

Following these analyses, the focus of the family intervention program was shifted to a group of families who had been specifically referred for the modification of stealing behavior. At the time of their report, Reid and Hendriks (1973) were able to reflect on some preliminary observations on their experiences with this group. What is immediately apparent is the low level of motivation for treatment that is shown by parents of boys who steal. Although 27 of these families had been referred to the project, only five of them had actually entered treatment. As pointed out earlier, boys who engaged in aggressive behavior at home make their parents sufficiently upset to motivate them to enter and remain in treatment while boys whose behavior at home is relatively tolerable but who commit antisocial acts, like stealing, away from home are troublesome to their parents only on the relatively few occasions when they get caught and the authorities contact their parents. At this point of crisis these parents contact the clinic and request help in order to placate the authorities but when it comes time to keep their first appointment they either fail to appear or cancel it. For this, according to Reid and Hendriks (1973), they give such reasons as that the problem has ceased to exist, that the child had been unjustly accused, or that one of the parents (usually the father) refuses to cooperate. It seems that once "the heat is off" the motivation to seek help dissipates. Even those families who actually enter treatment manifest this lack of motivation; they miss or cancel many appointments, are very slow in completing their assignments, and are otherwise quite difficult to treat. After contact with another five of these families, Reid and Hendriks (1973) report the further observations that the parents of these boys are disinclined to track or monitor their children's behavior and that they typically spend much more time than other parents in activities away from the home so that their children are left unsupervised for long periods each day. The most common factor, however, is the parents' failure to view their boys' stealing as theft. They either ignore these incidents or relabel the behavior, often accepting their sons' explanations that they had borrowed or found the item in question or that it had been given to them as a present. In this fashion the stealing not only fails to be aversive to the parents but the boy is also protected against the negative consequences of his behavior.

With these considerations in mind, Reid and Hendriks (1973) evolved a tentative approach to the treatment of such families that begins with establishing an external incentive for change. In one case they instituted a "parenting salary" of $60 per month, contingent on the parents' cooperation in treatment. In another case, arrangements were made to have the boy immediately taken to the local detention facility each time he was caught stealing. He was kept there, cleaning windows or washing walls, for periods of from 3 to 24 hours at the end of which his father had to come to retrieve him. Since this meant that the father had to leave work or home in order to do this, the experience was aversive enough for that parent to have him begin to monitor his son's behavior and to manage the prescribed therapeutic programs. In yet another case, the focus was shifted from dealing with the boy's more deviant behaviors to fairly elementary parent-skill training and only after the parents had learned to take control of their children in very simple, nonthreatening situations were they able to extend this to the son's stealing and aggression.

Confirming the conclusion based on the behavioral observations that families of boys who steal have a low rate of both positive and negative interaction, Reid and Hendriks (1973) report the clinical impression that these families have "an incredible level of family disorganization and diffusion, a near-total absence of enjoyable family activities, and a lack of general parenting skills" (p. 218). They therefore focused treatment initially on teaching the parents and their children to relate more closely and positively with each other. Only after this could the parents be taught to monitor or track their children and, finally, to implement programs to modify the stealing itself. To what extent this approach is effective in dealing with the problem of boys who steal remains to be ascertained in systematic research with a larger number of families but the difficulties involved in maintaining a valid record of the number of thefts poses a considerable challenge for such research. Beyond this, however, the fact that these boys are typically unsupervised for long periods each day because the working schedules of both their parents tend to keep them from spending much time with their children raises societal issues that may make intervention at the behavioral level a rather impotent approach to solving the problem.

STEALING IN CLASSROOMS AND INSTITUTIONS

Stealing is sometimes a problem among elementary school children where pens, pencils, toys, or money may be taken from other children or from the teacher. Similar complaints come from institutional settings where a variety of items, including food, may be the object of such thefts. While such behavior is clearly a violation of norms, the labeling process does not define the perpetrators as delinquents; hence the problem is taken up here rather than under the earlier rubric of juvenile delinquency. As will be seen, such behavior is also more logically viewed as a behavioral excess of an aggressive nature than as a problem of deficient internal controls.

Switzer, Deal, and Bailey (1977) worked with students in three elementary school, second-grade classrooms where, according to teachers' reports, as many as two or three items were often reported missing in a single day, having apparently been stolen by one or more of the children. Desiring to compare the effectiveness of lecturing to the class on the importance of honesty and ''not taking things that do not belong to you,'' with a group contingency, the investigators employed a multiple-baseline-across-classrooms design in the following manner. So as to have an objective measure of stealing that would not be confounded by the number of items available on any given day, 10 items such as five-cent pieces, felt-tip pens, and erasers were placed at various locations in each of the three classrooms at the beginning of each day. The placement of these tracer items was systematically varied, using locations where such items might ordinarily be found. Data gathering was conducted by an observer who also served as a teacher-aide and who would check on the presence or absence of the items at 15-minute intervals during daily class sessions of approximately 90 minutes.

The number of tracer items stolen during the baseline period averaged 1.46 items per day in Class 1, 2.87 items per day in Class 2, and 1.91 items per day in Class 3. In view of the multiple baseline design, the length of this phase was 41 days, 47 days, and 69 days respectively (see Fig. 14) so that the daily averages are derived from the stealing of 60, 135, and 132 items in Class 1, 2, and 3 respectively during these baseline days. The long baseline periods were necessitated by the fact that there was considerable variability in the amount of items stolen on each day, some days passing without any thefts while on other days as many as seven or eight items would disappear. At no time, however, did more than three days pass without any stealing having taken place.

The lecture on honesty was given to two of the classes once every five days for a total of three such lectures. No lectures were given to the third class which continued in the baseline condition. Although there was an increase in the mean number of items stolen during the lecture phase (3.36 in Class 1 and 4.00 in Class 2), this rise is difficult to interpret because a similar increase took place during the same time period in Class 3 where no lectures had been given

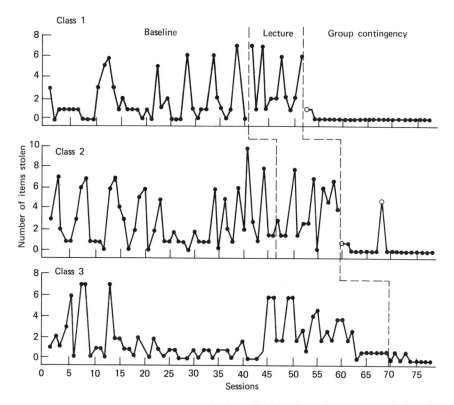

Figure 14. The number of items stolen per day in each of the three classrooms under baseline and experimental conditions. Open circles indicate that the stolen items were returned during the "return" phase of the group contingency. (Switzer, Deal, & Bailey, 1977. Copyright by the Society for the Experimental Analysis of Behavior, Inc.)

in order to control for a possible sequence effect. At any rate, it can be stated that the lecture method was totally ineffective in eliminating stealing.

The group contingency condition, instituted following the lecture phase in Classes 1 and 2 and after the 69th class session in Class 3, had the teacher announce to the children each morning that they could have 10 minutes of free time after their snack if she did not notice anything missing. When (according to the observer's signal to the teacher) none of the tracer items had been stolen by the end of the 90-minute session, the teacher would praise the class for not taking anything that did not belong to them and remind them of the free time they had thereby earned. If something had been stolen, on the other hand, the teacher would identify the item or items that were missing and say, "I am going to leave the room; if you return [the item] by putting it on my desk, then you will be able to talk during snack, as usual. If [the item] is not returned, then you will have to sit quietly while you eat your snack, and lay your heads down on your desks when you have finished" (Switzer et al., 1977, p. 269). The teacher would then leave the room for two or three minutes and institute the appropriate contingency upon her return. The investigators had taken certain precautions to assure that no undue social stress would be placed on individual students by this group contingency and none could be detected.

As reflected in Figure 14, the results showed that the group contingency procedure immediately reduced and eventually eliminated the stealing of the tracer items in all three classes. The teachers reported that the theft of other items had also decreased but the absence of a valid detection method makes it impossible to ascertain whether this represented true response generalization. In quantitative terms, the effect of the group contingency was that in Class 1 a single item was stolen on the first and on the second day. The item stolen on the first day was returned, the other item remained missing. After that, and for the remainder of the school year, no further thefts were observed. Quite similar results were reported for Class 2, except that in addition to the thefts on the first two days, five items were stolen and returned on the 17th day of the group contingency phase, with no further thefts thereafter. In Class 3, one item each was stolen and not returned on day 2 and day 4, followed by no further instances of theft.

Some aspect of the group contingency condition appears to have had a rather drastic effect on the stealing behavior of these second graders, at least as far as the known tracer items were concerned. What specific aspect of this contingency was responsible for the change in the children's behavior cannot be ascertained, given the research design that was used. As the investigators recognize, the contingency included positive reinforcement for no thefts, reinstitution of existing privileges for the return of stolen items, and punishment for failure to do so. There is, however, yet another aspect of the group contingency condition that may have played a role in its remarkable effectiveness. It is the sudden omniscience demonstrated by the teachers who always knew whether something had been stolen and, if so, specifically what it had been. This must have seemed quite awesome to a class of second-grade students and the one or two children who are likely to have been responsible for the many thefts during baseline may well have desisted from stealing because they knew that their action would be certain to be discovered in some mysterious fashion. The thefts of five of the ten "bait" items in Class 2 in the middle of the contingency phase almost seem as if the teacher's perspicacity was being tested. When it turned out that the teacher correctly identified every single one of the stolen items, they were quickly returned and no further thefts were dared after that. It would be informative to test this speculation by replicating the Switzer et al. (1977) study, adding a condition in which the teacher merely demonstrates such omniscience without employing any other consequences for the occurrence or nonoccurrence of stealing.

Theft is often a problem in institutional settings where residents or inmates steal items both from each other and from the staff. Wetzel (1966) reported a case study some years ago in which he successfully eliminated the stealing by a 10-year-old resident in a home for mildly disturbed children. In that case stealing was monitored by the staff who would search the boy's pockets, locker, and room for property belonging to others. When such an item was found, a form of time-out was instituted which consisted of the contingent withdrawal of the boy's valued privilege of talking to and visiting with the cook of the treatment facility.

A more systematic study of behavioral intervention in stealing by institutionalized individuals was reported by Azrin and Wesolowski (1974) who used an overcorrection procedure with profoundly retarded adults. This is here presented because the level of functioning of these adults was at or below that of most children and because the procedure can and has been used with young children for dealing with other problem behaviors (Foxx & Azrin, 1973a, b). Overcorrection is based on the principle that undesirable behavior which has disruptive effects can be discouraged if the person who has engaged in such behavior is not only made to correct the situation by repair or restoration but must also undertake additional corrective activity. Such overcorrection thereby restores the disrupted situation to a better state than existed before the disruption (Azrin & Wesolowski, 1974). In the case of stealing, the overcorrection principle suggest that the thief not only return the stolen item (which would be simple correction) but also give the victim more than had been stolen. When Azrin and Wesolowski (1974) applied this procedure with 34 severely and profoundly retarded residents of an institutional ward they were able completely to eliminate the targeted stealing behavior within four days.

The retardates in the Azrin and Wesolowski (1974) study had been provided with between-meal commissary periods during which such a high level of stealing took place that the staff questioned whether this routine could be continued. The commissary period consisted of having the residents enter a room one at a time. There they were allowed to select one of a number of displayed items such as a drink of soda, a candy bar, or a bag of potato chips. Upon having obtained the selection, the resident would walk to a small table to consume it while the next person entered the room to make his or her choice. Stealing usually took place while the residents sat at the table and took the form of grabbing the snack item from the hands of someone in a nearby seat. The investigators first assessed the effectiveness of simple correction which consisted of having the offender return the stolen item to its owner immediately after the theft. During the five days when this procedure was in effect about 20 stealing episodes occurred each day. At this point the overcorrection contingency was introduced. Here the trainer not only required the thief to return the item to the owner but also guided the offender back to the commissary display where an identical item had to be secured, brought back to the table, and placed into the victim's hands. Under both procedures, the intervention was accompanied by verbal reprimands, relevant instructions, and, where necessary, manual guidance.

As the data shown in Figure 15 reflect, the overcorrection procedure resulted in an immediate drop from 20 to 10 stealing episodes. On the second day of the theft reversal phase, only five episodes were recorded and on the third day only two. This represents a 90-percent decrease from the rate when simple correction was in effect. From the fourth day on and for the ensuing 16 days of observation no further thefts took place. It appears that in this application, overcorrection is a highly effective procedure that quickly reduces the undesirable behavior on which it is contingent. By definition, overcorrection is thus a form of punishment and it may well be that the aversive aspect of the procedure is entailed not only in being deprived of the stolen item, but also in the extra effort it requires of the person who is required to carry it out.

As described by Azrin and Wesolowski (1974), after returning the stolen item to the victim, the offender had to get up from the table, walk a few steps

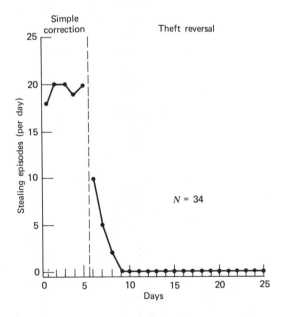

Figure 15. The number of stealing episodes committed each day by 34 adult retarded residents in an institution. During the five days of simple correction, the thief was required to return the stolen item. During the theft-reversal (overcorrection) procedure (subsequent to the vertical dashed line), the thief was required to give the victim an additional item identical to the one stolen, also returning the stolen item. The stealing episodes consisted of stealing food items from the other retarded residents during commissary periods. (Azrin & Wesolowski, 1974. Copyright by the Society for the Experimental Analysis of Behavior, Inc.)

to the display area, obtain the new item, return to the table, and place the item in the victim's hands. This activity also interrupted the offender's consumption of his own snack, thereby adding a time-out aspect to the procedure. The authors also stress the reeducative aspect of their procedure in that it involved practicing the positive action of giving snack items to another person. Moreover, since for many of the more persistent thieves the victims' annoyance upon losing their possession seemed to be a source of reinforcement, the overcorrection procedure eliminates this reinforcing consequence by changing the victim's reaction from suffering to pleasure. Azrin and Wesolowski (1974) believe that their procedure should be especially effective when the thief dislikes the victim so that the theft has aggressive overtones since, after overcorrection, the victim emerges in a happier state rather than in the usual bereft condition. The aggressive aspects of stealing were noted by these authors because when the thieves were required to return the item to the victim, "they often attempted to destroy it, rather than allow the victim to regain it, as if their goal were to cause distress to the victim, rather than merely to possess the item" (p. 579).

FIRE SETTING

Having defined the destruction of someone else's property as a form of aggressive behavior, brief mention should be made of the treatment of one form of such destruction, fire setting. Like stealing, this behavior tends to occur intermittently and surreptitiously, making it difficult to bring under control by the introduction of immediate consequences. Given the principle that it is best to treat undesirable behavior in the setting and at the time it occurs, a therapist will find it difficult to follow this principle in the case of the child who sets fires. Several approaches to treatment have been reported but, partly because fire-setting is a high-magnitude–low-frequency and relatively rare problem, controlled research is not available.

A case study by Holland (1969) dealt with a seven-year-old boy whose fire setting seemed to take place exclusively in the home so that he could be treated in that setting and by his father. Prior to treatment he had been setting fires whenever he found matches while his parents were either in bed or out of the house. Various punishments had been ineffective. At the beginning of treatment a new set of contingencies was announced. The boy was told that he would permanently lose his highly prized baseball glove if he set another fire and that he could earn a reward (money) if he immediately brought to his father any matches or matchbook covers that he found. The father then placed an empty matchbook cover conspicuously on the table. When the child brought this to him he was given five cents and urged to buy himself something at the store.

The following week the program was extended to include a combination of a response-cost and satiation procedure. The boy was given the opportunity to strike matches under his father's supervision. A full matchbook was made available with 20 pennies placed next to it. For each match that the child struck, one penny was to be removed from the pile, the boy having been told that he could keep any coins left over at the end of the session. He also received praise for desisting from the use of matches. The child struck 10 matches during the first session, three the following day, and one from the third day on when the ratio of matches to money was thinned out. Holland (1969) reports that all fire setting had ceased by the end of four weeks and that none had taken place over an eight-month follow-up period. In the absence of an experimental design it can of course not be determined whether the change in the boy's behavior had indeed been the result of the intervention and lacking the capacity to monitor his activity outside the home one cannot even be sure that the fire setting had not merely been displaced from the home, where it had been easy to discover, to other settings where it remained undetected.

Working with a 7-year-old boy who had started four fires within a three-month period just prior to the referral for therapy, Stawar (1976) added a cognitive component to an operant treatment approach. The principle used for this intervention was to teach the boy a response to finding matches that was incompatible with lighting them and starting a fire. It was to take any matches he might find to his mother or other adults without striking them. His mother was instructed to reinforce the boy's match-bringing behavior and occasions for learning trials were set up by placing books of (nonfunctional) matches in places around the house where the boy might readily find them.

The procedure thus bears considerable similarity to the approach used by Holland (1969) but instead of simply announcing the contingencies to the child, Stawar (1976) elected to use operant principles to teach the child a fable "to promote," as he puts it, "the development of more adaptive cognitive schemes" (p. 285). The story the child was to learn dealt with a boy who found matches and brought them to his mother whereupon he received praise and rewards for being such a good little boy. Stawar (1976) presumed that his "operantly structured fantasy" functioned "at the cognitive level as a mediating cue or prompt" where it potentially enhanced the acquisition of the new and desirable behavior (p. 286). The boy's mother was then instructed to rehearse the little story with him at least once a week, providing appropriate reinforcers and to continue to reward the child for bringing her any matches he might find. The fantasy aspect of this intervention and the unsupported speculations about mediating cognitive processes on which it was based may or may not have contributed to the outcome that Stawar (1976) reports as complete cessation of fire setting after a two-week period during which 23 training trials had taken place. A follow-up seven months later revealed no further incidents of fire setting. Again, as in the case study by Holland (1969), one is left to wonder whether the improvement was real or apparent and whether the described procedure was in fact the critical independent variable. Case studies are at best suggestive, particularly so in the case of fire setting and other surreptitious acts where it is so difficult to monitor the target behavior.

Recapitulation

Aggression is fruitfully viewed as a form of excess behavior that can be reduced by changing its reinforcing consequences. When these consequences are provided by the child's peers, time-out procedures that involve physically removing the offender from the scene has been shown to be an effective form of intervention. Time-out is a consequence that reduces the frequency of the responses on which it is contingent. It is therefore a form of punishment, as is the closely related procedure, social isolation. As in any other punishment, the onset of time-out serves to reduce the behavior then taking place and its offset is a negative reinforcer that will strengthen the responses then being emitted. For this and other reasons, the use of time-out requires detailed assessment and careful monitoring lest its use be counterproductive.

Complaints about a child's aggressive behavior are often linked to coercive interaction patterns within the family and a considerable amount of research has been devoted to treatment approaches that seek to alter this pattern. Characteristics of the child's parents and of the social support system available to the family appear to be factors related to the outcome of such intervention which, at this point, is best described as promising.

Stealing and fire setting are forms of aggressive behavior that are particularly hard to treat, partly because they tend to occur at relatively infrequent intervals, seem to carry their own, inherent reinforcers, and can often go undetected so that it is difficult to introduce therapeutic consequences. Like aggression in general, these problems continue to call for intensive research which should be given the highest priority, considering the critical social implications of aggression.

CHAPTER 10

Disruptive Behavior

Like other terms used as chapter headings, *disruptive behavior* is an imprecise expression that subsumes a variety of behaviors which have in common only that they create disorder in someone else's routine. There is no behavior excess, however, that does not upset someone else's composure in one way or another. The use of the term "disruptive behavior" is, therefore, usually limited to behavior that disrupts the routine of the classroom thereby interfering with the function of that setting, namely teaching and learning. To further restrict the definition of disruptive behavior one usually excludes direct physical aggression, stealing, inattentiveness, or hyperactivity, thus limiting the term to cover only those behaviors that are at times referred to as classroom-discipline or management problems, misbehavior, acting out, or unruliness. Operationally, disruptive behavior can take the form of unauthorized talking, getting out of the seat, walking about, throwing things, making noises, or similar activities.

Rarely does the relativity of the definition of a psychological disorder become more apparent than in a discussion of disruptive classroom behavior for it should be obvious that not every child who talks out of turn during class can be viewed as having a problem that must be treated. As usual, the difference between ordinary misbehavior and a psychological disorder is based on the frequency and intensity of the behavior in question as well as on the tolerance level and expectations of the evaluating adults (Ross, 1980). The content of this chapter will also remind us that only a vague boundary separates unreasonable or even irrational demands of adults, to which children should not be made to conform, from children's truly excessive behavior which responsible adults must attempt to reduce. This issue of children's rights and adults' responsibilities will be examined in the context of treating noncompliant behavior (Chapter 14). Lastly, this discussion of disruptive classroom behavior will bring us close to the gray area that is the interface between behavior therapy, the specific, systematic approach for treating psychological disorders, and behavior modification, the more general application of psychological principles for bringing about changes in behavior that need not necessarily fall into the realm of psychological disorders. To set an arbitrary limit to the scope of this chapter, we shall generally exclude discussion of studies that deal primarily with the application of behavioral methods to the management of entire classrooms, such as token economies. These applications have been authoritatively discussed by O'Leary and O'Leary (1976, 1977).

THE CONTROLLING EFFECT OF TEACHER ATTENTION

The potency of teacher attention as a reinforcer of child behavior has been recognized since the early demonstrations of Wolf and his associates showed that a young girl's social interactions could be influenced by the contingent use of her teachers' reactions to her behavior (Allen, Hart, Buell, Harris, & Wolf, 1964).

Teacher attention takes a variety of forms, ranging from smiles, pats on the back, and praise statements to frowns, criticism, and reprimands. The absence of teacher attention—ignoring—also belongs among this range of response-contingent consequences. As with all other consequences, however, these cannot be designated as positive, negative, or neutral unless their function with respect to a particular behavior has been carefully analyzed. Words of praise are not necessarily positive reinforcers, a reprimand may not be a punisher, and ignoring a behavior does not inevitably lead to its undergoing extinction. Paradoxical as it may seem to those who forget that the definition of a response consequence depends on its function with respect to that response, some children react to praise as if it were a punishment and to a reprimand as if it were a reward.

When planning an intervention based on the contingent use of teacher attention it is important to remember that in the context of a classroom, teacher attention is embedded in a social system; it is never an isolated event. When directed at an individual child whose behavior one seeks to change, teacher attention and that child's reaction to it may serve as a stimulus controlling the behavior of the other children and their behavior may, in turn, influence both the teacher and the targeted child. What is more, responses a teacher directs at an individual child must be viewed in terms of the educational approach used in that classroom and in the school. Such questions as what is being taught and how this is being taught, whether rules are clearly spelled out and how they are implemented, how the teacher operated in the past, and what experiences the child encounters in other classes and with other teachers must all be taken into consideration before an intervention is introduced and while it is evaluated. Lastly, adding to these complications, there is the relationship between school and home because the extent to which the child's parents support or sabotage the efforts of the teachers will have an important impact on the success or failure of any treatment approach that focuses on classroom behavior.

Rules, Praise, Ignoring

In one of a series of studies on the effect of teacher behavior Madsen, Becker, and Thomas (1968) assessed the relative contribution of rules, praise, and ignoring to the control of children's inappropriate classroom behavior. The subjects were three problem children in regular classrooms; two were attending second grade and one was in kindergarten. The two boys in second grade, Cliff and Frank, had been selected because they displayed a high frequency of problem behaviors. Cliff was described as constantly fiddling with objects in his desk, talking, not doing his work, or misbehaving by bothering other children and walking around the room. Of late, he had also been hitting others without apparent provocation. Frank displayed similar problems but in addition, his record included intense fighting on the playground. Both boys scored at or above the average level on intelligence tests and their academic performance was appropriate for their grade placement. Unlike Cliff and Frank, who came from stable family backgrounds, the kindergarten child, Stan, had a very disorganized home environment. His behavior was described as "wild" and uncontrollable. He would push and hit others, grab at objects, swear profusely, and steal school property. He often wandered around the room and frequently destroyed any work he produced rather than take it home.

Trained observers recorded the behavior of these children, using nine coding categories for inappropriate behavior and one category for the converse, appropriate behavior. The latter included such actions as answering questions, listening, raising the hand, and working on assignments. In addition to observations of child behavior, teachers' behavior was also observed and coded, furnishing a record of the teacher's reactions to the children's behavior along the dimensions of approval, disapproval and, the absence of either, ignoring.

The design of the study called for a phase* during which baseline observations were gathered. This was followed by the introduction of explicit rules for

---

*It is not possible to ascertain from their published report how long Madsen et al. (1968) maintained the various experimental conditions for they only present the number of days during which the teachers were observed and these varied both within and between conditions during the life of their study which began "in late November and continued to the end of the school year" (p. 140).

classroom behavior which were formulated and discussed with the class, posted in a conspicuous place, and repeated several times each day. After conclusion of this phase the teachers were instructed to ignore inappropriate classroom behavior unless a child was being hurt. In the second-grade class, this was accompanied by continued rehearsal of the rules, while the rules were not emphasized in the kindergarten class. After a period of time during which this phase was in effect, a combination of rule rehearsal, ignoring of inappropriate behavior, and praising of appropriate behavior was instituted and continued in kindergarten until the end of the study. In the second-grade classroom a reversal to the baseline condition was attempted, after which the rules-ignore-praise condition was reinstituted. Saying that reversal was "attempted" reflects the recognition by Madsen et al. (1968) that instructing a teacher to resume handling her class the way she had before the intervention had begun does not necessarily result in a return to the baseline conditions. Their data, in fact, show that this teacher was unable fully to adhere to these instructions. Before discussing the results of this study it should be noted that the various contingencies had been in effect for all the children in the classrooms but that behavioral observations were made only on the three targeted children and their teachers.

Madsen et al. (1968) report that the introduction of rules alone had little or no effect on the targeted children in either class. Ignoring-plus-rules led to an increase in disruptive behavior, while ignoring-without-rules resulted in little change. These data, however, are somewhat difficult to interpret because both teachers found it hard to be consistent in ignoring inappropriate behavior. What is clear is that all three children's inappropriate behavior decreased in frequency when the rules, plus ignoring, plus praise condition was in effect. The investigators concluded that this triple-contingency was a potent factor in obtaining better classroom behavior from the targeted children. It should be pointed out that this combination is essentially a DRO (differential reinforcement of other behavior) procedure inasmuch as undesirable behavior is placed on a relative extinction schedule while desirable behavior is reinforced. Whether a similar effect could have been achieved if the teachers had introduced praise for appropriate behavior while continuing their baseline behavior with respect to inappropriate behavior (expressing disapproval of it) cannot be determined from this study.

The changes in the behavior of the targeted children were reflected not only in the observer-recorded data but also in the impressions of the teachers who reported that the boys responded very positively to receiving praise. Frank sat quietly, finished his tasks, asked for extra assignments, and participated in class discussion as did Cliff, who worked harder on assigned tasks, learned to ignore the misbehavior of other children, and improved in his academic performance. Stan, the child in kindergarten, "changed from a sullen, morose, muttering, angry individual into a boy whose smile seems to cover his whole face" (Madsen, Becker, & Thomas, 1968, p. 150). He learned to follow rules, paid attention to teacher-directed activities for long periods of time, and inter-acted in a more friendly way with other children in the class. Since the teachers' praise appears to have been the key to these changes, it is useful to examine the instructions the investigators had given to the teachers when they asked them to "catch the child being good." Supplemented by individual con-ferences in which the written instructions were discussed and explained, the teachers received the following statement:

> The first phase included specifying explicit rules, writing them on the board and reviewing them 4–6 times per day. The second phase was designed to reduce the amount of attention paid to behaviors which were unwanted by ignoring them. This third phase is primarily directed toward *increasing* Appropriate Behaviors through praise and other forms of approval. Teachers are inclined to take good behavior for granted and pay attention only when a child acts up or misbehaves. We are now asking you to try something different. This procedure is characterized as "catching the child being good" and making a comment designed to reward the child for good behavior. Give praise, attention, or smile when the child is doing what is expected during the particular class period in question. Inappropriate Be-havior would not be a problem if all children were engaging in a great deal of study and school behavior, therefore, it is necessary to apply what you have learned in the workshop. Shape by successive approximations the behavior desired by us-ing praise and attention. Start "small" by giving praise and attention at the first signs of Appropriate Behavior and work toward greater goals. Pay close attention to those children who normally engage in a great deal of misbehavior. Watch carefully and when the child begins to behave appropriately, make a comment such as "You're doing a fine job, (name)." It is very important during the first few days to catch as many good behaviors as possible. Even though a child has just thrown an eraser at the teacher (one minute ago) and is now studying, you should praise the study behavior. (It might also decrease the rate of eraser throw-ing.) We are assuming that your commendation and praise are important to the child. This is generally the case, but sometimes it takes a while for praise to be-come effective. Persistence in catching children being good and delivering praise and attention should eventually pay off in a better behaved classroom.
>
> Some examples of praise comments are as follows:
>
> I like the way you're doing your work quietly (name).
>
> That's the way I like to see you work_____.
>
> That's a very good job_____.
>
> You're doing fine_____.
>
> You got two right_____, that's very good (if he generally gets no answers right).
>
> In general, give praise for achievement, prosocial behavior, and following the group rules. Specifically, you can praise for concentrating on individual work, raising hand when appropriate, responding to questions, paying attention to di-rections and following through, sitting in desk and studying, sitting quietly if noise has been a problem. Try to use variety and expression in your comments. Stay away from sarcasm. Attempt to become spontaneous in your praise and

smile when delivering praise. At first you will probably get the feeling that you are praising a great deal and it sounds a little phony to your ears. This is a typical re-action and it becomes more natural with the passage of time. Spread your praise and attention around. If comments sometimes might interfere with the ongoing class activities then use facial attention and smiles. Walk around the room during study time and pat or place your hand on the back of a child who is doing a good job. Praise quietly spoken to the children has been found effective in combination with some physical sign of approval.

General Rule: Give *praise* and *attention* to behaviors which facilitate learn-ing. Tell the child what he is being praised for. Try to reinforce behaviors incom-patible with those you wish to decrease. (Madsen, Becker, & Thomas, 1968, p. 145. Copyright by the Society for the Experimental Analysis of Behavior, Inc.)

Teacher Attention vs. Counseling

The impact teacher attention has on disruptive classroom behavior which Madsen et al. (1968) had shown to be so impressive with young, and academi-cally fairly well-achieving children, was demonstrated to have a similar effect with low-achieving, adolescent boys in seventh grade whose age (because they had repeated one or more grades) ranged from 12 to 16 years. Twelve such boys participated in a study conducted by Marlowe, Madsen, Bowen, Rear-don, and Logue (1978) which had been designed to compare the effectiveness of teacher attention (with and without token reinforcement) with two different approaches to counseling.

The 12 students had been selected from a classroom of 39 because of their high rate of inappropriate behavior. Following baseline observations of inap-propriate, off-task classroom behavior, the boys were divided into three groups, matched for average inappropriate behavior. These groups were then randomly assigned to one of three treatment conditions. One group received behavioral counseling consisting of 30-minute group sessions during which the counselor emphasized the importance of on-task behavior. The students re-ceived approval for positive behavior while inappropriate behavior was ig-nored. Sessions were controlled by the counselor who stressed adherence to rules and attempted to teach the boys how to correct themselves when they had behaved inappropriately and how to credit themselves for appropriate be-havior.

The second group of boys participated in 30-minute group counseling ses-sions based on client-centered principles. Here the emphasis was on developing a warm and friendly relationship with the students, maintaining respect for the students and their ability to solve their own problems, sensitivity to students' feelings, and on having the counselor behave in a genuine, authentic fashion. For both the behavior and the client-centered conditions the same individual served as counselor. The investigators thereby hoped to control for counselor personality and background variables but by so doing, they failed to equate counselor skill in the two approaches. This is a dilemma that invariably arises when two treatment methods are compared.

The two counseling groups, plus the third group, which as a no-contact control received no counseling, experienced six experimental conditions, as follows: A 10-day baseline, followed by 18 days of counseling sessions for the two counseling groups. After this, and while counseling continued, a teacher-attention phase was instituted for five days. This was similar to the approach used by Madsen, Becker, and Thomas (1968) and included explicit rules, praise for appropriate, and ignoring of inappropriate behavior. In the next phase, and again with concurrent counseling, a token reinforcement program was added to teacher attention and continued for seven days. Here, for appropriate classroom behavior, the entire class could earn tokens which were redeemable for doughnuts and soft drinks on the last day of the week. There followed four days' return to the baseline condition during which no counseling took place while the teacher attempted to reinstate her preexperimental approaches to classroom management. In the final phase of the study, lasting eight days, teacher attention plus token reinforcement were once again instituted but no concurrent counseling sessions were conducted. Their design thus permitted the investigators to compare the effect of counseling with no counseling, of teacher attention with and without counseling, and of teacher attention plus token reinforcement with or without counseling.

The results of this study showed that teacher attention in the form of approval for acceptable social behavior and good academic performance was highly effective in reducing the students' unacceptable, off-task behavior, particularly when the teacher accompanied her praise statements with the delivery of tokens. Apparently the use of tokens not only served the expected function of reinforcing the students' behavior but it also seemed to have served as a reminder to the teacher to give verbal approval since this reached its highest frequency during the token phase of the study.

As far as the effect of counseling is concerned, the data reported by Marlowe et al. (1978) show that the students who had received behavioral counseling reduced their off-task behavior more quickly than the students in the client-centered counseling and no-contact control conditions. The investigators suggest that the behavioral counseling experience had helped prepare the students for the teacher attention condition that was later implemented. It must be noted, however, that during the final phase of the study when teacher attention and token delivery were in effect, all students, including those who had received no counseling at all, reduced their off-task behavior considerably below the baseline frequency. While behavioral counseling may speed up the acquisition of positive, on-task behavior it may not be a necessary step and the investigators concluded that the best use of the time of a behaviorally oriented consultant may be in helping the classroom teacher focus attention on the positive behaviors of the students and to reinforce that behavior by the judicious use of praise and other rewards.

In examining some of the quantitative evidence that supports the above conclusions it may be well to be reminded that the work by Marlowe et al. (1978) suffers from a few defects that detract from the persuasiveness of their results, particularly insofar as the effect of the counseling experience is concerned. We have previously touched on the problem created by the investigators' desire to control the variables related to the person of the counselor by having the same individual serve as both client-centered and behavioral counselor. There is also the fact that the boys who were being exposed to the two counseling and the no-contact conditions were all in the same classroom. Some contamination was thus unavoidable and the investigators recognized this by pointing out that the boys whose behavior had improved and who were receiving reinforcement might have served as models for the others. This would be desirable from a practical standpoint but it does confound the results of an experiment. More importantly, one has to keep in mind that the control group against which the effect of counseling was to be compared received no contact during the counseling-only phase of the study. This leaves unanswered the question whether the difference in off-task behavior between the no-contact control and the two counseling groups was due to the counseling or to the special attention the boys in the counseling groups received when they met with the counselor in small groups of four. A placebo control group, given similar attention but no counseling, would have provided an answer to this question.

A word must also be said in defense of client-centered counseling which, as the data shown in Figure 16 reflect, had about the same effect on off-task behavior as no counseling at all. It may simply be that eight 30-minute sessions with highly disruptive adolescents are not enough to have an impact, though behaviorally oriented counseling appears to be able to do so in that amount of time. There is also the problem of the discontinuity between the client-centered approach with its relatively loose structure and the behaviorally oriented classroom management procedures with their stress on rules. The boys in the behavioral counseling group were essentially receiving pretraining for the structured behavioral intervention in the classroom that followed so that they were able to benefit from this sooner than the students in the other groups. Client-centered counseling, on the other hand, may have been quite irrelevant or even counterproductive for the later experience in the classroom. The procedure used by Marlowe et al. (1978) thus cannot be considered to have provided a fair test of the effectiveness of client-centered counseling. A more valid test would be to relate such counseling to a classroom intervention that is based on client-centered concepts. There the counseling might set the stage for the classroom experience, as the behavioral counseling seems to have done for the classroom experience based on behavioral concepts.

While the results of the study by Marlowe et al. (1978) are unconvincing regarding the differential effectiveness of the two counseling methods they compared, they leave little doubt as to the impact of differential teacher attention and token reinforcement on the classroom behavior of the 12 disruptive

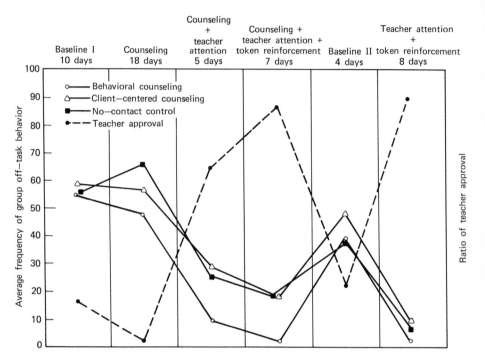

Figure 16. Average frequency of students' off-task behavior by group and condition shown in comparison with average teacher approval ratio. (Redrawn from Marlowe et al., 1978.)

adolescents who had been the targets of this intervention. As Figure 16 reflects, whenever teacher approval of positive student behavior was low, as in the baseline and the counseling-only conditions, student off-task behavior was high. Conversely, when teacher approval was high, as in the three conditions calling for teacher attention, the inappropriate classroom behavior of the boys was low. In that sense, Marlowe et al. (1978) replicated with disruptive adolescents the results that Madsen et al. (1968) had reported with much younger children, thereby lending further support to the statement that teachers' attention in the form of praise and other approval of desirable behavior, combined with the ignoring of undesirable behavior, is a potent tool for the reduction of disruptive classroom behavior. Such differential teacher attention seems most effective in controlling disruptive behavior when it is applied in combination with explicit rules, classroom structure, and the use of token reinforcements (O'Leary, Becker, Evans, & Saudargas, 1969). Yet one must also recognize that there are instances in the course of a teacher's day when certain kinds of behavior simply cannot be ignored or where the teacher's tolerance for disregarding disruptions has become exhausted. In order to accommodate to this reality, Madsen, Becker, and Thomas (1968) had provided for the use of some mild negative consequences, such as having the teacher turn out the lights, stop to talk, send a child to the office, or deprive a child of some privilege. The same consideration led O'Leary, Kaufman, Kass and Drabman (1970) to examine the effect on disruptive behavior of delivering different kinds of reprimands. We turn to this issue next.

The Use of Reprimands

In studies designed to demonstrate the effectiveness of behavioral intervention for decreasing disruptive behavior in classrooms such investigators as O'Leary, Becker, Evans, and Saudargas (1969) usually instruct teachers to praise appropriate behavior and to ignore disruptive behavior. While this is effective, it leaves the teacher without a means to respond to instances of undesirable behavior that, in the teacher's opinion, cannot be ignored. Under ordinary circumstances, one of the responses teachers resort to most frequently when they notice a student misbehaving is to issue a verbal reprimand that is intended to call the student back to the task. Such reprimands are usually issued while the teacher is some distance away from the offending child so that the statement, being said loud enough for that child to hear, will also be heard by the other children in the classroom. This not only distracts the children who are working on their task but it also singles out the disruptive child for special public attention which may account for the fact that the use of loud reprimands tends to lead into a vicious cycle in which an ever-increasing number of such reprimands are needed to control ever-increasing disruptive behavior. This observation motivated O'Leary, Kaufman, Kass, and Drabman (1970) to investigate whether teachers might be able to use an effective alternative to the loud reprimand that did not have these characteristics. Their alternative was a soft reprimand, a verbal corrective statement, delivered in such a manner that only the offending child was able to hear it.

The study comparing the differential effect of loud and soft reprimands (O'Leary et al., 1970) was carried out with two children in each of five classrooms. The children had been selected because of their high rates of disruptive behavior such as not remaining seated, making noises, talking out of turn, touching another's property, and engaging in behavior incompatible with pursuing assigned tasks. An observation code composed of nine classes of such behavior was employed by trained observers who recorded the frequency of disruptions for 20 minutes per day over a four-month period. The design followed an ABAB reversal pattern where the base period (phase A) consisted of having the teacher use her customary ways of reprimanding disruptive behavior which, for all five teachers, consisted of corrective statements delivered in a loud fashion. After collecting baseline records for one month, the investigators instructed the teachers to maintain their previous rate of reprimands but to make them in a soft manner, that is, in such a way that only the child to whom the comment was addressed could hear it. This mode of reprimanding was to be used with all the children in the classroom, not only those targeted for the study, and it was to be maintained throughout the day. After the soft-reprimand condition had been in effect for a month, baseline conditions (phase A) were reinstituted, that is, the teachers were urged to return to their usual (loud) mode of delivering reprimands. Finally, during the last month of the study, the soft-reprimand condition was reinstated and maintained until the end of the school year.

Before we examine the results of this study which, to anticipate, showed soft reprimands to be more effective than loud reprimands in reducing the mean frequencies of disruptive behavior, it is important to acknowledge that the intervention did not work equally well with all children and that not every teacher was able to implement it in an effective manner. With one teacher, who is described as having been very skeptical about the possibility of soft reprimands being capable of influencing disruptive behavior, the two targeted children showed an increase in disruptive behavior when soft reprimands were instituted whereupon the focus of the study was changed for that classroom. In another class, one of the two target children showed an increase in disruptive behavior under soft-reprimand conditions. Here too the teacher seemed less than enthusiastic about the procedure and used it in an inconsistent fashion. She feared that soft reprimands were a sign of weakness and found it too strenuous to walk over to the child's seat for the purpose of whispering a reprimand. That teacher reported that her patience became exhausted as the day wore on so that her "natural tendency to shout like a general" would take over. As with any other method of treatment or intervention, soft reprimands work only when they are used correctly and consistently by a person who has some expectations that they can be effective.

The results of the study by O'Leary, Kaufman, Kass, and Drabman (1970) are summarized in Table 1. Classes A and B were at second-grade level, the others were third-grade classes. The descriptions of the children show all of them to have presented management problems for their teachers. Child D in Class A, for example, was described as "nervous and restless." He bit his nails, drummed his fingers on his desk, and stuttered. He would often be out of his chair, bothering other children. Child S was uncooperative and silly, often giggling and talking. Children Z and W were described as aggressive, often hitting or kicking other children, while children V and B were disrupting the class by their excessive talking. The rest of the children were described in similar terms. As can be seem from Table 1, the experimental effect of changing from loud to soft reprimands was clearly shown in classes A, B, and C although the disruptive behavior of the child identified as V did not show the ex-

Table 1 **Frequencies of Disruptive Behavior under Various Conditions of Reprimand (summarized from O'Leary et al., 1970)**

Class A	Loud I	Soft I	Loud II	Soft II
Child D	1.1	.8	1.3	.9
Child S	1.4	.6	1.1	.5
Class B				
Child Z	1.0	.9	1.3	.8
Child V	1.7	1.4	1.3	.6
Class C				
Child E	.9	.6	1.1	.4
Child W	1.6	.8	.9	.3
			Double Soft	Double Loud
Class D				
Child B	1.6	1.3	1.1	1.8
Child R	1.5	1.9	2.0	2.0
Class E				
Child D	.9	1.0	—	—
Child J	.4	.8	—	—

Note: Entries represent mean frequencies of disruptive behavior for Class A and average of mean frequencies of disruptive behavior during the last 5 days of each condition for the other classes.

pected increase when the loud reprimand condition was reinstituted. The results from the classes labeled D and E reflect the difficulties the investigators had encountered in having the teachers follow their instructions. Although the teachers in these classes had been requested to hold the number of reprimands approximately constant regardless of condition, the teacher in class D markedly reduced the number of reprimands she delivered during the first soft-reprimand condition. For this reason, she was asked to double the number of reprimands delivered during the next two conditions (shown as double-soft and double-loud in the table). She succeeded in doing this with child B but not with child R since a record of the number of reprimands delivered by that teacher during the various conditions shows that she gave that child almost no soft reprimands and the observers noted that even those were rarely if ever soft in intensity. This was the teacher who had admitted to her natural tendency to shout like a general. As for the children in class E, it can be seen that for them soft reprimands had the effect of increasing disruptive behavior, leading the investigators to change the focus of their approach with this teacher.

Looking at the results obtained with the ten children by O'Leary et al. (1970) it can be concluded that when teachers succeed in using soft reprimands in a proper fashion they can often, though not always, succeed in reducing disruptive behavior thereby reducing the need for such reprimands. This statement must be coupled with the investigators' own qualification to the effect that soft reprimands should not be viewed as an alternative to praise. An ideal combination, they propose, would probably be frequent praise combined with some soft reprimands and very occasional loud reprimands.

That soft reprimands are effective in reducing disruptive classroom behavior is, in some respects, a paradoxical result. The finding that loud reprimands are ineffective and do, in fact, serve to increase disruptive behavior has been explained by viewing the reprimand as a form of adult attention that serves as a reinforcer for the behavior on which it is contingent. If the attention represented by a warning or criticism shouted from the front of the room is reinforcing, one should expect that the teacher coming over to the child's seat, bending down and whispering a reprimanding statement should be even more reinforcing since the attention is now more personal. Yet, in terms of its function of reducing undesirable behavior, such soft reprimands are a more effective form of punishment than the loud reprimand. Why? One could take refuge in the pragmatism of the functional analysis of behavior by stating that if a stimulus can be shown to serve a punishing function by contingently weakening behavior, it is not necessary to ask why this is the case. Yet because this is not a satisfactory answer for most people, some speculations seem in order.

One of the reasons for the effectiveness of soft reprimands might be that, unlike the loud reprimand, it is less noticeable to the other children in the classroom. This point is made by O'Leary et al. (1970) and it seems to imply that the loud reprimand, noticeable to the entire class, has a reinforcing effect because it provides peer attention that may outweigh whatever punishing aspects the reprimand itself might possess. In this respect it is interesting to note that three of the four children (S, V, and B), whose mean frequencies for disruptive behavior had increased under the first loud-reprimand condition, were described as enjoying having other children laugh at them, acting as a clown, and loving to be with other children. At the same time this explanation raises the question whether the circumstance that the observations for this study had been made during the arithmetic lesson inadvertently contributed to the effectiveness of soft reprimands. While attending to arithmetic problems in their workbooks children might be less aware of the teacher's walking over to an individual child to deliver a soft reprimand and, conversely, more aware of the sudden interruptions caused by a loud reprimand. The effect of loud versus soft reprimands might be worth investigating in a classroom situation where children's attention is focused on the teacher standing in front of the class so that her walking to a child's desk to deliver a soft reprimand would be highly noticeable.

A second explanation O'Leary et al. (1970) offer for their findings is that soft reprimands are presumably different from the reprimands children ordinarily receive at home or in school, where "being yelled at" tends to be the norm. Loud reprimands, they reason, might thus elicit conditioned emotional reactions that, in turn, activate further disruptive behavior. There is little evidence to support this speculation and it would have to be put to an explicit test before it could be accepted with confidence. If loud reprimands do indeed serve as a stimulus for emotional reactions one might expect this to affect not only the child at whom the reprimand is directed but also the other children in the room most of whom would have been similarly conditioned since "being yelled at" is not the exclusive privilege of disruptive children. Yet in the classrooms where these investigators sampled the disruptive behavior of the entire class they found no relationship between the behavior of the nontargeted children and the reprimand conditions.

In addition to the two explanations advanced by O'Leary et al. (1970) another possible explanation presents itself.* It has to do with the adaptation effect to repeated stimuli or, in conditioning terms, with extinction of a conditioned stimulus when it remains unpaired with the unconditioned stimulus over the course of many trials. A disruptive boy is likely to have heard loud verbal reprimands (e.g., "Sit down!" "Stop that!" "Be quiet!" "Behave yourself!") both at home and in school so many times that he has eventually learned to ignore them; they have lost their effectiveness as stimuli capable of suppressing behavior. The effectiveness of such verbal statements presumably stems from the fact that in the earlier conditioning history of such children the statements had been paired with more concrete physical punishments or, at least, that the loud volume at which they are emitted did, at one time, have aversive qualities. Either because the child adapts to this volume so that the statements are no longer aversive, or because they are no longer paired with physical punishment, the reprimands have lost their effectiveness as punishers. If, in addition, being given a loud reprimand in the classroom carries some positive reinforcement value in terms of peer reactions one would expect the effect that is so often observed; loud reprimands increase rather than decrease disruptive behavior. The effectiveness of the soft reprimand might then be explained by the fact that its stimulus characteristics are sufficiently different from the loud reprimand that the adaptation effect has not generalized to it and/or that the teacher's proximity while delivering it carries sufficient threat of physical punishment that the soft verbal reprimand is capable of suppressing disruptive behavior, functioning as an effective punishing stimulus. This formulation would predict that soft reprimands will eventually lose their potency, just as repeatedly used loud reprimands seem to do.

While O'Leary, Kaufman, Kass, and Drabman (1970) have demonstrated that soft reprimands are more effective than loud reprimands with certain chil-

---

*There is also the explanation once offered by a frivolous student who suggested that teachers whose soft reprimands are effective might have bad breath or body odor so that their proximity when whispering a reprimand has aversive qualities that make such reprimands serve as effective punishers.

dren under specific conditions, the explanation for this effectiveness calls for further study as does the question whether this form of intervention in disruptive behavior can be used under other conditions with older children.

CONTINGENT SOCIAL ISOLATION

Studies dealing with the use of reprimands to control disruptive behavior had usually been conducted in regular classrooms where the range of unacceptable behaviors is relatively limited. The more extreme forms of disruption that may be found in special-education settings often require additional or other forms of intervention. One of these is often erroneously referred to as time-out. In the technical sense, as used in the experimental analysis of behavior, time-out refers to a response-contingent period of time during which no positive reinforcement is available and which results in a reduced frequency of that response. As pointed out in the previous chapter, time-out is a response-suppression procedure and thus a form of punishment by removal. In order to use time-out it is necessary that one have identified the positive reinforcer that is maintaining the response one seeks to suppress. If one has not identified the reinforcer, one cannot speak of withholding it. In applied settings, such as a classroom, it is usually very difficult to ascertain what it is that serves as the positive reinforcement of a child's disruptive behavior. It is often assumed, but rarely demonstrated, that the reactions of a disruptive child's classmates contribute to the reinforcement of such behavior. These reactions, however, are not under the direct control of the teacher so that it is not possible to withhold them from the offending child. What is usually done, therefore, is to remove that child temporarily from the classroom, thus removing the child from putative reinforcers instead of removing unidentified reinforcers from the child. This should not be called time-out (from positive reinforcement). As suggested by Drabman and Spitalnik (1973a), it is more appropriate to speak of such intervention as *contingent social isolation* and to view it as punishment by application. Like other forms of punishment, social isolation should be used with circumspection and only in combination with explicit contingencies of positive reinforcement for acceptable, disruption-incompatible, alternative behaviors. Such positive reinforcement should then continue beyond the point where the disruptive behavior has been suppressed and then only gradually faded so that the acceptable behavior can eventually be maintained by the natural reinforcers available in the child's environment.

In order to conduct research on the effect of contingent social isolation on disruptive classroom behavior it is necessary to employ a design that guards against a number of pitfalls which, as Drabman and Spitalnik (1973a) pointed out, have plagued most studies of this topic. Clearly, if one desires to test the effectiveness of contingent social isolation one must take steps to assure that this variable is not confounded with other treatment techniques being used at the same time. Furthermore, the contingency under investigation must be employed in a consistent manner and implemented in consequence of clearly defined criteria for disruptive behavior. One methodological problem that had not been recognized by anyone until Drabman and Spitalnik (1973a) pointed it out stems from the social isolation procedure itself. If the dependent variable is a specified disruptive behavior that is observed and counted during baseline phases in order to compare its frequency there with its frequency during the social isolation phase of the study, the very fact that the disruptive child is not in the classroom while in social isolation would reduce the frequency of observed disruptions.

To deal with this dilemma, Drabman and Spitalnik (1973a) created a new observational measure which they called "pseudo-timeout." This entails having the observers record during baseline conditions the periods of time during which the observed child *would* have been absent from the classroom *if* the social isolation condition had been in effect. This permits not only a calculation of a baseline frequency that compensates for the artifact potentially created by the difference in time a child spends in the classroom during baseline and during social isolation conditions but it also provides information on the characteristics (topology) of the child's behavior in the period immediately following a disruptive response.

Working with disturbed children who were residents in a psychiatric institution, Drabman and Spitalnik (1973a) used the procedure just described to observe the classroom behavior of five children every day of the week during an entire 55-minute period. Three forms of disruptive behavior had been targeted for the purpose of this study: out-of-seat, aggression, and nonpermitted vocalization. The first two of these behaviors were subjected to intervention while vocalization served as a control in a multiple baseline design. Treatment consisted of response-contingent social isolation that took the following form. As soon as one of the targeted behaviors had reached the predetermined criterion (one occurrence of aggression or three consecutive 20-second observation intervals of out-of-seat behavior), the observer would give an unobtrusive signal whereupon the teacher would instruct a teaching assistant to take the child out of the class, address the child and say "You have misbehaved. You must leave the class." The teaching assistant would then immediately escort the child to a small, empty, dimly lit, sound-resistant music practice room in which the child had to remain for 10 minutes. It is noteworthy that isolation was terminated on a fixed-time basis, regardless of what the child was doing at that time. This, as we shall see later, has implications that other investigators have considered in their use of contingent social isolation.

The results reported by Drabman and Spitalnik (1973a) demonstrate that their use of contingent social reinforcement was effective in reducing the frequency of the behaviors that had been thus punished. During the first baseline phase which lasted for 11 days the mean percentage of out-of-seat behavior for the five children was 34. During the 16 days that contingent social isolation was in effect this behavior was significantly reduced to a frequency of 11 percent. When that contingency was removed during the second baseline phase, lasting 10 days, the mean frequency of this behavior increased to 15 percent which, it will be noted, is significantly below the frequency for the first baseline phase. Aggression, a less frequent form of disruptive behavior for these children, had a mean frequency of 2.8 percent during the first baseline, fell to .37 percent while social isolation was in effect, and remained at .40 percent when that intervention ceased. For both of these phases the reduction in frequency below the first baseline is statistically significant. For the third observed disruptive behavior, vocalization, which had not been punished, the mean frequencies remained relatively unchanged throughout. The mean frequency had been 32 percent during first baseline, became 28 percent while social isolation was in effect for the other two behaviors, and was 27 percent during the second baseline. These minor fluctuations fail to reach the usually accepted level of statistical significance.

Aside from the fact that theirs is probably the only controlled study of the effect of contingent social isolation on the disruptive classroom behavior of individual children, the work by Drabman and Spitalnik (1973a) is also noteworthy in that they were able to demonstrate maintenance of improved behavior over a period of 10 days following cessation of their intervention. As we shall discover shortly, other investigators were not able to maintain the effect of social isolation beyond the phase during which it was employed. Whether this is due to the highly consistent, rigorous, objective, and rapid manner in which Drabman and Spitalnik implemented their isolation procedure or to some other factor peculiar to their procedure, setting, or persons is, unfortunately, an imponderable.

A Method with Pitfalls

We turn now to an examination of two other studies that investigated the effect of contingent social isolation on disruptive behavior and which are probably best viewed as examples of what not to do. Ramp, Ulrich, and Dulaney (1971) reported a case study of a 9-year-old boy who was attending third grade of an elementary school and who had been described as a "disciplinary problem" in that he would disrupt the class by talking out of turn and getting out of his seat. The teacher's usual methods for controlling such behavior, such as having him stay after school, keeping him in the classroom during free time, not permitting him to go to gym, or sending him to the principal's office had failed to reduce this disruptive behavior. When an observer was placed in the classroom to count the number of 10-second intervals per 15-minute observation session during which out-of-seat and talking-out behavior took place, the record showed that during the 18-day baseline phase, the boy averaged 23.7 out-of-seat and 17.1 talking-out intervals per session. At this point an instructions procedure was introduced that consisted of having the teacher request the boy to ask for permission before speaking or getting out of his seat. During the eight sessions this condition was in effect, the average number of disruptive responses increased, out-of-seat reaching a mean of 29.6 and talking-out a mean of 22 intervals per session.

On the 27th day the investigators instituted what they call a delayed time-out procedure (Ramp et al., 1971). For this, the boy was informed that the following conditions would henceforth be in effect. Every time he was out of his seat or talking without permission a red light, mounted on his desk for this purpose and operated by the observer, would be briefly illuminated and that for each such episode he was to spend five minutes in a "time-out booth" later in the day during a period usually allotted for recess or gym. The time-out booth was located in the hallway, measured 4 × 3 × 5 feet high, and contained a chair and a table. The booth was open on top so that air and the normal light from the hallway could easily enter and the walls were painted a light gray. Thus, while the booth isolated the child from contact with the surrounding environment, it and similar arrangements should not be viewed as a "black hole" or a "sweat box" as inflammatory newspaper accounts have at times suggested. In line with our earlier discussion regarding the definition of time-out, it should be noted that it is incorrect to use that term for the procedure here employed since recess and gym from which the boy was excluded could hardly have been the reinforcing consequences that maintained his disruptive behavior.

Whatever its function, the effect of this contingency on the boy's behavior was very dramatic. In the very first session he talked without permission but once and left his seat only twice, thus having to spend 15 minutes in the time-out booth. Note that on this day the boy had not yet experienced the social isolation so that the reduction in his disruptive behavior seems mediated solely by the signal light. Ramp, Ulrich, and Dulaney (1971) regretably failed to employ a control for the effect of the light alone, before it had been designated as a signal for later social isolation. It is thus impossible to tell whether the boy responded to the light's reminding him of the teacher's injunction against talking or getting out of his seat without permission or whether the association of the light with the impending aversive consequence resulted in the suppression of the disruptive behavior. Nor is it clear, of course, whether the isolation in the booth was in itself an aversive consequence or whether and to what extent the concomitant deprivation of the privilege to go to gym or recess contributed to the suppression of the disruptive behavior. At any rate, during the following 22 days during which the so-called time-out contingency was in effect the boy never again left his seat without permission and spoke out of turn only on five separate occasions. However, as soon as the light was removed from his desk and the contingency was no longer in effect, the boy's disruptive behavior quickly returned to baseline proportions, with six out-of-seat intervals and 21 talking intervals on the very first day and an average of 25.4 out-of-seat intervals per session during the remaining 17 sessions of the study.

As a demonstration of the temporary effectiveness of the intervention they had decided to use, the work by Ramp, Ulrich, and Dulaney (1971) is of interest, but as a model to be applied in working with disruptive children it must be rejected. Like any other punishment, social isolation alone serves only to suppress the behavior on which it is made contingent; it cannot produce disruption-incompatible, desirable behavior to take the place of the response being punished. As this study so clearly demonstrates, as soon as the punishment contingency is removed, the undesirable behavior returns when no constructive alternative has been taught. For that reason it is ill-advised to use social isolation or other forms of punishment without concomitantly undertaking systematic efforts to strengthen desirable behavior. Yet, when using social isolation, one faces a peculiar dilemma, for how is one to teach constructive behavior to a child who is alone in a room?

The fact that a social isolation procedure maintains its effect only as long as the contingency is in force was also apparent in a study reported by Lahey, McNees, and McNees (1973) who used this method of intervention with a 10-year-old boy who had been placed in an elementary level class of so-called educable mentally retarded children because of his disruptive behavior. This behavior consisted of repeatedly uttering obscene words and phrases, accompanied by facial twitches. This problem is sometimes referred to as a verbal tic or as Gilles de la Tourette's syndrome. During a baseline phase lasting four days, the objectionable behavior occurred approximately twice per minute during one-hour periods of classroom observation.

The intervention introduced by Lahey et al. (1973) began with an eight-day phase during which they tried an approach generally known as "negative practice" but which they prefer to call "instructed repetition." It consisted of having a teacher take the boy to another room four times a day for 15-minute sessions during which he was to repeat his most frequently used obscene word over and over again. This method has at times been employed in the treatment of involuntary muscle movements (tics) on the assumption that bringing the response under voluntary control will enable the person to suppress it or that such massed practice will somehow satiate a postulated "need" to engage in the behavior. Whatever the theoretical rationale, negative practice is also likely to be an aversive procedure so that whatever effect it may have could well be due to its function as a punisher. In fact, Lahey et al. (1973) report that they discontinued this procedure because both pupil and teacher "strongly disliked these sessions." Nonetheless, the frequency of the target behavior in the classroom fell to about half its baseline level during this phase though the rate of one incident per minute was still considered to be intolerable.

At this point Lahey et al. (1973) instituted what they refer to as a "time-out contingency" even though they had made no attempt to identify the consequences that might have been reinforcing the boy's objectionable behavior. They used a well-lighted 4 × 10 foot room, adjacent to the classroom for their purpose. All objects had been removed from that room and it had a door that could be locked when they boy was inside. Following every occurrence of the target behavior the child was immediately placed in that special room for a minimum of five minutes and until he had been in there quietly for one minute. The latter condition is an important part of a time-out or social isolation contingency because the termination of this aversive event will function as negative reinforcement of any behavior that is taking place just prior to release from the room. Thus, if a boy should be kicking and screaming when the door is opened to release him, it will be kicking and screaming while in that room that is strengthened by the procedure. In general, the onset of an aversive event can serve as a punishment for the reponse that immediately precedes it while, conversely, its termination can serve as a (negative) reinforcement, strengthening whatever behavior is taking place at that moment.

With the introduction of the "time-out" contingency, which was in effect during the entire school day, the behavior of the boy in the Lahey et al. (1973) study underwent a marked change. The rate of his obscene utterances dropped to about one every 5 minutes during the observation hours and his parents reported that he had gone an entire weekend without his objectionable habit so that they had been able to take him out in public for the first time in two years. Unfortunately, and as we had seen in the Ramp, Ulrich, and Dulaney (1971) study, the improvement could be maintained only for as long as the social isolation contingency was in effect. When it was discontinued after 14 days, the obscene utterances once again rose to the baseline level of approximately two per minute and they could only be held to the acceptable level of about one per hour by reintroducing the aversive consequence. The teacher continued to use the isolation procedure successfully for the remaining four weeks of the school year but a noteworthy sidelight appears in the teacher's report. It seems that the room that was being used for isolation was not available for one hour each day during the third and fourth weeks. While the boy's objectionable behavior was kept under control during the rest of the day when the room was available, his utterances returned to baseline level during that one hour of each day! This is a reflection of the fact that social isolation serves a punishing function so that its effect generalizes to stimuli associated with it, such as the available room or a red signal light, which come to elicit avoidance responses in their own right. As soon as these stimuli are removed or unavailable, these avoidance responses cease and the punished behavior returns to baseline levels.

On the basis of these case studies one can conclude that social isolation, at least as used here, is an ineffective procedure for obtaining long-term benefits. This is one reason why it should be used sparingly and with circumspection. Other reasons are that while a child is in the isolation or time-out room he or she misses the academic activities going on in the classroom and that, with any but rather docile, cooperative, or small children, removing a child to the isolation room can entail considerable physical struggle that is not only undesirable as such, but also further disruptive of the activities of other children in the classroom, especially if that child then screams and bangs on the door of the room. Lastly, as with any other form of punishment, the use and advocacy of social isolation in a responsible, therapeutically sound context can easily lead to abuse by persons who, either because they misunderstand the principles involved or in order to provide a euphemism for their cruelties, will lock children in dark closets for long periods of time and call this time-out. Justified public outrage over such perversion of a therapeutic procedure has caused the procedure itself, even when used appropriately, to have become suspect in the eye of the public. As O'Leary and O'Leary (1976) have urged, time-out and social isolation should be used "very, very discriminately and usually only after other methods have been tried" (p. 490).

POSITIVE PRACTICE PROCEDURES

One very promising alternative to the use of such a controversial procedure as social isolation is *positive practice*, a procedure Azrin and his colleagues have successfully used in treating enuresis (Azrin, Sneed, & Foxx, 1974), stealing (Azrin & Wesolowski, 1974), self-stimulatory behavior (Foxx & Azrin, (1973b), and messy eating (O'Brien, Bugle, & Azrin, 1972), among other problems. As pointed out in connection with discussions of these difficulties and disorders, positive practice is based on the principle that when an error or disruptive action takes place, the individual must practice the correct way of behaving. A teacher's or therapist's demand that the child engage in such practice probably makes it an aversive consequence as far as the child is concerned. At the same time, positive practice has definitive educative functions in that it enhances the establishment of desired behaviors even while it may serve as a punisher for the undesired behaviors that set the occasion for such practice. Thus, while other forms of punishment, such as reprimands, social isolation, or loss of privileges merely suppress the undesirable behavior, necessitating a separate effort at teaching the desirable alternative, positive practice encompasses both of these goals, punishing the disruptive behavior while teaching its positive alternative. Azrin and Powers (1975) recognize the aversive aspect of positive practice when they state that in order to minimize "the connotation of vindictiveness of the required practice" (p. 526) the teacher or therapist should, in each instance, explain to the child that the additional practice is required only because he or she had not yet learned the proper skill.

In order to implement positive practice procedures one must ask oneself what the desired alternative of the changeworthy behavior should be. When disruptive classroom behavior consists of getting out of one's seat or speaking without permission, a desired alternative might be asking the teacher for permission before leaving the seat or before talking (and to desist from these behaviors when permission is not granted). Working with six boys who had been designated by their teachers as extremely disruptive and who were attending a special education class during summer because of their severely deficient academic skills, Azrin and Powers (1975) studied the effectiveness of positive practice by comparing it with two other procedures: the delivery of a reminder-reprimand for each act of disruptive behavior, and forfeiture of recess for misbehavior. Positive practice itself was applied under two conditions. In the one used first it was delayed until the recess period, in the other the child was required to engage in one trial of positive practice immediately after the offense and to finish the required number of practices during recess. Using recess for engaging in positive practice meant, of course, that positive practice also entailed a loss of recess time so that these two conditions were confounded. In all conditions, the teacher stated the rules about not talking and not leaving one's seat at the beginning of each class period and consistently praised all positive behavior.

Azrin and Powers (1975) describe the positive practice procedure as follows. Any student who broke the rule that had been announced at the beginning of the class period was required to remain quietly in the classroom during the 10-minute recess and to follow the positive practice procedure. For this, the teacher would first ask the student what the correct procedure was for talking in class or leaving one's seat and the student had to recite that procedure to the teacher. The student was then required to raise his hand and to wait until the teacher acknowledged him by name whereupon the child was to ask the teacher for the desired permission. The teacher would then acknowledge that the child had practiced correctly, and say, "Let's practice again." The entire procedure was then repeated for several trials. The length of time for which positive practice was carried out depended on the number of students who were required to participate in this procedure during any given recess period. If only one or two students were scheduled, the duration was 5 minutes with the first student having to remain quietly in the classroom while the other went through the procedure. When more than two students had been scheduled, the 10-minute recess period was divided equally among them. As soon as a child finished his required practice, he could join the other children at recess, thus motivating quick cooperation. During a 5-minute period about five to ten positive practice trails would usually take place and if a student's performance was incorrect or where procrastination ensued, the teacher would demand that the practice be begun anew.

In the delayed condition of positive practice Azrin and Powers (1975) gradually reduced the duration of the procedure. This fading was accomplished by decreasing the time devoted to positive practice by half each day if the number of disruptions the previous day had been two or fewer. When this number exceeded two on any given day, the duration of positive practice was again increased to 5 minutes. A similar fading process had been employed in the immediate condition where positive practice was gradually reduced on successive days until the student was required only to recite the rule upon having broken it.

The results reported by Azrin and Powers (1975) and shown in Figure 17 reflect the effectiveness of their procedure in reducing the disruptive behavior of the six boys with whom it had been used. During the first three days when the students were merely reminded of the rules and reprimanded for breaking them there was an average of 29 disruptions per day. When a loss-of-recess contingency was imposed for the next four days, disruptions decreased significantly and immediately to about 11 per day. With the instituting of positive practice in its delayed form, the frequency of disruptions showed an immediate drop to about two per day, a significant reduction from baseline of about 95 percent. This level was maintained for 12 days at which point positive practice was changed to the immediate condition and maintained for the next six days. Here, it will be recalled, a child was required to engage in the procedure once as soon as he had violated the rule and complete it later during the recess period. Disruptions now fell to an average level of about 0.4 per day but these data are based on only four children because two of them were absent during all or some of the time.

While the ABCD design used in this study limits the confidence with which a conclusion can be drawn from it, the fact that the statistically significant reductions in disruptive behavior took place immediately upon a change in the conditions from reminder-reprimand to loss of recess to positive practice does lend support to the authors' contention (Azrin & Powers, 1975) that the changes were brought about by their interventions and not by the children's increasing familiarity with the teacher or other uncontrolled factors. The investigators describe the atmosphere in the classroom at the beginning of their study as one of general chaos and confusion with students continuously walking and running about, hitting, talking, shouting, and otherwise interfering with those

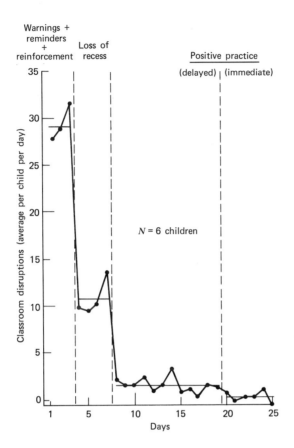

Figure 17. Changes in average frequencies of classroom disruptions. (After Azrin & Powers, 1975. Copyright by Academic Press, Inc.)

trying to study. This, of course, was at the beginning of a six-week special summer school class for children who knew neither each other nor the teacher. Seven days later, when positive practice had been instituted, the class is described as relaxed and attentive, with the children showing consideration for others and none of them shouting or walking about. While some of this change may have been due to a general "settling down" of the group, the fact that the change coincided with the introduction of the positive practice contingency does suggest that it was an important, if not the critical variable. It is also of interest that these children, who had been referred to this special session because they had been extremely disruptive in their regular classrooms during the school year, seemed to maintain their improved behavior after returning there at the start of the new term. The teacher who had been in charge of the summer class instructed the regular classroom teachers in the use of positive practice and maintained telephone contact with them regarding the children's behavior. The anecdotal report, presented by Azrin and Powers (1975), states that the children were no longer a problem and were behaving well.

THE USE OF TOKENS

We have discussed interventions in the disruptive classroom behavior of children by the use of differential teacher attention, praise, reprimand, contingent social isolation, and positive practice. We turn next to a consideration of the effectiveness of tokens as either generalized positive reinforcers or when employed in the context of a response-cost procedure. A token, as was pointed out in other contexts, is any object or symbol that has acquired the capacity to serve as a reinforcer because the person receiving it has previously learned that the token can later be used to obtain an object or privilege, the back-up reinforcer, that has some value in its own right. Tokens have the advantage of being readily delivered when reinforcement is most effective—at the time the desired response is emitted. Also, by virtue of the fact that the same object, such as a poker chip that is used as a token, can be traded for one of a variety of back-up reinforcers, reinforcement is personalized and thus of optimal potency.

The principle of using tokens as reinforcers is familiar to everyone inasmuch as the money we earn for the services we render or the goods we sell is no more than a symbol that derives its reinforcement value from the fact that we can use it to purchase things we need or desire. Just as is the case in the exchange of money, so the use of tokens calls for an explicit set of rules regarding their economy that is communicated to and understood by everyone involved in the transaction. In order for tokens to be used effectively, each child in the program must possess the answers to the following questions: "How many units of what behavior must I emit in order to earn how many tokens and how many tokens must I accumulate before I can exchange them for the back-up reinforcer of my choice and what are the items from which I may make that selection?"

In institutional settings tokens have been used successfully with groups of children in comprehensive programs that place all or many of their activities under token contingencies, a so-called token economy (Kazdin, 1977). In such situations, back-up reinforcers can range from favorite foods or snacks, to special privileges or activities that can be obtained within the institution itself. When tokens are used with individual children whose disruptive classroom behavior is the target of intervention a number of issues must be considered and we turn to these in the following.

Effect on Other Children

In a study conducted by Drabman, Spitalnik, and Spitalnik (1974) it was shown that disruptive classroom behavior can be significantly decreased by the use of token reinforcement contingent on constructive behavior. Using a regular first-grade class of 23 children, these investigators studied the differential effectiveness of four types of token reinforcement programs. Tokens took the form of points that could be earned for "good behavior" and these were used to earn free time, one point being equal to one minute. Free time consisted of access to art supplies, felt-tipped pens, tumbling mats, modeling clay; the kind of material readily available in most classrooms and requiring no extra expenditure inasmuch as it was neither consumed nor taken home by the children.

These were the four token programs investigated: (1) Individual reinforcement where each child in the group earned tokens depending on his or her own behavior; (2) group reinforcement where the number of points earned by the group was determined by the behavior of the most disruptive child; (3) group reinforcement where the number of points earned by the group was determined by the behavior of the least disruptive child; and (4) group reinforcement of a randomly selected member of the group. While the contingencies involved groups of children, the focus of the study was on the behavior of four, individually targeted disruptive children. It was found that the behavior of these four children improved significantly under each of the four token programs examined and that the manner in which the tokens were dispensed made no difference in their improvement. In terms of deciding which type of program to use for classroom application, the choice must thus be based on considerations other than effectiveness.

One of these considerations is the effect of a group contingency not only on the behavior of the nondisruptive children in the class but also on their attitude toward the child who earns (or loses) back-up reinforcers "for them." Spitalnik et al. (1974) obtained data relevant to both of these issues. A sociometric device was used to assess the attitude question. It revealed that the children came to view a disruptive child as a more responsible person when that child's behavior has the basis for the number of points earned by the group. It therefore seems that if one wishes to use a token program to increase the respect the rest of the class has for a disruptive child, the reinforcement contingencies for the group should be based on the behavior of that child. That system, however, turned out to be the least preferred of the four when the class was asked for their opinion about this. As far as the children were concerned, the most popular system was the one in which earning free time was based on the behavior of the least disruptive member of the group, yet this system was disliked by the teacher whose preference was for the one in which the behavior of randomly selected children determined the reinforcement. Since this system was the second most popular with the children, it is probably the most likely candidate for adoption.

Regarding the effect of the token reinforcement program on the behavior of the nondisruptive children, Spitalnik et al. (1974) report that children who had been selected for observation because of their good behavior neither improved nor became significantly worse during any of the four token programs. This information is useful in that parents and teachers are sometimes concerned lest their efforts to reduce the undesirable behavior of one child by the use of tokens will have untoward consequences on the behavior of other children. It must be remembered, however, that in the investigation just discussed, the back-up reinforcements were available to all children; hence the disruptive child was not singled out as the only one for whom the contingencies were in effect. How do other children react when they are not sharing in the positive reinforcements earned by a child who is the target of individualized attention? The following study conducted by Christy (1975) provides an answer to this question, as does a report by Drabman and Lahey (1974) that will be presented later.

Working with two groups of preschool children who were attending a remedial program for youngsters with such problems as hyperactivity, oppositional or overly demanding behavior, withdrawal, and speech disorders, Christy (1975) investigated whether children who observe one of their peers receiving reinforcement for specified behavior will exhibit changes in their own behavior. The study took place during periods when the children were supposed to be in their assigned seats, working with modeling clay. During a baseline period one observer recorded the in-seat behavior of each of the five or six children in the group, while other observers monitored children's aggressive and disruptive behavior and the actions of the teacher. Following this, the teacher announced to the class that she was going "to make a deal" with one of the children that entailed his receiving "a goody" if he was in his seat when a tape recorded whistle sounded at variable intervals. When earned, small edible reinforcers were then dispensed to that child, accompanied by the statement, "Here's your goody for sitting." This procedure resulted in a marked increase of in-seat behavior on the part of children who were targeted for this intervention at different points in the study.

When people first hear about a token program of this nature, they often ask whether other children, observing the "bad" member of their group receiving reinforcement and the special attention associated with it, won't reason that in order to obtain similar treatment they too have to be "bad." The study by Christy (1975) provides an interesting answer to this question. Not only did the other children who saw one of their peers receiving reinforcement for in-seat behavior not get out of their own seats more often, but by the end of the study all of them were found to be in their seats more frequently or more consistently. Nor was there an increase in either aggressive or disruptive behavior. Complaints such as "It's not fair" or "I'm sitting too!" or comments regarding the procedure, like "There went the whistle," were heard with some frequency from a few of the children on the first day of each treatment phase but the teacher, as instructed, ignored these verbalizations and they quickly ceased.

This study thus demonstrates that children who observe another child earning tangible reinforcers for reducing the frequency of some undesirable behavior will not necessarily begin to engage in that behavior in the expectation that they too will then be rewarded for reducing it. Christy (1975) suggests that her findings may be a function of the fact that throughout the study the teacher maintained a high frequency of positive attention and praise statements for the children's work (but not for sitting down). It may be that children who are receiving plentiful reinforcement for desirable behavior do not view one child's receiving some additional reinforcement as a major inequity, suggesting that individualized reinforcement should be used only in a setting where there is a high base rate of reinforcements for everyone.

Home-based Reinforcement

Viewed from the perspective of school administrators, the handing out of rewards for good behavior in the form of food or other tangibles in school may be a questionable or, at least, unorthodox procedure. In fact, beyond the early primary grades, even the students might consider such a procedure inappropriate. Parents, too, may object to their children receiving such rewards especially when they consist of candy about which many have legitimate concerns based on nutritional considerations. In addition to these potential constraints on a school-based program of rewards, there is the further limitation that a classroom teacher has available only a limited range of potential reinforcers. Available backups for tokens may not contain an item that a particular child finds reinforcing and even such naturally available consequences as additional time for recess may not always serve a reinforcing function. Finally, when a treatment program is focused on only one child in a classroom, teachers may resist introducing a procedure that involves giving rewards to that child alone because they are apprehesive about the reactions of the other children. Research results, such as those we have just reviewed, which should allay these concerns, may not be very convincing to teachers who justifiably question the generalizability of these findings to their own classes. All these considerations lead one to look for a way of implementing a systematic program of reinforcement for desirable behavior that fits into the social ecology of the school.

There is, of course, a consequence for behavior that has long been a part of the manner in which schools operate; it is report cards and notices to parents regarding their child's behavior. Both are based on the assumption that by giving parents feedback on their child's performance and behavior they will praise or reprimand their child. From the standpoint of the principles of learning, report cards, coming as they do on a thin, fixed-interval schedule, are delayed, hence very ineffective consequences for day-to-day classroom behavior. The reproving notice on the other hand, though a more immediate consequence, calls attention only to unacceptable behavior in the expectation that the parents will react by punishing the child. Missing from the school's usual repertoire of instigating parents to administer a consequence for their child's classroom behavior is a notice that informs them of the desirable things their child has done that day so that they might reward these at home. Parents have available to them a wide range of potential reinforcers that are appropriate both to their individual child and to their own system of values. "Good behavior notices," systematically given to a child at the end of the class period or the school day, would therefore answer all the objections to a school-based reinforcement program we have mentioned above.

A home-based reinforcement system in which students received daily "report cards" from the teacher so that the home could provide the back-up reinforcers in terms of privileges granted or withheld, was evaluated by Bailey, Wolf, and Phillips (1970) and found to be very effective. That study, however, had been carried out in the context of the Achievement Place project where the home was supervised by trained teaching-parents so that the question whether typical parents without special training could also support such a home-based program remained to be investigated. Such an investigation was undertaken by Ayllon, Garber, and Pisor (1975) who worked with a third-grade class of children from an economically disadvantaged background who were highly disruptive and of low academic achievement. A single two-hour meeting was held with the parents of these children to explain the home-based reward program to them. The program functioned as follows: In class the students would earn one point for each 15-minute interval during which they did not engage in disruptive behavior. Points were lost when disruptive behavior did take place. At the end of the day those students who had not exceeded two disruptions per 15-minute period throughout the school day received a "good behavior letter." This letter was to be taken home where the parents were to use their own style and judgment in supplying suitable rewards. Appropriate sanctions were to be brought to bear when the child did not bring such a letter home since this was to be taken as an indication that the child's behavior had not merited such recognition.

The results presented by Ayllon et al. (1975) show that their procedure was highly effective. Disruptive behavior that had averaged 90 percent of observation intervals during baseline was reduced to an average of 10 percent when the letter-home contingency was in effect. During an experimental phase when the "good behavior letter" was handed to the children when they came to school in the morning so that it was not contingent on classroom behavior, disruptive behavior rose to an average of 50 percent. When the letter was once again made contingent on the children's behavior, their disruptive behavior was immediately reduced to zero.

Reinforcement or Information?

In the studies that we have discussed thus far in which tokens were used to increase constructive classroom behavior, the assumption has always been that the token or the object for which it could later be traded served the function of reinforcing such behavior. Drabman and Lahey (1974) asked the important question whether behavior change necessarily requires that children receive a tangible item as a reinforcer or whether all that is needed is some feedback that informs them when a desired response has been emitted. In studying this issue these investigators also looked at the effect their intervention with one child had on the behavior of other children in the classroom. Unlike Christy (1975) who had dealt with preschool children in small groups, Drabman and Lahey (1974) worked with a 10-year-old girl in a regular classroom whose inappropriate, disruptive behavior was of the kind that typically results in clinic referrals. Their study then is not a contrived analogue but an investigation in a "real life" setting.

The study conducted by Drabman and Lahey (1974) entailed four phases in an ABAB design. During the first baseline phase which covered 10 school days of observations the frequency of disruptive behavior of the targeted girl, Charlotte, and of her classmates was recorded, using a coding system similar to the one developed by O'Leary and his associates (O'Leary, Becker, Evans, & Saudargas, 1969). In this system an observer watches for 20 seconds and then enters his or her observations on the coded record for the next 10 seconds before returning to another 20-second observation, continuing this observe-record alternation for the entire class period. As used in the study under discussion, the categories of disruptive behavior cover being out of the chair, touching another's property, playing in a manner incompatible with learning, making noise, failing to comply with a request by the teacher, not attending to the assigned task, vocalizing without permission, turning around, and coming into contact with another person. Each of these categories is objectively defined and the observers are trained in their use so that they achieve a high level of reliability which, expressed in terms of agreements, averaged 86 percent for the 37 observation days in the Drabman and Lahey (1974) study.

After the baseline phase, this study entered the first treatment phase, lasting 18 school days, during which the following contingencies were in effect. A timer was placed in the classroom and set by the teacher to ring at regular intervals four times during a class session. The teacher had privately explained to

Charlotte that each time the timer rang she would be given a rating depending on her behavior at that moment, ranging from zero for very poor, to 10 for very good behavior. Each time the timer rang the child was quietly informed of her rating and the total score for the day was given to her at the end of the class. None of the other children was informed of this arrangement although the ringing of the timer must have been apparent to them. A second baseline phase, during which the timer was removed, followed this treatment phase. It lasted for eight school days and Charlotte was given no feedback, being told simply that she was expected to continue "to be good" even though the timer was not going to be used. Finally, there followed another treatment phase of 11 school days during which the contingencies involving timer and feedback were again in effect.

It should be stressed that the numerical ratings that had been given to the target child as feedback on the acceptability of her behavior were based on the teacher's judgment and not on the frequency count the observers were maintaining concurrently. Furthermore it is important to note that these ratings were in no way related to any other consequences. Unlike the conditions obtaining in the typical token program, the ratings did not represent a back-up reinforcer for which they could later be traded. With nothing more than subjectively determined, but systematic feedback on her behavior available to the child, her disruptive behavior revealed a remarkable change. Charlotte's average number of disruptive behaviors had been 1.39 per 20-second interval during the first baseline phase. This dropped to 0.498 during the first feedback phase, returned to 1.77 when baseline conditions were reinstituted, and fell again to 0.370 during the second feedback phase. These results strongly suggest that the effectiveness of a system of token reinforcement derives in large part from the information the delivery of a token provides as to the acceptability of one's behavior. It may be that regular feedback is sufficient for modifying a disruptive child's behavior even when it is given only four times per class period.

There were several other aspects to the investigation by Drabman and Lahey (1974). As mentioned, they had also gathered data on the disruptive behavior of Charlotte's classmates. While Charlotte had been the most disruptive child in the class, the other 12 students also engaged in some of the behavior on which the O'Leary code is focused. During the first baseline phase, their disruptive behavior averaged 0.714 per observation interval and this decreased to 0.550 while the feedback to Charlotte was in effect. It rose to 0.780 during the second baseline phase and returned to 0.503 when the feedback procedure was again introduced. Compared with the behavior of her peers, that of the targeted child, Charlotte, was more disruptive during baseline and less disruptive during treatment phases but the changes displayed by the nontargeted peers nonetheless attained statistical significance.

This finding then, provides yet another answer to the question about the effect on the other children in the classroom when one of them is singled out for the special attention entailed in a treatment procedure. The behavior of the other children, it seems, parallels the changes displayed by the targeted child. Given the fact that the intervention used with Charlotte was relatively unobtrusive, with feedback given so quietly that only the ringing of the timer was clearly obvious to the others in the class, it would appear that at least some of the effect on her classmates' behavior was due to the change in the behavior of Charlotte. One highly disruptive child may stimulate others in the class to engage in disruptive behavior of their own so that, when the disruptive child settles down and this instigation is removed, the other children's behavior also improves. A look at some of the categories of disruptive behavior used in this study lends support to this speculation. If the disruptive child touches another's property, that other child may well retaliate in some fashion and the same should hold true with the category labeled Aggression where the child "makes a movement towards another so as to come into contact with him." It would be an unusually well-behaved child who did not counter this with a similar movement of his or her own. That Charlotte's peers noticed the improvement in her behavior seems reflected in the fact that they addressed significantly more positive comments to her and rated her more highly on a sociometric device during treatment than during baseline phases. Drabman and Lahey (1974) chose not to speculate about the reason for their finding that the classmates' behavior underwent changes that reflected those of Charlotte's but they do make the important point that the effect they demonstrated makes it questionable whether classmates can be used as untreated controls in studies on the effectiveness of a treatment procedure that is applied to selected children in a classroom.

PEER-ADMINISTERED CONSEQUENCES

Thus far we have discussed programs designed to modify the behavior of disruptive children that called for the teacher or a teaching assistant to monitor the children's behavior and to institute the delivery of the reinforcing consequences. This places demands on the teaching staff that may be greater than their other responsibilities may allow. The question thus arises whether a child's classmates can play a role in reducing disruptive behavior.

It has been demonstrated (Solomon and Wahler, 1973) that when a child engages in disruptive behavior other children in the classroom will attend to that behavior thereby providing one of the reinforcing consequences that maintain it. The rationale for the time-out procedure whereby the disruptive child is removed from the classroom contingent on unacceptable behavior is, of course, based on the assumption that it is the peer reaction that serves as a positive social reinforcer. If peer attention can maintain disruptive behavior, might it not also be used to strengthen desirable behavior? Solomon and Wahler (1973) demonstrated that this is indeed possible. They asked five children in a sixth-grade class of 30 students to help selected target children improve their school performance. It was explained that these children's poor performance was due to their disruptive behavior and that this could be altered by ignoring the disruptive and attending to appropriate behavior. In a brief training session these change agents were then taught how to discriminate between disruptive and appropriate behavior and how to respond to each. The results were striking. Classroom observations showed that during baseline all of the children in the class directed 100 percent of their social attention to the target children's disruptive behavior which occurred at a very high rate. When the five change agents then used the DRO procedure they had been taught, this disruptive behavior decreased while the desirable behavior increased. A reversal design permitted the investigators to demonstrate that the changes in the target children's behavior coincided with the introduction and termination of the treatment procedure.

The peer therapists who participated in the study just cited had been selected on the basis of their popularity among the children and the teacher's perception of their potential willingness to cooperate with the adults. In an investigation reported by Sanders and Glynn (1977) peers with both high and low popularity were trained to be therapists for their disruptive classmates. This showed that both types of peers can succeed in improving the behavior of the children to whom they are assigned. One might wonder whether the role of peer therapist has a negative effect on these children's acceptance by their classmates; whether they come to be seen as "teacher's pet." Sanders and Glynn (1977) looked into this by examining the sociometric preference scores of peer therapists before and after their project. They found that those whose scores had been low showed significant improvement (became more popular), while those with initially high scores remained high. Using peers as therapists thus seems to have the desirable by-product of increasing the popularity of initially unpopular children. The approach seems to have much promise, particularly in treating behavior that occurs in situations where adult influence is limited. Interestingly, it does not seem necessary that the peers chosen to assist as therapists be particularly intelligent because Drabman and Spitalnik (1973b) report an instance where a 14-year-old with an IQ score of 42 served as contingency manager and was as effective as a teacher in reducing the disruptive behavior of two of his peers.

SELF-MANAGEMENT

If improvement of classroom behavior does not require the ongoing presence of a trained therapist but can be placed in the hands of teachers, teacher-assistants, and other children, the obvious next step is to ask whether the disruptive children themselves might be able to learn how to control their own behavior. This question has been raised both by investigators who work in the operant tradition (e.g., Drabman, Spitalnik, & O'Leary, 1973) and by those who approach the modification of behavior from a cognitive point of view (e.g., Meichenbaum, 1977). Both approaches suggest that this might be a promising direction to pursue.

Self-monitoring

In order to teach children to control their own disruptive behavior it is first necessary to induce them to monitor their own actions and to do so in an accurate manner. As with other covert behavior, the person trying to teach this must have a way of checking the self-monitoring so that the child must be asked to keep a record of the behavior in question that someone else can inspect. There is some indication that the very act of keeping a record of one's own behavior may result in a change in the frequency of that behavior. For example, Broden, Hall, and Mitts (1971) instructed an eighth-grade boy to keep a record of the number of times he talked in class without permission by making a check mark on a small card. When this procedure was first introduced it seemed to result in a decrease of the target behavior which increased again when recording was discontinued. Upon subsequent reinstatement of the recording, however, there was only a slight, insignificant improvement, leading to the conclusion that merely keeping a record of one's own behavior may have a positive, but transitory effect on that behavior. In the case of a girl who recorded whether or not she was studying in class, Broden et al., (1971) found that her study behavior increased and remained high. Here, however, the records were turned in at the end of the week to the counselor who would then praise her for improved performance. With the girl, then, the self-recording was tied to a positive consequence while in the case of the boy it was an end in itself. This, plus the fact that the girl had asked for help with her problem while the boy had not expressed any concern about his may well have been responsible for the different effect in the two cases. It is noteworthy that with neither of these children was there much correlation between the records they kept themselves and those maintained by classroom observers. The changes in their behavior must have been more a function of the act of self-monitoring than of the accuracy of their records. Conceivably, it is not so much the keeping of a record as the focusing of attention on one's own actions that leads to the observed changes in behavior. The accuracy of self-recording is nonetheless an important issue, particularly when a child is to receive reinforcement on the basis of that record.

Keeping a record of one's own behavior entails two steps, either of which may lead to an inaccurate record. First one must be able to evaluate one's own behavior correctly, to know, as in the two cases just cited, whether one is or is not studying, is or is not talking out of turn. If the self-evaluation is accurate the question of accurate recording essentially becomes a function of honesty or, to put it in more behavioral terms, of the consequences one anticipates for keeping a valid record. If a child is reinforced for a record that ostensibly shows improvement in behavior whether or not this has taken place, there is a likelihood that the record will be falsified in the direction of improvement. On the other hand, if there is some way of checking so that turning in a falsified record has aversive consequences, the validity of the records should increase. Drabman, Spitalnik, and O'Leary (1973) demonstrated in an after-school program for disturbed children that it is not only possible to teach honest self-evaluation but that such evaluation, when incorporated in a token reinforcement program, can significantly reduce disruptive classsroom behavior. A replication of this study, conducted by Turkewitz, O'Leary, and Ironsmith (1975), showed that the improvement in behavior brought about by such a procedure can be maintained after the back-up reinforcers are withdrawn. Unfortunately, the improvement held only in the special setting where it had been acquired and did not generalize to the children's regular classroom. We shall return to a discussion of the issue of generalization and maintenance of improvement after looking at one other aspect of self-management, the self-delivery of reinforcers.

Self-reinforcement

In a completely self-contained program of self-management, an individual would first have to determine that his or her behavior should be changed. Following this, the person would have to set the direction and goal of such change, record his or her responses, evaluate the progress made, and then provide the reinforcers for such progress. There is no report of such a program ever having been carried out by a disruptive child; in fact, it would be difficult to imagine how a report of such solitary self-treatment by a child could find its way into the literature. For that matter, when O'Leary and O'Leary (1976) reviewed the topic of self-management of classroom behavior, they found no study where disruptive children themselves had determined the goals of an intervention.

As far as the self-delivery of reinforcers is concerned, we have a report by Bolstad and Johnson (1972) who compared self-regulation and externally imposed regulation procedures in the treatment of disruptive children in first- and second-grade classes. They selected the four most disruptive children in each of 10 classrooms and, following baseline observations, taught two of these children in each classroom to observe their own disruptive behavior. This began with a phase in which the children's records of their self-observations were compared with the records of observers and where reinforcement was contingent on obtaining an accurate match between the two records. Following this, the children continued to maintain their own records and awarded themselves points contingent on the limited frequency of their disruptive behavior. Although the back-up reinforcers for these points continued to be dispensed by an adult so that the children may not have perceived the reinforcements to be entirely under their own control, the value of the back-up reinforcer was clearly a function of the points they had awarded themselves. In the final phase of this study back-up reinforcers were no longer available and one group of children who had monitored their own behavior was asked to continue their self-observations.

Of the various comparisons made by Bolstad and Johnson (1972) that of particular relevance to this discussion is the one between the children who had monitored their own behavior and the children whose behavior had been monitored by adults. While the disruptive behavior of both these groups decreased relative to a control group, the children who had monitored their own behavior behaved slightly better than those who had been externally monitored and this advantage persisted during the extinction phase when back-up reinforcers were no longer available. As these investigators conclude, self-regulation procedures are not only capable of reducing disruptive behavior, but even young children are able accurately to observe and record their own behavior. Not unlike the finding reported by Drabman and Lahey (1974), the present study also disclosed that the behavior of untreated disruptive control children improves while their peers participate in a systematic program designed to reduce disruptive behavior. This spread of effect thus appears to be a real phenomenon and not an artifact of one study, suggesting that in a classroom with several disruptive children it may not be necessary to treat each one of them in order to improve the behavior of all.

Self-punishment

Self-management procedures reviewed thus far all involved the delivery of positive reinforcement for increases of appropriate or decreases of inappropriate classroom behavior. In the study by Bolstad and Johnson (1972) children could award themselves eight points for having fewer than five disruptive episodes per session, four points for fewer than 10, and none for more than 10. In that sense, disruptive behavior resulted indirectly in the loss of reinforcers but such loss was implicit in the economy by which the points were dispensed. It is also possible to arrange a contingency where disruptive behavior leads directly to a loss of something of value, such as points or tokens that are already in the child's possession. This would be a response-cost contingency and when such a contingency reduces the disruptive behavior it would have to be considered a form of punishment. To use a more familiar expression, it is a fine for misbehaving.

If children can be taught to be in charge of rewarding themselves for appropriate behavior, can they also be put in charge of fining themselves for inappropriate behavior? Kaufman and O'Leary (1972) examined this issue in a study of disruptive adolescents who, as residents of a psychiatric hospital, attended the hospital school. In a teacher-managed program these investigators had found no difference in the effectiveness to reduce disruptive behavior and increase academic performance between systems where the boys earned rewards for positive or were fined for negative behavior. After three months, the evaluations of behavior that led to these consequences were turned over to the boys themselves and it was found that this procedure was as effective as the teacher-managed system, regardless of whether it involved reward or response-cost. This is particularly interesting in view of the fact that the boys' self-evaluations bore little resemblance to the evaluations that the teacher continued to maintain. The boys were found to give themselves the highest ratings possible but despite the fact that their records were inaccurate they continued to exhibit low rates of disruptive behavior. It is thus not clear whether the self-evaluations and their consequences were indeed instrumental in maintaining the improved behavior that had originally been established when the teacher was in charge of the system. What would have happened if the self-evaluations had come at the beginning of the program? A study by Humphrey, Karoly, and Kirschenbaum (1978) addresses this question.

Working with nine boys and nine girls, 7 to 9 years old, and attending a second-grade reading class of 22 children in an urban public school, Humphrey et al. (1978) compared the effectiveness of self-reward and self-imposed response-cost in facilitating increased academic and decreased disruptive behavior in the classroom. Reward and response-cost contingencies were based only on the children's performance with their reading workbooks; no contingencies were applied directly to disruptive behavior. Under the response-cost condition, the children began the session with a supply of tokens, equal to the maximum number that could be earned by the self-reward group running concurrently. The children would fine themselves for inaccurate or incompleted work by removing a designated number of tokens from their supply and placing them in a "bank." The reverse of this procedure was in effect for the children working under the reward condition. There, the child would take possession of tokens depending on the quality and amount of work he or she had done. All tokens, those still owned by the response-cost children and those earned by the reward children, could be exchanged for back-up reinforcers later in the day. There was little opportunity for manipulating these consequences dishonestly because the rate and accuracy of the work performed was easily checked by the teacher who also knew how many tokens the children had in their possession at the end of each session. The research design led one group of children to experience the response-cost condition before the reward condition while the other group followed this sequence in reverse. A baseline condition, when neither contingency was in effect, preceded the first intervention phase and was interposed between the two forms of intervention.

The results of this study by Humphrey et al. (1978), show that regardless of the order in which they occurred, both self-reward and self-imposed response-cost procedures improved the children's reading rate and accuracy but that reward was somewhat more effective than response-cost. Disruptive behavior which, as pointed out, had not been the direct target of intervention, decreased by about 34 percent from baseline regardless of whether self-reward or self-imposed response-cost procedures were in effect. There was, however, considerable variability in the rate of disruptive behavior so that, from the point of view of disruption as a target of intervention, this study is at best suggestive.

An approach that combined response-cost with a self-instruction procedure was reported by Kendall and Finch (1976) who consider their treatment to be based on a cognitive approach. Though they refer to the 9-year-old boy with whom they worked as an impulsive child, the description of him as "an aggressive, feisty, and uncooperative child" and the fact that he was "a behavior problem in the classroom" suggests that a discussion of this case under the rubric of disruptive behavior is not inappropriate. The focus of the treatment was on the boy's pronounced tendency to switch conversational topics, activities, and rules of play in an inappropriate and untimely manner. He was trained in verbal self-instruction, following the procedure pioneered by Meichenbaum and Goodman (1971), which, in this child's case, focused on finishing a task or a topic before switching to a new one. The therapist would first model self-instruction and then have the boy verbalize it aloud. After an additional modeling by the therapist the boy was instructed to perform a task while saying the instructions silently to himself. The child was then given five dimes which, in line with the self-instructions, he was allowed to keep if he completed the task without switching but from which he had to pay a 10-cent fine for each instance of inappropriate switching. Employing a multiple-baseline design across targets (topics, games, and rules) these investigators were able to demonstrate that the frequency of switching decreased to near zero as a result of the treatment procedure. What is more, the boy's behavior and performance in school improved and the gains he had made were maintained over a six-month follow-up period. Given the fact that this boy's treatment had consisted of eight 50-minute sessions, this result is indeed remarkable.

GENERALIZATION AND MAINTENANCE

The success Kendall and Finch (1976) had with their intervention can probably be attributed partly to their effort to build generalization into the treatment procedure. This, as O'Leary and O'Leary (1976), among others, have pointed out, must be considered an essential part of any treatment program for it is not sufficient to teach children to behave appropriately in but one setting and only during a limited period of time. Explicit steps must be taken to assure that this improvement in behavior is also manifested in other settings (generalization) and that it lasts beyond the termination of the treatment program (maintenance).

The method Kendall and Finch (1976) had employed to achieve generalization was to conduct treatment in a variety of rooms, on a variety of tasks and topics, and under the direction of two different therapists. This probably prevented the newly learned responses from coming under the control of a limited number of stimulus conditions so that the appropriate behavior was more readily generalized to such other settings as the classroom. In addition, the self-instructions the boy had been taught can be presumed to have functioned as covert stimuli that he carried with him from place to place although there is no evidence that this is indeed what happened. By combining the response-cost procedure with self-instruction Kendall and Finch both here (1976) and elsewhere (1978) are unable to ascertain which of the ingredients of their treatment package is primarily responsible for the behavior changes they demonstrate or whether it is only in combination that they produce the observed effect. While it is intuitively attractive to expect training in self-instruction to have a high potential for facilitating generalization and maintenance of treatment benefits, thus far this procedure lacks convincing evidence that it does indeed possess that capacity (Meichenbaum & Asarnow, 1979). When Varni and Henker (1979) introduced self-instruction, self-monitoring, and self-reinforcement in sequential fashion with three disruptive ("hyperactive") boys they found that self-instruction failed to improve performance unless an adult was in the room monitoring the behavior of the child and that self-monitoring did not significantly affect responding. But when a combination of self-monitoring and self-reinforcement techniques was introduced (on top of the previously taught self-instruction) all three children showed improved levels of academic performance and a reciprocal decrease in their disruptive behavior. By conducting their treatment both in the clinic and in the children's classroom, these investigators were able to attain improvement in both settings but that, of course, is not evidence for generalization.

Among other methods that have been tried in order to enhance generalization and maintenance of treatment effects are those which Walker and Buckley (1972) incorporated into their experimental strategy. These involved having the peers of the disruptive child selectively attend to his appropriate behavior, establishing common elements in both the regular and the experimental classrooms, and giving teachers explicit training in techniques based on behavioral principles. While the research design of that study had certain flaws (Cone,

1973), it did demonstrate that any of the three methods employed resulted in generalization and maintenance over a two-month follow-up period. The problem with these interventions is that each calls for deviation from typical classroom procedures, thereby providing the disruptive child with a so-called prosthetic environment that supports his or her improved behavior. The same was true of the case study reported by Epstein and Goss (1978) where a 10-year-old disruptive boy continued to need the teacher's special attention in order to maintain improvement based on a self-control procedure. Ideally, as O'Leary and O'Leary (1976) have pointed out, a child's appropriate classroom behavior should be controlled and maintained by the stimulus and reinforcement conditions that are naturally available in the typical classroom situation. One should not expect to "reprogram" the peers or the teacher for the benefit of an individual child though one might hope that as the basic principles of reinforcement theory come to be more generally incorporated in the training of teachers they would routinely enhance desirable and reduce undesirable behavior by selectively reinforcing the former and ignoring the latter.

Recapitulation

Behavior that interferes with the classroom missions of teaching and learning is a problem of considerable concern to those responsible for children's education. Such actions as not remaining in one's seat, talking out of turn, throwing objects, or making noise have therefore been the focus of much study intended to devise effective methods for reducing this disruptive behavior so that constructive studying can take its place and be strengthened. Relatively mild forms of disruptive behavior can be controlled in the classroom by having the teacher differentially attend to desirable and ignore undesirable behavior, but teachers often find that the latter cannot be ignored. In that case, occasional reprimands, delivered so that only the offending child can hear them, may serve to maintain a classroom atmosphere conducive to learning. When disruptive behavior reaches proportions where in-class procedures are ineffective, social isolation imposed contingent on the occurrence of such behavior can be a powerful intervention but the many potential pitfalls inherent in the use of this method make it a procedure of last resort to be used with great circumspection. Positive practice is a negative consequence that has much to recommend it because it has a strong educative component. It is a recently developed procedure that shows much promise for reducing disruptive and other inappropriate behavior. Thus far, however, the most frequently used and extensively studied procedure for the reinforcement of desirable classroom behavior entails the use of tokens. Among the questions relating to their use that have been investigated are their effect on other children in the classroom who are not covered by the token procedure, alternatives such as home-based programs, and the feasibilty of having a child's peers administer the reinforcing consequences.

Having moved the responsibility for inducing behavior change with disruptive children from the outside therapist, to the child's teacher, parents, and peers, the next logical step was to explore whether the disruptive children could be taught to control their own behavior. Research has show that children can indeed learn to monitor their own actions and to use reinforcers so as to increase the behavior adults deem desirable. Since most of the studies dealing with the reduction of disruptive behavior have taken place in specialized settings and over relatively short periods of time, the question whether improvements thus obtained will generalize to the child's natural environment and remain effective over an extended time span is currently a priority item on the agenda of investigations in the field of child behavior therapy.

11

Excessive Avoidance Behavior: Fears and Phobias

GENERAL CONSIDERATIONS

Avoidance responses that are regularly emitted in the presence of specific stimuli or classes of stimuli are usually attributed to fear and when these responses are so vigorous as to interfere with a person's functioning the condition may be labeled a phobia. These avoidance responses are often accompanied by facial and verbal expressions that we call fearful and with specialized laboratory equipment it is sometimes possible to demonstrate that physiological changes in breathing, heart rate, or skin conductance are correlated with the observed behavior. Thus, while fear is an inferred internal state it has sufficient observable correlates to make the term useful in a discussion of behavior disorders and their treatment. Nonetheless, because the observable correlates do not always appear together, often varying from individual to individual, a therapist is well-advised not to assume that all avoidance behavior is a reflection of fear.

In the discussion of social skill deficits (Chapter 2) we encountered children whose withdrawal from peers seemed the result of their lacking the skills needed for appropriate peer interaction. For these children, the treatment focus was on establishing the skills in which they were deficient. A casual observer might have attributed the social withdrawal of these children to fear and the picture is complicated by the fact that deficient approach skills and excess avoidance responses may be presented by the same child. Not possessing the skill needed for adaptive interaction with peers, a child may be teased or attacked by them and thus come to fear and avoid other children. On the other hand, a child who had once interacted with other children but had a number of aversive experiences in the course of such interactions may have come to fear peers and, avoiding them, failed to maintain the age-appropriate skills needed for adaptive interaction. This relationship between fear and skill is probably often entailed in the refusal to attend school, which is usually labeled *school phobia*. Afraid of school and therefore avoiding it, a girl falls behind in the school work and then fears returning even more because in going back to school she might encounter academic failure. Conversely, a boy who is not doing well academically may find school so aversive that he refuses to go there, whereupon the extended absence results in even greater academic retardation. In either instance the children would need help not only in overcoming their fear of school but also in catching up with the academic skills appropriate for their grade level.

Whatever form the treatment of fears and phobias may take and, as we shall see, there are many, the goal must always be to enable the child to approach the previously avoided people, situations, animals, or objects and to be able to interact with them in an age-appropriate, constructive manner. This often calls not only for fear reduction but also for skill training and the most effective forms of treatment have usually been those which focus on both of these goals, often by using a combination of several methods.

The rigorous requirements of careful research often demand that only one treatment method be used in order to test its effectiveness, but the requirements of good clinical practice call for a far more flexible use of various methods, often making it impossible to know which of these represents the effective ingredient of the treatment combination. This dilemma was recognized as long ago as 1924 when Mary Cover Jones published her pioneering study on the elimination of children's fears (Jones, 1924b). Having tried to remove the marked fears of 70 individual children, ranging in age from 3 months to 7 years, using such methods as distraction, ridicule, exhortation, extinction, and exposure, Jones found that what we would now call counterconditioning and observational learning alone resulted in unqualified success. At the end of her report, Jones (1924b) states, "It should be noted that apart from laboratory analysis we have rarely used any of the above procedures in pure form. Our aim has been to cure the fears by the group of devices most appropriate at any given stage of treatment" (p. 390). This previously cited statement is quoted here again because in what follows, the material has been organized around discrete treatment approaches, many of which should, in practice, be combined in such a fashion as to provide maximum benefit to the child in treatment.

SYSTEMATIC DESENSITIZATION

The origin of behavior therapy with children may be traced to the early work of Jones who, in the classical case of Peter (Jones, 1924a), employed a method she called "direct conditioning." Based on the principles of respondent conditioning, it entailed the paired presentation of a fear-arousing stimulus (a rabbit) with a stimulus presumed to elicit a fear-incompatible response (food). The treatment is described in the following words:

> During a period of craving for food, the child is placed in a high chair and given something to eat. The fear-object is brought in, starting a negative response. It is then moved away gradually until it is at a sufficient distance not to interfere with the child's eating. The relative strength of the fear impulse and the hunger impulse may be gauged by the distance to which it is necessary to remove the fear-object. While the child is eating, the object is slowly brought nearer to the table, then placed upon the table, and finally as the tolerance increases it is brought close enough to be touched (Jones, 1924b, p. 388).

Treated by this method daily or twice daily for a period of two months, Peter (aged 2 years, 10 months at the time) was eventually able to fondle the rabbit affectionately and to let it nibble at his fingers. The fear response had apparently been replaced by fearless behavior that had presumably been elicited by the favored food, a sequence that would now be labeled counterconditioning or, since it also entailed graded exposure, systematic desensitization.

We qualified the above summary by the words "apparently" and "presumably" not in order to minimize the remarkable contribution of Jones but because this case study lacks the necessary controls that would permit one to have confidence that the observed result was, in fact, due to the principles on which the treatment was based. Circumspection is called for, in particular, because Jones (1924a) reports that occasionally other children who did not fear the rabbit were brought in to help with the "unconditioning." It is of course not known to what extent Peter's improvement was the result of this modeling of approach behavior. Before turning to a discussion of more recent work, it is well to quote Jones's important cautionary note regarding the pairing of fear-evoking with fear-incompatible stimuli. She writes:

> This method obviously requires delicate handling. Two response systems are being dealt with: food leading to a positive reaction, and fear-object leading to a negative reaction. The desired conditioning should result in transforming the fear-object into a source of positive response (substitute stimulus). But a careless manipulator could readily produce the reverse result, attaching a fear reaction to the sight of food (Jones, 1924b, p. 389).

Behavioral methods of treatment are often straightforward and seem easy to apply but Jones's caveat should be heeded by anyone who seeks to change the behavior of another, whether by this or any other procedure, because the change may not always be in the desired direction. Intervening in the lives of others is a grave responsibility, not to be undertaken lightly nor without appropriate training.

Putative Principles and Practical Procedures

In what Jones (1924a) called the "method of direct conditioning," she paired the presentation of the feared rabbit with the ingestion of a favored food on the assumption that the food would elicit an emotion, such as pleasure, that would become associated with the rabbit and replace the fear that had previously been elicited by such an animal. This approach to treating fears entails the further assumption that pleasure and fear are mutually exclusive, incompatible emotions so that once pleasure has become the conditioned response to the stimulus of the rabbit, this stimulus will no longer elicit the fear. This notion that one emotion is replaced by another, more desirable emotion led Wolpe (1958) to speak of *therapy by reciprocal inhibition* and to give currency to the term *counterconditioning*.

Because fear is an internal state that is usually inferred from observing such behavior as avoidance responses or verbal statements, it is not known whether the theoretical formulation based on the principles of respondent conditioning is, in fact, what accounts for the frequently documented improvement that follows treatment by what is now usually called *systematic desensitization*. By omitting reference to conditioning, this term leaves open the question about the process that underlies the procedure, stressing instead the systematically graded, gradual exposure to the feared object. Yet, as Davison and Wilson (1973) have pointed out, it is not even clear whether that is the crucial ingredient of this form of treatment. All we really know on the basis of what can be observed is that clients who had avoided a given object are able to approach that object following exposure to a multifaceted experience labeled treatment. Have such clients simply learned previously missing approach skills? Have they acquired the means for controlling their own fears as Goldfried (1971) among others suggests? How much of the change in clients' behavior is due to the positive social reinforcement provided them by the implicit or explicit approval they receive from the therapist for making approach response to the previously avoided (feared) object? Given all of these imponderables, therapists in clinical practice rarely worry about the theoretical niceties that might explain what makes systematic desensitization work but do what Jones (1924b) did so long ago, combine various techniques in more or less systematic fashion. A case in point is the work by Obler and Terwilliger (1970), highlighted by the critique (Begelman & Hersen, 1971) and rebuttal (Terwilliger & Obler, 1971) it engendered.

From among a group of 150 neurologically impaired children who exhibited severe phobias, Obler and Terwilliger (1970) selected 30 who were extremely fearful either regarding the use of a public bus or about seeing a live dog. Fifteen of these children were randomly chosen for individual treatment, while the remaining 15 served as controls, matched for age, sex, intelligence, and phobic object. Fifteen college graduates who had received 10 hours of training in the application of a modified form of systematic desensitization served as therapists, each working with one child who was assigned on a random basis. The intervention consisted of a five-hour-long session per week for 10 weeks. At the beginning of treatment the therapist would ask the child to look at pictures or models of the stimulus (dog or bus) that was the object of the child's phobia. Once the child seemed able to tolerate exposure to these representations of the phobic object, the therapist would gradually proceed to expose the child to the actual object, continuously offering encouragement for moving closer to the bus or dog. Eventually the children were able to touch the previously feared object. At this point each child was given the opportunity to be exposed to the stimulus without the therapist being present. Reinforcement was now shifted from the therapist's encouraging praise statements to the presentation of a concrete prize such as toys, books, pets, or candy. These were dispensed immediately upon the child's having successfully completed the defined task, such as talking to the bus driver, placing a token in the fare box, or remaining in a room together with a dog.

The effectiveness of this treatment was measured by a parent rating scale that had been administered prior to and again at the end of the treatment. Among 10 questions dealing with the child's functioning in school, peer relations, and other aspects of behavior, one dealt specifically with the child's bus or dog phobia. This asked whether the child had recently been able to ride a bus (touch a dog) and if so, whether with the help of another person or completely alone. Since the investigators assumed that the parents did not know that their child was to be treated or had been treated for the phobia, they viewed the responses to these questions as providing them with a valid measure of treatment outcome. At the beginning of treatment, none of the children had been able to approach the phobic object but at the end all but one of the 15 children had improved, eight now able to make the approach unassisted and seven able to do so when accompanied by another person. Only two of the children in the untreated control group showed some improvement in that they were able to make contact with the phobic object with the assistance or in the company of another person.

Obler and Terwilliger (1970) ascribe the significant change in the treated children's phobic avoidance behavior to what they call their "modified systematic desensitization method'' but, as Begelman and Hersen (1971) pointed out in their critique of that study, the treatment of these children included several distinguishable techniques beyond systematic desensitization. As originally introduced by Wolpe (1958) in work with adults and modified by Lazarus and Abramovitz (1965) for work with children, graded approximations of the feared object are presented by instructing the client to imagine these while either in a state of relaxation (Wolpe) or while visualizing pleasant scenes, as in the method of "emotive imagery" (Lazarus & Abramovitz). Believing that the relatively nonverbal, unimaginative, intellectually retarded children with whom they were working would not be able to follow the verbal instructions needed to evoke such images, Obler and Terwilliger (1970) developed the modification of using models or pictures and then the phobic object itself, thus placing the child in "direct confrontation with the fear-producing stimulus, but with the therapist acting as a buffer between the two" (p. 316). Of course such *in vivo exposure* (or *active participation*, as Hatzenbuehler and Schroeder [1978] call it) was not originated by Obler and Terwilliger (1970), inasmuch as Jones (1924a) had gradually exposed Peter to a live rabbit, employing the dimension of distance. As had Jones, Obler and Terwilliger also mixed procedures in order to help the children for whom they had assumed therapeutic responsibility.

Begelman and Hersen (1971) observe rather critically that the Obler and Terwilliger (1970) method contained a distinct operant component in that the therapist sought to reinforce the child by praise statements and tangible rewards for moving closer and closer to the feared object. This, of course, is the process of successive approximation or shaping that is used in work based on the principles of operant learning (Skinner, 1953). In addition, the fact that the therapist accompanied the child in approaching the feared object may well have introduced aspects of observational learning in that the therapist served as a fearless model. Begelman and Hersen (1971) list several additional elements that might have played a role in the treatment of these phobic children and question whether its effectiveness was indeed a consequence of systematic desensitization, as Obler and Terwilliger (1970) had assumed.

In their rebuttal to the criticism Begelman and Hersen (1971) had raised about their work, Terwilliger and Obler (1971) highlight an issue that plagues almost all research on clinical procedures. It is the dilemma based on the fact that the requirements of rigorous research and the demands of clinical practice are often incompatible. Investigators must often choose between doing well-controlled research on problems with relatively little direct clinical relevance or studying meaningful clinical problems with somewhat loose research methodology. Even the best clinical research usually is a compromise in which some methodological rigor has to be sacrificed in order to study a problem under conditions where some constraints must be placed on the therapists' flexibility. These constraints may entail the use of a therapy manual that all therapists are expected to follow, with the investigator taking steps to assure that they do, so that the independent variable can be clearly specified.

When 15 different individuals are given 10 hours of training and then work with phobic children in weekly five-hour meetings over a 10-week period without a check on whether they are really following the instruction "not to deviate from the training procedures through the course of treatment" (Obler & Terwilliger, 1970, p. 316), it calls for an act of faith to accept the investigators' description of their therapeutic procedure as a veridical statement of what transpired during the contact between the children and their therapist. Terwilliger and Obler (1971) acknowledge this when they write, "The aim was not to do in vivo desensitization per se, but to do therapy on brain-injured patients. That consideration rather than methodological concerns determined the use of 'in vivo' tactics" (p. 15).

Obler and Terwilliger (1971) also agree that variables other than desensitization, such as shaping and modeling, were highly likely to have played a role in the treatment of the children. It can be argued that whenever a therapist and a client work together in the course of treatment, their social interaction may contribute to the client's improvement, whether by the therapist's modeling coping behavior, by the therapist's implicit approval of the client's adaptive responses serving as reinforcement that shapes behavior, or by other subtle (and possibly still unknown) factors. Obler and Terwilliger (1970) should not be faulted for having failed to use a pure distillate of systematic desensitization as their treatment method but they can be taken to task for not having recognized that they were dealing with an amalgam of procedures that, by design, contained a large proportion of operant aspects inasmuch as they had "intensively instructed [their therapists] in how to dispense the rewards in attempting to decondition the monophobia" (p. 316).

Variations and Combinations

As originally developed by Wolpe (1958) for use with adults, the counterconditioning method for reducing fears and phobias requires that the client be able to imagine fear-eliciting scenes so that these can be paired, in a carefully graded sequence, with a fear-incompatible state of relaxation which the client has previously been taught to assume at the therapist's request. Therapists working with young children have reported that their clients have difficulty learning to relax, imagining appropriate stimuli, or following the instructions for the procedure. Tasto (1969), for example, though able to teach a four-year-old boy relaxation, was unsuccessful in getting him to experience anxiety to imagined loud noises, which were the object of his phobia. Like others, he turned to an *in vivo* procedure, presenting a series of noises in gradually increasing volume thereby overcoming the child's problem.

Wish, Hasazi, and Jurgela (1973) report similar experience with an 11-year-old boy whose fears centered around loud sounds, such as thunder, fire-crackers, or jet engines. This boy was not only able to learn muscle relaxation but he also participated in establishing a fear hierarchy, a list of various sounds arranged in the order of the discomfort (anxiety) they elicited. These sounds were then recorded on tape and the boy was instructed to listen to them after first having relaxed himself. This "automated direct deconditioning" as the authors call it, combined with reinforcement for each completed session, succeeded in eliminating this child's phobia within eight days and a follow-up nine months later showed that his tolerance for the previously feared noises was maintained.

In their review of the use of desensitization procedures in the treatment of fearful and phobic children, Hatzenbuehler and Schroeder (1978) differentiate between methods based on passive association and those involving active participation. The case of Peter (Jones, 1924a) is an example of passive association in that the therapist brought the feared stimulus to the child. Active participation, on the other hand, is exemplified by the study by Obler and Terwilliger (1970) where the children were taken to the feared stimulus, such as a bus. While the distinction between passive association and active participation might be useful in making plans for treatment, it probably does not represent a true dichotomy. As Hatzenbuehler and Schroeder (1978) themselves recognize, the two types of desensitization are probably best construed as two processes on a continuum of gradual exposure to the feared stimulus. In the case of Peter, for example, the therapist at first brought the feared rabbit closer and closer to the passive child but once Peter was playing with the rabbit, he was obviously engaged in active participation. It may be true, as these reviewers further state, that a child who exhibits severe avoidance behavior might best be started in treatment with a method involving passive association but that, as the child's tolerance for the stimulus increases or with children whose problem is less severe, active participation becomes the method of choice. Active participation is, after all, the ultimate goal of any treatment aimed at permitting a person to interact with a stimulus that had previously elicited fear and avoidance responses.

There are many case reports in the literature that deal with the treatment of fearful or phobic children by using direct participation. The problems include a 4-year-old's water phobia (Pomerantz, Peterson, Marholin, & Stern, 1977), and the fear of high buildings by a seven-year-old (Croghan & Musante, 1975). In the latter case, the therapist would take the child on walks during which they approached high buildings while engaging in various games. This playful interaction with the therapist presumably furnished the positive emotional response that was being paired with the fear-eliciting tall buildings but here, as in most of these studies, the basis of the child's improvement can only be surmised, especially since the child also received rewards and praise at the end of each session. A mixture of methods that are presumably based on respondent conditioning principles with various forms of reinforcement that are typically used in operant approaches can be found in almost every report of the treatment of fears and phobias in children. Tasto (1969), for example, had the child's father place a coin inside a balloon so that, when the child popped the balloon, tolerating the noise this made, he was able to obtain and keep the coin. Like Obler and Terwilliger (1970) who, as we have seen, had also confounded respondent and operant principles, Tasto (1969) referred to his approach as systematic desensitization. One need not make a shibboleth of conceptual purity or proscribe from clinical practice any procedure that does not fit a particular theoretical framework, but knowledge will not be advanced so long as we are unable to identify the ingredients of the treatment procedures being used. As Hatzenbuehler and Schroeder (1978) concluded from their review of desensitization procedures in the treatment of childhood disorders, "data on desensitization have advanced little past anecdotal records and offer little improvement over the case study level of investigation" (p. 841).

One of the few instances where the investigators explicitly recognized that they were using both respondent and operant approaches was a report by Lazarus, Davison, and Polefka (1965) who treated a 9-year-old boy's *school phobia*. They first reduced this boy's intense fear of school by exposing him to school-related stimuli in gradually more difficult steps that were accompanied by the presentation of anxiety-reducing stimuli. In the company of a therapist whom the boy seemed to like and who might thus be viewed as an elicitor of responses that were incompatible with anxiety, he took his first walk to school on a Sunday. The following day, he and his therapist walked together from the house to the schoolyard while the therapist sought to elicit from the boy anxiety-reducing, pleasant ideation. On subsequent days, the boy visited the empty classroom after school hours, then entered the classroom with the therapist for a brief chat with the teacher, and only after a week of such in vivo desensitization did the child spend the entire morning in the classroom while the therapist waited outside. Throughout all this, approaching the school was actively reinforced by the therapist's praise and attention. Since, at the same time, as many as possible of the reinforcements attendant on staying at home during school hours were removed, the operant contingencies had, in effect, been reversed. Before treatment, the boy had received a great deal of attention and parental solicitude while staying home. Now he received praise and attention for going to school. While this case report differs from most others in the fact that the investigators made explicit what principles of learning they were using, it still lacks any experimental controls that might enable one to ascertain what aspects of the treatment (if any) were responsible for the reported improvement. There is, in fact, only one study of the effect of systematic desensitization on the treatment of fears and phobias of children in which the problem was approached in a well-controlled fashion. It is the work of Miller, Barrett, Hampe, and Noble (1972) and its follow-up by Hampe, Noble, Miller, and Barrett (1973).

Evaluative Research

In order to compare the effect of treatment on children's phobias, Miller, Barrett, Hampe, and Noble (1972) randomly assigned 67 phobic children between the ages of 6 and 15 to one of three conditions. One group received systematic desensitization, another play therapy, and the third remained untreated as a waiting list control. The fears and phobias of the majority of these children (69 percent) centered on school, some (9 percent) feared sleeping alone, 6 percent feared the dark, and the rest had diverse fears of such things as dogs, heights, and deep water. The number of fears per child ranged from seven, exhibited by one child, to one, the latter representing the mode (26 children). Each type of treatment was conducted by one of two therapists to whom the children were assigned on a random basis. Following an initial assessment, treatment sessions of one hour took place three times a week for a period of eight weeks.

Miller et al. (1972) present a fairly detailed description of how they proceeded with the children who had been assigned to the systematic desensitization condition which, though conducted in the context of an experimental design, nonetheless permitted the therapist enough flexibility to respond to the demands of the clinical situation. Thus, no constraint was placed on the therapist in coordinating the treatment with school personnel or other significant persons in the child's life. One of the parents was usually seen together with the child for the first 15 minutes of the session and on occasion the therapist would spend an entire session with the parent present "in order to deal with resistance problems, parental guilt, or other clinical phenomena that the therapist judged to be likely to threaten continuation of the child in treatment" (p. 271). Where necessary, the contingencies the parents were using with their children were modified, assertiveness training was given, or the parents received concurrent treatment from another therapist. Against this somewhat variable background, systematic desensitization proceeded in a fairly structured fashion which the investigators describe as follows.

> In the first session, the therapist established rapport, explained the rationale of the treatment, taught the parent to relax as a model for the child, started relaxation training with the child, and assigned a homework task of relaxation practice

10 min. a day. By the fourth session, relaxation training was usually complete as was construction of initial fear hierarchies. From this point, systematic desensitization proceeded as with adults . . . A relaxed child was asked to imagine a scene that he had listed as arousing little anxiety. If he could imagine the scene comfortably, he was asked to switch to a pleasant scene. Then he was asked to imagine the next scene in the hierarchy. If imagining a scene caused the child to signal anxiety, the therapist asked that the scene be "switched off" and that the pleasant scene be imagined again. At this point, the therapist either repeated the scene or revised the hierarchy to provide an item that aroused less anxiety. Periodically, the child was asked to describe scenes as a check on the vividness of imagery. When all items of a fear hierarchy could be imagined comfortably, an "in vivo" test was arranged. If unsuccessful, systematic desensitization continued (p. 271).

Noteworthy in this description is that these investigators seemed to have had no difficulty in teaching children as young as six years the muscle relaxation technique that Wolpe (1958) had introduced in his treatment of adults and that these children, some of whom had intelligence test scores in the 75–79 range, had been able to help construct fear hierarchies and to respond to instructions to imagine fear-arousing and pleasant scenes. All this would throw doubt on the oft-voiced assertion (e.g., Gelfand, 1978) that young children are not usually able to perform these demanding actions.

All children were reevaluated after eight weeks and again after 14 weeks, using various checklists and behavioral measures applied by a member of the research team who had not been involved in the treatment. The results showed that all three groups, those who had received either systematic desensitization or play therapy *and the no-treatment control*, showed a marked reduction of the phobias that had been the targeted problem. This discouraging finding regarding the value of the clinical treatment of children's phobias is not much improved by the fact that when the reports of the children's parents were used as the basis for outcome evaluation, those whose children had been in the treatment groups reported the remaining phobias to be significantly less severe than those whose children had been in the waiting list control. As has been shown in other studies (e.g., O'Leary, Turkewitz, & Taffel, 1973), parents tend to perceive treatment outcome more favorably than other, more objective criteria would seem to warrant. Support for the effectiveness of therapy is provided, however, when the outcome results of Miller et al. (1972) are analyzed so as to separate the data for younger (ages 6 to 10) from those of older (ages 11 to 13) children. This showed that for the young phobic children either kind of therapy had been highly effective and superior to the waiting list control. Of the 24 children in that age group, 23 had successful outcome and only 1 was a treatment failure based on severity ratings by the independent evaluator. Among the 14 young children in the waiting list control group, on the other hand, 8 were scored as improved and 6 as unimproved. The 20 older children who had received treatment showed outcomes that differed little from those of the control group. Treatment success was found with 9, failure with 11, while of the 9 children in the control group, 4 had improved and 5 had remained unchanged.

One and two years later Miller and his associates (Hampe, Noble, Miller, & Barrett, 1973) reevaluated the condition of 62 of the children who had participated in their original study. By that time many of the children who had been on the waiting list as well as those who had shown no improvement after the first eight-week course of treatment had received some form of therapy. By now, 80 percent of the children were either problem free or significantly improved and only 7 percent continued to have a severe phobia. Reflecting on the results of their study and its follow-up, Hampe et al. (1973) concluded that the justification for the treatment of children's phobias "comes from the fact that treatment greatly hastens recovery" (p. 451) but that "it is necessary to devise differentiated treatment procedures for different age groups" (p. 452). This latter statement is, of course, based on the fact that the children who were 10 years old or younger had responded to treatment so much more favorably than those who had been 11 years or older. Differentiating, in fact individualizing the treatment for different children, is typical of good clinical practice and such practice should be reflected in the design of studies on the effect or effectiveness of treatment. As Paul (1969) pointed out in his discussion of clinical research, the question to be asked is not "Does therapy work?" but, "What treatment, by whom, is most effective for this individual with that specific problem, under which set of circumstances, and how does it come about?" (p. 44).

It is very likely a mistake to assume that all avoidance behavior that someone has labeled a phobia is sufficiently alike to enable one to treat all cases by a standard method. What has been called school phobia is a case in point. The common feature of most of these cases is that the child refuses to go to school. Some of these children may do so because they have an overwhelming fear of another child at school, of a particular teacher, of failure when called upon to recite, or of the school as a physical building. Other cases of school refusal may relate to the child's fear of leaving home, separating from mother, getting on the bus, or passing a specific corner on the way to school. Still other children may find activities away from school, whether at home or on the street, so much more reinforcing than being in school, which may in fact be aversive to them, that they engage in the behavior (truanting) that is more immediately reinforcing. Only a thorough assessment of the individual case can help a therapist ascertain the most appropriate method of treatment. One reason for the remarkable success Kennedy (1965) obtains with his method of rapid treatment for school phobia may well rest, in part, on the fact that he differentiates between two distinct types of this problem. One, which he designates as Type I, has among a number of characteristics that the school refusal has an acute onset and that the child is in the first few years of school. Type II, on the other hand, is found in cases where similar episodes have occurred several times before and where the youngster is usually in the upper grades. The treatment method Kennedy (1965) describes has been successful in all of 50 Type I cases but it does not seem suitable for Type II. Since this method entails forced school attendance and parental reinforcement for such attendance it is outside the realm of systematic desensitization and entails forced exposure to which we shall turn next.

FORCED EXPOSURE

Forced exposure to the feared object is found in two treatment methods that are occasionally used with phobic children. One method, *implosion*, has the client imagine exposure to the phobic object in greatly exaggerated form (Stampfl & Levis, 1967). In the other method, *flooding*, clients are exposed to the actual situation or object that is the focus of their phobia. In both methods, anxiety is thus purposely raised under controlled conditions of treatment with the intention of helping the client overcome the phobia. The theoretical rationale for this seemingly paradoxical procedure is based on the formulation that the phobic avoidance response is acquired in terms of the avoidance learning paradigm. As outlined by Baum (1970), the fear is originally learned through respondent conditioning, possibly by the pairing of the conditioned stimulus (phobic object) with an unconditioned aversive stimulus. Subsequent encounter with the phobic object will elicit fear. The feared object is then avoided and the avoidance response is thus negatively reinforced and maintained by fear reduction. This avoidance prevents the fear response from undergoing extinction since extinction of a conditioned response requires that the individual be exposed to the conditioned stimulus under circumstances where the aversive stimulus with which it had been paired in the original conditioning situation does not appear.

Forced exposure is designed to permit the fear response to undergo extinction by providing the client with the opportunity for meeting the feared object, unpaired with the aversive stimulus that had presumably been present when the phobia was first acquired. This formulation, reflected in the folk wisdom of immediately getting back on the horse after one has fallen off, might be viewed as giving the fearful person an opportunity to discover that there is really nothing to be afraid of. Forced exposure as a method of reducing avoidance behavior has long been studied in animal laboratories (Solomon & Brush, 1956), but in clinical practice, particularly with children, it is rather rarely used because therapists are justifiably reluctant to use a procedure where "the cure may be worse than the disease." Aside from the understandable reluctance of clinicians to require children to experience the high level of stress that exposure to the phobic object would demand, there is the considerable risk that, unless the procedure is carried out with great care and skill, the child, instead of learning not to fear the phobic object, associates the therapist with the fear and henceforth refuses to cooperate with or return to treatment.

Aside from the work by Kennedy (1965), whose approach to school phobia includes aspects of flooding, forced exposure has also been used by Smith and Sharpe (1970) who treated a 13-year-old school-phobic boy. He had been absent from school for seven weeks when he began treatment. The boy was instructed to imagine highly anxiety-arousing scenes involving his worst apprehensions regarding school. After one such session, he was able to attend math, the most anxiety-arousing class for him, and after a total of four treatment sessions he returned to school full time. Smith and Sharpe (1970) report that this boy's gains were maintained and that his peer relationships and grades improved.

Another report of the clinical use of forced exposure comes from Yule, Sacks, and Hersov (1974) who worked with an 11-year-old boy with a phobia about loud noises. They began their intervention with a more benign form of treatment, *in vivo* desensitization, and only when this had failed to reduce his fears of all sudden loud noises did they turn to the more radical flooding. This took the form of having the boy agree to join the therapist in a room with a large number of inflated balloons whose bursting noise he greatly feared. The therapist then burst a number of these balloons, much to the child's distress. As the therapist continued to burst balloons, the boy's startle response diminished and he could finally be pursuaded to push balloons against a nail held by the therapist, thus creating the feared noise himself. In the first session, a total of 200 balloons were burst but the boy agreed to return for a second session on the following day when 320 balloons were noisily destroyed. By the end of this session the child had come to enjoy the procedure, enthusiastically bursting the rubber spheres. A follow-up two years later revealed that this child had exhibited no further fear of noises and that his peer relationships had improved.

Four points are noteworthy in the report of the above case study. One is that flooding was resorted to only after a less drastic form of treatment had failed. A second point is that this child was disconcerted about having his fears, desired to be relieved of them, and agreed to participate in what had been described to him as an unpleasant experience. The third point is that the boy experienced not only a forced exposure to the feared noises but that he was induced to produce these noises himself, thus gaining control over the fear-arousing stimulus and being able to anticipate its appearance. Giving the child mastery over the feared stimulus may be a useful, though not always feasible method for helping young children overcome a fear. Lastly, it should be noted that the boy's experience with bursting balloons began with the therapist modeling that behavior, thereby introducing an aspect of observational learning which, in itself, seems a potent method for the reduction of avoidance responses. We turn to this topic next.

OBSERVATIONAL LEARNING

When Jones (1924b) tested a variety of approaches for the reduction of children's fears, she found that of the methods she tried, only counterconditioning and observational learning led to unqualified success. When used to reduce a child's fear, observational learning basically entails having that child observe an adult or child model approach the feared object or engage in the feared behavior. Because the model plays such a crucial role in observational learning, the procedure is at times referred to as *modeling* though, to avoid confusion, it would seem best to limit the use of that term to describe what the model is doing in the presence of the fearful child whom one calls the observer.

Bandura (1969) who, with numerous associates and students, has contributed much of the research on which the application of observational learning to the treatment of fears and phobias is based, has suggested that its effect derives from a disinhibition of approach responses. According to this view, the avoidance responses, from which the presence of fears and phobias is usually inferred, represent an inhibition of approach responses that the individual is presumed to have in his or her repertoire but fails to emit. In a more recent formulation Bandura (1977a) supplements this conditioning view of observational learning in cognitive terms, asserting that the individual's expectations of personal efficacy are modified as a result of mastery experiences.

As pointed out earlier, a fearful child may be avoiding the feared object not only because this results in fear-reduction but also because he or she does not have the skills needed to make appropriate approach responses that might lead to reinforcement. In such instances the avoidance response would represent not merely an inhibition of available approach responses but also (or solely) a lack of required skills so that observing a model would not only serve to disinhibit but also to teach a skill. Take, for example, the case of a girl who is afraid of dogs. Observing another girl approach and play with a dog may not only result in the vicarious extinction of the avoidance response (Bandura, Grusec, & Menlove, 1967) but may also represent a demonstration of how one goes about playing with a dog, that doing so does not lead to harm, and that one can enjoy oneself in this activity. When, following these observations, the fearful girl approaches and plays with the dog she not only practices those skills but also discovers for herself that doing so is not dangerous and, in fact, fun. This would be the mastery experience that provides the individual with the expectation of personal efficacy of which Bandura (1977a) has spoken.

As research on the use of modeling procedures in the reduction of children's fears has progressed over the years, it has become customary to differentiate among three approaches: *vicarious modeling, symbolic modeling,* and *participant modeling*. In vicarious modeling children observe a live model while they themselves are not engaged in an activity related to their fears. In symbolic modeling, fearful children are shown a film or videotape that displays a model or models engaging the feared object. In participant modeling, finally, the fearful child joins a model in making a graded sequence of approach responses to the feared object or situation.

Vicarious Modeling

In one of the first studies of the use of models to reduce the avoidance behaviors of children, Bandura, Grusec, and Menlove (1967) worked with 48 nursery school children, ranging in age from three to five years all of whom had demonstrated fear of dogs in a behavioral assessment situation requiring approach to a tame and friendly dog, a cocker spaniel named Chloe. The children were divided into four groups, equated for fearfulness, each of which was exposed to a different treatment condition. Children in the first condition observed a 4-year-old boy who fearlessly modeled approach behavior toward the dog in the context of a highly enjoyable party attended by four children at a time (modeling-in-positive-context). In the second condition, the party was omitted and the children, again in groups of four, merely observed the model's approach behavior (modeling-in-neutral-context). The third condition was a control, consisting of having the children attend a cheerful party while the dog was present but nobody modeled approach behavior (exposure-in-positive-context). Lastly, a further control condition entailed having the children participate in a party where neither dog nor model was present (positive-context condition). Each of these four conditions required eight treatment sessions lasting 10 minutes and held on four consecutive days. On the fifth day and again one month later, all children were given the performance test that had been used at the beginning of the study and which assessed their willingness to approach the dog. Generalization of approach responses to another dog, a mongrel named Jenny*, was also tested during these posttreatment and follow-up sessions. Since the results demonstrated the clear superiority of the two modeling conditions, regardless of context, over mere exposure or simply having a party, it is well to examine the model's behavior in some detail.

Two different 4-year-old boys had served as models for different groups of children. Accomplices of the investigators, they were unknown to most of

---

*In a footnote to their article Bandura et al. (1967) express their gratitude to Chloe and Jenny "for their invaluable and steadfast assistance with a task that, at times, must have been most perplexing to them." These names undoubtedly belong in the annals of child behavior therapy alongside those of Jones's Peter, Risley's Ricky, Burchard and Tyler's Donny, and Lovaas's Chucky and Billy.

the children and had been chosen because they completely lacked any fear of dogs. After Chloe had been placed in a playpen across the room from where the children were seated, the model would perform a prearranged sequence of interactions with the dog, lasting approximately three minutes per session. It is noteworthy that the model's approach behaviors followed a *graded sequence*, a procedure that is analogous to the fear hierarchy used in systematic desensitization. This grading may be the critical difference between a therapeutic model and a model observed in everyday life where children with a fear of dogs can frequently observe fearless children playing with dogs without this having a therapeutic effect on their fears. Grading of the approach behavior of the model was accomplished by varying the physical restraints on the dog, the directness and closeness of the model's approach responses, and the duration of the model's contact with the animal. Thus, on the first day the dog was confined to the playpen and the model would merely express a greeting and pet her occasionally. On the following days, the model exhibited progressively longer and more active interactions with the dog, contacting her with both hands and feet, feeding her and giving her milk from a baby bottle. During the fifth session, the dog would be on a leash outside the playpen with the model walking her around and playing with her. Later the leash was removed and during the last two sessions, the model would climb into the playpen with the dog where he petted, hugged, and fed her.

   As previously stated, the results of the posttest and follow-up showed that the two modeling groups (with and without party context) improved significantly more than either of the two control groups. On a terminal performance test that required a child to remain alone in a room where the dog was confined in the playpen, 67 percent of the children who had been in the modeling groups were able to do so while only 33 percent of the children in the control groups could tolerate such exposure. A similar significant difference in favor of the modeling groups was reflected in the follow-up phase of the study where the requirement of successfully performing the described criterion task with both the familiar dog, Chloe, and the unfamiliar Jenny, was met by 42 percent of the treated but only 12 percent of the control children.

Symbolic Modeling

The use of a live model has a number of disadvantages that limit its clinical application to some extent. There is, first of all, the problem that the model must be carefully trained so that the behavior displayed is therapeutically effective. That means that the model must approach the feared object in a very gradual manner and demonstrate pleasure at making that contact. Since, as Kornhaber and Schroeder (1975) have demonstrated, similarity between model and observer on the dimension of age is important for successful therapeutic use of modeling, one would have to train a young child to be a model when similarly aged children are to be treated for their fears. Young children who can easily learn how to serve as models may not be readily available. There is the further problem that *in vivo* modeling calls for the availability of a fear-arousing stimulus appropriate to the fearful child's particular problem. In the case of the fairly frequently encountered fear of dogs, for example, a therapist would need access to a friendly dog who permits himself to be played with and petted without making sudden vigorous movements, barking, or engaging in other unexpected behavior that would only serve to confirm the fearful child's apprehensions. In order to circumvent these difficulties several investigators have resorted to using filmed or videotaped displays showing a carefully graded sequence of a model making approach responses to a feared object, such as a dog. This not only permits one to make a careful selection of model and dog but it also facilitates the repeated presentation of the same sequence which can be watched by one child or by groups of children.

While symbolic modeling has the advantages just enumerated, a comparison of the relative effectiveness of live versus filmed models in reducing young children's avoidance behavior toward dogs showed that the degree of improvement is considerably greater when a live model is used (Bandura and Menlove, 1968). These investigators had also compared a film showing multiple models (several children playing with a dog) with a film in which only a single model's behavior was displayed. In comparison with a control group that watched a film containing no animals, both modeling conditions reduced the observers' avoidance behavior but the film with the multiple models was somewhat more effective than the one where only a single model was shown. This study thus suggests that where live models are not available, filmed models may be a feasible, though less effective substitute.

Filmed models may be particularly useful in reducing children's anticipatory fear of impending dental treatment (Adelson, Liebert, Poulos, & Herskovitz, 1972) or hospitalization and surgery (Melamed & Siegel, 1975). In those situations the use of a live model, though not impossible (White & Davis, 1974), may be highly impractical and a carefully produced and edited film a feasible alternative. Melamed and Siegel (1975) studied 60 children between the ages of 4 and 12 who were admitted to a pediatric hospital for surgery of a nonemergency nature. Matched for age, sex, race, and type of operation, these children were divided into an experimental and a control group. Prior to their admission, the youngsters in the experimental group watched a 16-minute film showing a 7-year-old boy prior to, during, and after a hernia operation. The children in the control group were shown a film of a boy on a nature trip in the country. The dependent measures were self-reports, parental reports, and a physiological measure of sweat-gland activity. These were taken before and after the showing of the film, the night before the surgery, and again during a one-month postsurgical examination. The analysis of the results showed that the children in the group who had seen the modeling film evidenced lower sweat-gland activity, fewer self-reported medical fears, and less anxiety-related behavior than the children who had watched the control film. These differences obtained both before surgery and at the follow-up one month later. Inasmuch as only the children in the control group were reported by their parents to have manifested an increase in behavior problems following hospitalization, the procedure used in this study may have important preventive implications.

The model, who had been depicted in the film used by Melamed and Siegel (1975), was a 7-year-old white male, who was different in age, skin color, and sex from many of the children who watched the film since these ranged in age from 4 to 12 and included girls and boys of various races. While the data analysis did not address itself to possible differences along these demographic characteristics, it does not seem that they are important variables unless there is a wide discrepancy in the ages of model and observer as would be between an adult and a child. Kornhaber and Schroeder (1975), having studied this issue, reported child models to be far superior to adult models in helping reduce the avoidance behavior of children. There is yet another dimension along which model and observer can differ that may be an important variable in the effectiveness of a model—it is the dimension of fearfulness.

Meichenbaum (1977) distinguishes between *mastery models* and *coping models*. A mastery model displays highly competent, fearless behavior throughout the modeling sequence while a coping model at first displays some fear and hesitation then gradually approaches the feared object and behaves in a fearless, confident manner only at the end of the sequence. In these terms, the boy in the film used by Melamed and Siegel (1975) was a coping model. At the beginning of the film he exhibited signs of anxiety and apprehension but was then able to overcome his initial fears and finally completed each stage of his hospital experience in a successful and nonanxious manner.

While Kornhaber and Schroeder (1975) had found no difference between mastery and coping models in their ability to facilitate the reduction of children's avoidance responses on a behavioral test that required approaching the feared object (a harmless snake), they did report a significant difference in favor of the coping models on a measure that assessed the children's attitudes toward snakes. In general, it would seem that where the choice is between presenting a mastery model or a coping model, available evidence points to a coping model as potentially more effective in helping children overcome certain fears.

Participant Modeling

Thus far we have presented fear-reduction methods based on observational learning where the observer is a passive participant, that is, where the fearful child merely sits by passively and observes a model engaging in a graded sequence of approach behaviors. A potent improvement over this procedure appears to be *participant modeling* (Rosenthal & Bandura, 1978), where the fearful child actively joins the model in making the approach responses. When it was first developed participant modeling was called contact desensitization. Ritter (1968) compared this method with vicarious modeling, using a group of children between the ages of 5 and 11 who had been selected on the basis of their moderate fear of snakes. In this, as in most other laboratory studies using models to reduce fear, the subjects were selected by giving school children a behavioral test to determine how close they would approach an animal such as a snake or a dog. Those who demonstrated marked avoidance behavior on this test were then exposed to the treatments to be tested. It is noteworthy that these children were thus not the extremely phobic cases whose parents seek professional help on their behalf. Ritter (1968) divided children selected in this manner into three groups. One was a no-treatment control, another experienced vicarious modeling, while the third engaged in a mixture of vicarious and participant modeling that Ritter called contact desensitization. In this method, the fearful child first watched the therapist and a child model play with a harmless snake after which the observing child was encouraged to join the two in touching the snake. Following two 35-minute treatment sessions, 80 percent of the children in the participant modeling but only 53.5 percent of the vicarious modeling group were able to complete a terminal task that called for sitting in a chair with arms at the sides while the snake remained in the child's lap for 30 seconds. None of the children who had been in the control group were able to do this.

Participant modeling provides the fearful child with the experience of observing a model demonstrate approach responses to the feared object and then, following the model's example, to make direct contact with the feared object. The therapist also plays a more active role here than in vicarious modeling, particularly in a treatment situation where the therapist also serves as the model. In the study by Ritter (1968) just cited, the therapist demonstrated the target behavior together with the child model but she then encouraged the fearful child to hold on to her hand while they practiced the approach response together. This *guided participation* was then gradually faded out as the child continued to practice the approach responses more and more independently.

As Leitenberg (1976) has observed, in participant modeling the function of the therapist is quite complex since the role requires the therapist not only to be instructive and reassuring but also motivating, by virtue of the encouragement and prompting that is involved. It is very likely that such a procedure not only serves to reduce the child's fear but that it also develops approach skills and, as Bandura (1977a) would have it, expectations of personal efficacy. Lastly, when the therapist implicitly or explicitly praises the child for making approach responses and for succeeding in contacting the feared object, potential reinforcers are provided that should serve to strengthen the newly acquired behavior. As we shall see later, the addition of explicit and systematic reinforcement to participant modeling provides a powerful treatment that Leitenberg (1976) calls *reinforced practice.*

An early comparison between traditional systematic desensitization, participant modeling, self-administered symbolic modeling with and without relaxation, and a no-treatment control (Bandura, Blanchard, & Ritter, 1969) had shown that with individuals of a wide range of ages (13 to 59), all of whom displayed a fear of snakes, participant modeling was by far the most effective. The results of that study revealed that 92 percent of the group that had been given that form of treatment were able to tolerate the terminal test of having the snake crawl around their lap while they sat motionless in a chair for 30 seconds. When Blanchard (1970) conducted an experiment designed to isolate the relative contribution of merely observing a model interact with a snake, receiving information and reassurance about its harmlessness, and graded contact with the snake in the context participant modeling, he found that observing a model accounted for most of the improvement but that direct participation added a significant increment in facilitating approach behavior and reducing fear. On the other hand, being merely told that the snake was harmless and receiving reassuring explanations of its behavior did nothing to increase approach behavior and may, in fact, have counteracted the positive effect of direct experience to some extent.

The work on participant modeling discussed thus far has demonstrated its superiority over other methods for reducing fears but because the subjects in these studies had either been children selected from a school population on the basis of a screening instrument or, as in Blanchard's (1970) study, a self-selected sample ranging in age from 14 to 50 years with a median age of 22, we must look elsewhere for data directly relevant to the kind of children whose incapacitating fears lead their parents to seek professional help. Data of this kind are provided by research conducted by Lewis (1974) who worked with a group of children whose fear of water prevented them from taking part in swimming instructions. Such a disabling fear of a normally encountered, generally useful, and ordinarily enjoyed activity is far more representative of the kinds of problems typically seen in clinical practice than is a moderate fear of snakes which the majority of children may never encounter.

When treatment by observational learning includes guided participation, as in the study reported by Ritter (1968) that was discussed above, the therapist's modeling the approach behavior and the child's direct participation are confounded so that one cannot tell whether it is the modeling or the participation or the combination of the two that is responsible for the increase in the child's approach responses and the concomitant fear reduction. Lewis (1974) sought to separate the components of participant modeling in order to ascertain whether modeling alone or participation alone were as effective as the combination of the two and superior to a control condition. The children with whom she worked were 40 boys between the ages of 5 and 12 who were attending a summer camp for economically disadvantaged youngsters. They had been selected for participation in the study from among a larger group that, on the first day of camp, had displayed fear of water during preliminary swimming tests. All 40 of these boys had also received low scores on the subsequently administered behavioral test of swimming-related items. These ranged from getting into the 3-foot-deep pool, through putting the face in the water while holding on to the side of the pool, to floating 6 feet from the side of the pool with the face in the water. After this assessment, the boys were assigned to one of four groups that were equated for age and test scores.

Each of the children in the first—modeling plus participation—group was shown a brief, eight-minute film depicting three boys, age 7, 10, and 11, who, individually, performed graded tasks in the swimming pool that were similar to those used in the swimming test. These boys were coping models in that at first they displayed some fear and hesitancy, gradually increasing in competence as they completed the more difficult tasks. After their individual performances, the three models were shown together in the pool, playing with a ball and ostensibly enjoying themselves. The film was accompanied by voice recordings in which the models described what they were doing and how they were feeling, praised themselves, and expressed pride at successfully completing the activities in the pool. Immediately after a boy who had been assigned to this experimental condition had been shown this film by one female experimenter, another took him to the pool for the participation phase. This consisted of their spending 10 minutes at the pool where the experimenter would encourage the boy to attempt the items on the assessment test. The experimenter entered the pool after the child, doing no modeling but lending physical assistance when necessary, and giving social reinforcement for any activity he attempted and completed. This condition thus separated modeling, done by the boys in the film, from participation, which was guided by the female adult.

The boys in the second—the modeling-only—group, were individually shown the same modeling film after which they would spend 10 minutes at the side of the pool, playing checkers with the second experimenter. They were always allowed to win and received social reinforcement for doing so. Each of the boys in the third—the participation-only—group was shown an 8-minute cartoon film that had nothing to do with water and was accompanied by popular music. Immediately after this the boy would be taken to the pool to be exposed to the participation that had been used with the modeling plus participation group. Finally, in the control group each boy viewed the cartoon film and then played checkers with the second experimenter at the side of the pool.

Lewis (1974) assessed the effectiveness of these four experimental conditions at two points in time. The first evaluation took place on the day after the intervention and consisted of repeating the behavioral swimming test that had been used for the initial assessment. Beginning on the following day all overnight campers participated in swimming lessons in a different pool for five consecutive days after which the behavioral test was repeated once again and the swimming instructor, a male not otherwise involved in the study, rated each boy's swimming skill and degree of fear of swimming. Because not all of the 40 boys who had been in the experimental groups were overnight campers, only 29 received these swimming lessons and of those only 25 were available for the follow-up assessment. This attrition affected the different groups somewhat differently and circumscribes the conclusions one can draw on the basis of the last assessment but the differences between the pre- and postintervention scores on the behavioral test are quite robust and reveal the clear superiority of the modeling–participation combination over the other conditions.

At the time of the preintervention assessment, the average of the mean scores for the four matched groups was 33.26 on the behavioral test on which the maximum possible score was 64. It will be recalled that this score was based on the boys' willingness to engage in a graded series of activities in the swimming pool. Immediately following the intervention phase of the study, the control group in which the boys had watched cartoons and played checkers revealed no change in mean score while the mean score for the modeling plus participation group had increased to 51.60. The modeling-only and participation-only groups had means of 43.40 and 43.15 respectively. An analysis of variance performed on these data revealed that all boys who had been exposed to participation showed significant improvement in their behavior and that participation was a stronger treatment component than modeling in increasing approach behavior. The most effective intervention for inducing behavior change, however, was the combination of modeling and participation.

The somewhat attenuated data from the follow-up assessment conducted after the five days of swimming lessons revealed that the children who were available for this evaluation not only maintained their achievement but actually showed significant improvement over their postintervention scores. The ratings provided by the swimming instructor give an indication of the degree to which the children's increased approach responses to water had generalized from the pool where the testing and participation had taken place to the other pool where the swimming lessons had been conducted. An analysis of these ratings showed that in comparison with the boys in the other three groups, those in the modeling plus participation group showed more improvement in their swimming abilities, fewer signs of fear about participating in swimming activities, and less avoidance of swimming activities.

These trends suggest that the boys in the modeling plus participation condition generalized and maintained the intervention-induced changes more than those in the other groups (Lewis, 1974).

Skill Training or Fear Reduction?

The fact that participation was such an important component in the effective-ness of the procedures used by Lewis (1974) not only confirms the observation offered by Rosenthal and Bandura (1978) that "nothing succeeds like success" but it also suggest that one aspect of children's avoidance behavior in the case of swimming pool activities is a lack of skill and an unfamiliarity with the aquatic environment. Though Lewis (1974) does not report this, the black chil-dren in the Boys-Club-sponsored summer camp near a major midwestern city may never have had an opportunity to acquire familiarity with and appropri-ate skills for swimming pool activities. Modeling and participation may well compensate for this lack of experience so that the treatment may have been as much a form of skill training as a process of fear reduction.

At the beginning of this discussion of observational learning as a method of fear reduction we pointed out that this procedure seems to combine training in approach skills with reduction of fear. While, as Gelfand (1978) has pointed out, modeling may well be the most effective single method currently available for the treatment of phobic behavior, it is by no means clear just what is re-sponsible for the effect of this treatment. Positive results with modeling ther-apy are usually reported without providing information on whether there was evidence that the children involved had at one time possessed the requisite skills for approaching the feared object or situation. Possession of these skills would have to be present if the observation of a model merely served to free in-hibited approach responses, as Bandura's (1969) original formulation sug-gests. In the case of the fear of swimming and most likely in studies involving snake phobias and fear of surgical procedures the approach skills may simply not be in the child's repertoire so that the success of modeling therapy may largely be based on providing these skills with which the child can then more competently cope with the previously avoided activities or events.

The issue about the relative contributions of skill training and fear reduc-tion could be investigated by examining the effect of modeling therapy on two groups of children. One of these groups would have to be composed of chil-dren who had never approached a given phobic object and could thus be as-sumed never to have learned the requisite skills. The other group would con-tain children who at one time in their lives had demonstrated these approach responses but had then developed the avoidance responses from which one in-fers the presence of fear. If modeling is really such a powerful means of fear reduction, it should be effective with both of these groups of children.

School phobia might also provide a test of the skill-training versus fear-re-duction question since children who exhibit this problem have usually attended school at one time, but then ceased to go there with verbalizations of fear and other phobic manifestations. It can thus be assumed that these children have school-approach responses in their repertoire and that these responses need only be disinhibited in order to permit them to return to school. If the observation of a model who engages in relevant approach responses can provide this disinhibition, modeling therapy should be capable of treating school-phobic children but we know of no study in which modeling therapy alone was used in the treatment of school phobia.

OPERANT PROCEDURES

One of the procedures Lewis (1974) had included in her treatment of children fearful of entering the swimming pool was to have the adult who involved the child in guided participation provide social reinforcement in the form of praise and encouragement for any approach responses that the child emitted. Her research design did not permit a differentiation of the effect of reinforcement from that of other components of the procedure but a number of investigators have demonstrated that children's avoidance responses (fears) can also be treated by an explicit manipulation of reinforcing consequences.

Therapists who approach fears and phobias from the point of view of respondent conditioning as well as those who do so from the perspective of observational learning tend to speak of excess avoidance responses that they set out to reduce by a reciprocal increase in approach responses. Theoretical and practical considerations lead investigators working in an operant frame of reference to define the problem as one of zero or low probability of approach responses that they then attempt to increase by such methods as stimulus fading, shaping, prompting, differential reinforcement, or combinations of these. The theoretical considerations that lead to this approach are of course based on the fact that fear is an inferred emotional state about which those choosing operant formulations prefer not to speculate. On the practical level, available operant methods are designed to strengthen or weaken observable responses by the systematic manipulations of their antecedents and consequences. The target of intervention must therefore be defined in terms of observable responses and this precludes consideration of constructs like fear and phobia.

Fear, as Lang (1969) has pointed out, is a complex construct that has behavioral, cognitive, and physiological components. The behavioral component is found in overt avoidance responses; the cognitive component is expressed by verbal statements that refer to the individual's subjective feelings of distress and apprehension; the physiological component is manifested by heart rate changes and other indices of autonomic activities. It is not that therapists of an operant persuasion categorically deny the existence of the cognitive and physiological components of what is commonly labeled as fear; they simply choose, as a matter of strategy, to focus their interventions on the behavioral aspects (just as therapists of other persuasions choose to focus on cognitive or physiological aspects). It appears that when approach responses to previously avoided stimuli have been established by operant techniques, changes also can be found in the cognitive and physiological realms.

One of the advantages of treating such avoidance behavior as school phobia by operant means is that the preintervention assessment often reveals that there are contingencies operating in the child's environment that reinforce and thus maintain the avoidance responses. An operant formulation permits the intervention to focus not only on increasing the approach responses by positive reinforcement but concurrently to decrease the incompatible avoidance responses by placing these on an extinction schedule or by introducing aversive consequences. Analysis of cases of so-called school phobia often reveals that the children are being reinforced for staying away from school by various pleasant and attractive things that take place when they remain at home (Hersen, 1970). This was the case with Valerie on whose treatment Ayllon, Smith, and Rogers (1970) presented a detailed report.

A Case of "School Phobia"

Valerie was an 8-year-old girl who, in second grade, had begun to have increasingly more frequent absences from school until, in third grade, she came to school only for the first four days and then refused to attend altogether. Though she had never given the impression of being unhappy or afraid, her mother described that whenever she attempted to take the child to school, Valerie would throw such violent temper tantrums, screaming and crying, that it was nearly impossible to move her from the house. It was then that pediatricians at a local hospital diagnosed her as a case of school phobia. When the behavioral intervention was undertaken, detailed assessment, including observations in the girl's home and neighborhood, revealed that the consequences of her refusal to go to school were indeed quite positive. The mother, having given up all hope of getting Valerie to school, simply allowed her to sleep for another hour after the other children (aged 6, 9, and 10) had left for school. Until the mother had to leave the house to go to work, Valerie would follow her around and when the mother had to leave, she took the girl to a neighbor's house for the day. There were indications that the girl was loath to have her mother leave but once at the neighbor's she was free to do whatever she pleased for the rest of the day. She would play a variety of games and make occasional trips to the corner store where she bought candy, gum, or soft drinks with money that she had in her possession. It was clearly a comfortable routine for both child and mother who thereby avoided Valerie's tantrum behavior.

Ayllon et al. (1970) concluded that Valerie's school refusal was being maintained by the pleasant manner in which she was allowed to spend her day, regardless of how the refusal might initially have started. They therefore decided to reverse the contingencies such that being at school would result in positive consequences while staying away from school would be unrewarding or, indeed, unpleasant. As part of their behavioral assessment, these investigators had ascertained that Valerie reacted well to books and school-related work when these were presented to her by a female therapy aide who visited the home. They had also found that the child was willing to leave the house with that assistant, and that she was able to attend class when the aide took her to school. For a few days the therapy aide remained in Valerie's classroom, gradually decreasing her presence to five minutes. At the end of the days on which Valerie had attended school she was given some small prize by the teacher and much praise from both the teacher and the aide. While this assessment procedure had helped to determine that Valerie had all the skills necessary for going to school it was not sufficiently powerful to maintain voluntary school attendance. Ayllon et al. (1970) therefore embarked on a systematic program designed to reach the target of having the girl attend school independently, voluntarily, and regularly. This took the form of a home-based motivational system.

Charts were prominently posted in the home for each of the children in the family and a star was to be affixed to these at the end of each day on which the child had voluntarily attended school. Five such stars, reflecting perfect attendance for the week, were to result in a special treat or trip on the weekend and, in addition, three pieces of candy were to be dispensed at the end of each day to every child who had earned a star. A child who had to be taken to school, instead of attending voluntarily, failed to earn a star but was given one piece of candy because it was felt that some reward value had to be attached to any kind of school attendance. Putting up the stars and handing out the candy were accompanied by verbal praise and that occasion was to be made into a special event when the mother returned home from work in the evening. Ayllon and his colleagues (1970) do not explain why they had decided that Valerie's siblings, who had been attending school quite regularly, were to be included in the reward program. Contrary to the misgivings voiced by Levine and Fasnacht (1974) who feared that the introduction of explicit reinforcement for behavior that is already being emitted might disrupt that behavior, it did not seem to have resulted in untoward consequences as far as the siblings were concerned.

With the reinforcement program in place, but Valerie not leaving the house voluntarily with her siblings when these set out for school, the mother was instructed to leave the house 15 minutes later and to take the girl to school. The only exception to this was to be made if Valerie had a temperature above 100 degrees Fahrenheit since the girl had pleaded illness in the past when she did not want to go to school. Under this procedure, Valerie attended school for 10 consecutive days but she still had to be taken there and failed to go voluntarily. Recognizing that they had still not arrived at an effective approach to

Valerie's problem, Ayllon, Smith, and Rogers (1970) decided on a further modification. This entailed the introduction of a mild aversive consequence for the mother if Valerie failed to go to school. This was based on the assumption that having her mother accompany her to school was reinforcing Valerie's refusal to go there on her own. With the token system involving stars, candies, and treats still in effect, the mother was now instructed to get ready for work and to leave the house 10 minutes before the children had to leave for school. Mother was to go to the school and to wait there for the children who, upon their arrival, were to be given a reward. If Valerie failed to show up at school with her siblings, mother was to return home and escort the girl to school. Since there was about a mile between home and school, this scheme required that mother walk a total of three miles if Valerie failed to go to school. The therapists reasoned that by having Valerie's behavior result in such an aversive consequence for the mother it would lead her to become more active in conveying to the child the importance of going to school.

This change in procedure had a dramatic effect. On the first day, mother had to return home to get Valerie because she did not come to school with her siblings. Once the mother had taken Valerie to school the child remained there all day. In the evening, the siblings received their stars and candies but Valerie was given only one piece of candy and the reason for this was explained to her. On the second day, Valerie left home with her siblings and arrived with them at school where the mother who was waiting for them was much pleased and gave each a piece of candy. All received a star and three pieces of candy that evening but on the next day Valerie again stayed home when her siblings left for school and, after having waited at school for 15 minutes mother had to go back to the house to retrieve her. Since it was raining, this was a considerable inconvenience for the mother who, to judge by the following description, must have been furious.

> Once she reached home she scolded Val and pushed her out of the house and literally all the way to school. As Val tried to give some explanation the mother hit her with a switch. By the time they arrived at school, both were soaking wet. That evening, Val received some candy but no stars as she had not gone to school on her own. This was the last time Val stayed away from school (Ayllon et al., 1970, p. 135).

After this the mother continued going to school ahead of the children in order to reward their arrival there for another six days. On the fifth day Valerie had accumulated enough stars to have earned the special treat she had chosen; to have her cousin visit and stay overnight with her which she reportedly enjoyed. The child then continued to go to school regularly and voluntarily even after the mother no longer waited for the children at school. The star–candy–treat system was kept in force for another month but even when that was withdrawn, Valerie's school attendance remained unaffected. Follow-up for the next nine months revealed not only that Valerie was attending school regularly but that her academic performance had improved and that she was cooperative and socially skilled and outgoing. Even the experience of having another child snatch her money from her on the way to school and the family stress associated with her mother's initiating divorce proceedings against her husband failed to disrupt Valerie's now well-established pattern of going to school.

Like any other case report, the one presented by Ayllon, Smith, and Rogers (1970) does no more than illustrate the use of a treatment procedure; it does not prove its effectiveness. In the absence of controls, understandable though these are, one can only assume that it was the procedure and not some other factor that served as the independent variable. Why then present this report in such detail? It was to illustrate the sometimes tortuous path that treatment must follow in real-life clinical situations, to underscore the importance of careful assessment, and to show that treatment success depends on the therapist's readiness to introduce changes in the procedure as soon as it appears that one approach fails to result in improvement. That, of course, is possible only if the therapist has available carefully kept records of observable behavior that can reflect whether or not changes are taking place. Lastly, the case of Valerie provides a good illustration of the importance of conducting treatment in the environment where the problem behavior is displayed, in this instance, the home and the school.

The Teacher's Role

In order to be able to conduct treatment of children's school-related problems in the school, the therapist must be able to enlist the cooperation of teachers and other school personnel who then come to function as surrogate therapists. Such was the case in the treatment of a child whose refusal to participate in any classroom activity requiring verbal communication was successfully overcome by Bauermeister and Jemail (1975) through the application of operant principles. These investigators describe an excessively timid, fearful 8-year-old boy who spoke freely with members of his family but failed to interact verbally with his teachers or classmates. This problem, identified as *elective mutism*, was treated by having the boy's teachers shape his behavior by selectively praising classsroom participation or any reasonable approximation thereof. Such specific behaviors as hand-raising, answering the teacher's questions, reading aloud, and completing classroom assignments were targeted for intervention and their frequencies were recorded by the teachers. One of the teachers was instructed to set goals for these target behaviors at the beginning of each class period. This teacher then praised each occurrence of such behavior and rewarded the boy at the end of the period if he had met the specified criterion. The reward took the form of a star and for every 15 stars he had thus earned, the boy's mother would present him with a bigger star with the understanding that he would receive a bicycle once he had earned three of these. After approximately 20 school days during which this procedure had been in effect, the boy's behavior had undergone a signal change. He now raised his hand when questions were addressed to the class, answered teachers' questions, and read aloud whenever that was asked of him. Though these behaviors had not been targets of the intervention, he now also requested help when he was unable to complete some part of his work and interacted actively with his peers during recess. Bauermeister and Jemail (1975) also report that this child's grades improved and that his various fears abated. A follow-up, conducted a year later, revealed that the boy had maintained his level of classroom participation and that this behavior had generalized to other teachers in other classes and with other subject matter.

Stimulus Fading

When operant methods are applied in attempts to change children's behavior, the intervention is almost always focused on the consequences of the child's responses. In the case reported by Bauermeister and Jemail (1975), for example, the teacher presented praise statements and stars contingent on the boy having emitted specified desirable behaviors. Therapists using these procedures by and large ignore the other end of the behavior chain, the antecedent, discriminative stimulus that is to become the occasion when the desired response should be emitted.

Working with a child whose problem had also been identified as elective mutism, Wulbert, Nyman, Snow and Owen (1973) focused on both the antecedent and the consequent conditions by combining stimulus fading with contingency management. They thus succeeded in modifying the fearful behavior of a 6-year-old girl who while speaking freely at home, had refused to talk in the presence of strangers. This girl had not spoken during one year of preschool and was not talking in kindergarten where she behaved in an extremely passive fashion. She did not participate in any classroom activities but, when she carried the craft material home, she would make there all the things that the other children had constructed at school.

Treatment took place at a clinic where the mother brought the child three times each week. There the two of them would interact in various games and activities that required both motor and verbal responses from the child. With the girl thus engaged in an activity, a therapist who was a stranger to the girl was brought on the scene in a series of 25 graded steps of increasing closeness. At first the stranger was only audible, then visible and audible while standing in the hall, then very gradually present inside the room. On succeeding days.

the stranger was brought closer to the table where mother and child were sitting, eventually joining mother in reading questions with her in unison, then taking over from mother while she remained in the room, and finally remaining alone with the girl while her mother gradually withdrew. Throughout all this, the mother (and later the therapist) would dispense reinforcers and praise to the child.

During the first six days of treatment, as the stranger was moved closer to the child, her motor behavior dropped slightly below what it had been when she and mother had been alone but her verbal behavior ceased altogether. At this point an additional contingency was introduced that consisted of having the girl spend one minute in a time-out room whenever she failed to respond to a request for verbalization. With that combination of positive reinforcement, time-out, and stimulus fading the stranger's presence ceased to disrupt the girl's behavior.

Once the first therapist had acquired stimulus control over the girl's verbal and motor behavior, that is, the child would interact with that therapist in the absence of her mother, a second therapist was similarly faded in, and finally a third. Following this, four other persons were gradually introduced, including the girl's first-grade teacher. Just before school reopened in the fall, several children from her class were faded in, the actual classroom being used as the site for these last steps. With this preparation, the girl was able to begin school without difficulty and to participate in classroom activities, giving answers to the teacher's questions in a loud, clear voice.

Although a study of a single case, the investigation by Wulbert et al. (1973) included control conditions in that sessions with the strangers who were gradually faded in were alternated with sessions where a stranger who had not been faded in took the place of the mother. During these control periods the girl did not respond even when the time-out contingency was introduced as a consequence for such failure. This permitted the investigators to conclude that their fading procedure had been a necessary component of the treatment process.

Operant or Respondent? An examination of the details of the above case report raises the question how stimulus fading differs from the graded exposure to a feared stimulus that is used when treatment is based on the principles of respondent conditioning. Wulbert et al. (1973) seem to have conceptualized their approach as derived from operant principles. This is apparent both in the terminology they use and in their choice of an operant publication as the outlet for their report. Yet when one considers that the child they treated was playing games with, talking to, and receiving candy from her mother while the stranger was gradually moved closer and closer until that person was able to replace the mother, the parallel to the approach used by Jones (1924b) in desensitizing Peter to the presence of the rabbit cannot be denied. It is obviously unproductive to engage in an argument whether a given form of treatment is based on operant or on respondent principles. As pointed out earlier in this chapter, avoidance behavior that is mediated by fear responses is probably best construed as having both operant and respondent components. It is therefore likely that every treatment must entail features of both operant and respondent components in order to be effective. If that is the case, it might be most productive to build both components into a treatment plan in an explicit and systematic fashion. In practical situations encountered in the clinic, therapists often approach their cases in such comprehensive fashion. MacDonald (1975), for example, successfully treated an 11-year-old boy with an extreme fear of dogs by applying a combination of systematic imaginal and *in vivo* desensitization, modeling, skill training, and social reinforcement in what she called multiple impact behavior therapy. A similar combination of approaches has been developed and studied by Leitenberg (1976) under the label *reinforced practice*.

Reinforced Practice

A series of studies with phobic adults had enabled Leitenberg (1976) to isolate four major therapeutic elements which he combined in the method of reinforced practice. That method, in turn, was evaluated in a controlled study of fearful adults and children (Leitenberg & Callahan, 1973). The elements combined in reinforced practice are (1) repeated, graduated, *in vivo* practice in approaching the phobic stimulus; (2) delivery of social reinforcement for small improvements in performance; (3) trial-by-trial feedback on performance based on precise measures; and (4) the therapist's verbal statements designed to provide the client with expectations of gradual success (Leitenberg, 1976). Leitenberg and Callahan (1973) assessed the effectiveness of this method in the treatment of seven preschool children whose fear of the dark required that a light be kept on in or near their bedroom at night. These children, and an equal number who were assigned to a no-treatment control group, had been recruited from among youngsters enrolled in nursery schools and kindergartens. The parents of these children considered the fear to be a minor one and expected their child to overcome it with increasing age, but they were nonetheless willing to permit the child's participation in a study.

For pre- and posttest measures, the investigators timed how long a child was willing to remain alone in a dark room. The test was structured as a game in which one could win a prize with each child instructed to enter the room alone, shut the door, and come out as soon as he or she felt the least bit afraid. At pretest, the mean time the 14 children were willing to remain in a completely light-proof room with the door shut was 21.92 seconds. Children were matched on the basis of their pretest scores and randomly assigned to a treatment and control group. This process of matching unfortunately resulted in the mean age of the treatment group (6.0 years) being 8 months higher than that of the control group, a difference which, at that age level, might be deemed critical. At any rate, at the end of treatment (described below) the control group was willing to remain in the test room for a mean of only 27.71 seconds while the treatment group tolerated this exposure for a mean of 198.85 seconds. This difference is statistically significant but since Leitenberg and Callahan (1973) fail to report whether the treated children were now willing to sleep without a nightlight, one cannot tell whether it is of practical significance.

The treatment of these fearful children had proceeded as follows. Each child was seen individually for two sessions per week for a maximum of eight sessions. There were five trials in each session. Treatment was terminated when a child was willing to remain in the dark room for five minutes on two consecutive trials. The room used for treatment, a small photographic darkroom that was different from the one used for the pretest, adjoined a lighted hallway and had some light filtering in underneath the door. At the beginning of the first session, the therapist instructed the child to enter that room, shut the door, and remain until the least bit of fear was felt, whereupon he or she was to come out. The children were told that this procedure would be repeated a number of times and that for each time they remained longer than their previous longest time they would be able to select a prize from among a collection of trinkets, crayons, and candies. In order to provide the children with feedback on the length of time they had remained in the room, a "thermometer" was drawn on a sheet of paper and marked off in units of 10 seconds. After each trial, increases in elapsed time were shown on this graph by shading in the appropriate units with a pencil. Improvement was praised and resulted in the award of a prize. If the time spent in the room was less than on the previous trial, the appropriate degrees of shading on the graph were erased and the child informed that he or she had not done as well this time. Upon reaching the criterion of success or after eight sessions, the child and the matched control were given the posttest in both the treatment room and in the pretest room, thus providing some measure of generalization.

The published description of reinforced practice as applied to children (Leitenberg & Callahan, 1973) reflects the graduated practice, the social reinforcement for improvements, and the feedback of performance; three of the four elements Leitenberg (1976) views as the components of this form of treatment. The fourth component, the therapist's statement of expectation of success, is not explicitly mentioned in that part of the publication by Leitenberg and Callahan (1973) which describes their work with children although it is included in the discussion of their work with phobic adults. Leitenberg (personal communication, February 21, 1979), however, recounts that the children too had been informed of the therapist's intent to try to help them become less afraid of the dark.

In a "treatment package" such as is represented by the reinforced practice procedure, it is impossible to know, pending research aimed at this question, which of the ingredients or combination of ingredients is critical to its effectiveness. What, for example, is the function of the induced expectation of success? This clearly falls into the realm of cognitive processes. Could it be that expectations of success alone can help fearful children overcome their problem? This leads us to a study that might provide an answer to this question.

SELF-STATEMENTS

It is not unlikely that a boy who observes a model approach a fear-arousing object will say to himself something like, "Gee, it's not dangerous after all," or that a girl experiencing the effects of systematic desensitization will think, "Wow, I can do it." We do not know to what extent these cognitions contribute to therapeutic progress but recent years have seen a number of attempts to base therapy of children on the direct induction of self-statements designed to modify their behavior (Meichenbaum, 1977). Such self-statements or *verbal controlling responses* might, in fact, be taught to children before they encounter a potentially fear-arousing stimulus, thus "immunizing" them to fears instead of later having to expose them to a feared stimulus as a part of treatment.

A well-controlled study of the effectiveness of verbal controlling responses in helping children cope with their fears of the dark was conducted by Kanfer, Karoly, and Newman (1975), who compared two versions of that approach with a control condition. Forty-five children between the ages of 5 and 6 who were attending kindergarten had been selected from among a larger group on the basis of their being unable to remain alone in a dark room for at least three minutes. Five children who displayed signs of intense discomfort and crying were excluded from the study so that, as is so often the case in research on treatment procedures, the sample was not representative of the kind of children whose parents seek help for them from clinical resources.

Despite this drawback, this study made an important contribution to the evaluation of the cognitive approaches to the treatment of children that have come to be known by the somewhat incongruous term of *cognitive behavior therapy*.

The pretest, training, and posttest took place in a schoolroom that could be totally darkened. The children had become familiar with the experimenter during the previous week and had seen the room before they were asked to help "find out some things" about children their age. The room was equipped with a dial rheostat with which the child could control the level of illumination and it contained a two-way intercom system through which the child was able to speak to the experimenter, stationed immediately outside the room. A separate loudspeaker facilitated the delivery of the experimenter's instructions. For the pretest the child was taken to this room, familiarized with the rheostat, and told to try to stay in the dark for as long as possible. The child was also told that the experimenter would return when called over the intercom system. After turning off the lights and leaving the room, the experimenter timed how long the child was able to tolerate the dark.

For the training phase, which immediately followed the pretest, the children were divided into three groups of 10 boys and 5 girls each on the basis of their pretest performance. It was explained to each child that what was to follow would be a little different in that the experimenter would speak to the child through the "talk box" and that the child would have to repeat some words after the experimenter. These words, different for each of the three groups, represented the independent variable of the study. The children in the *competence group* were told to say, "I am a brave boy (girl). I can take care of myself in the dark." Those in the *stimulus group* were instructed to say, "the dark is a fun place to be. There are many good things in the dark." For the *neutral group* the phrase was, "Mary had a little lamb. Its fleece was white as snow." Each child was rehearsed in the appropriate sentence until it was reproduced for three consecutive errorless trials (Kanfer et al., 1975).

Once the child had learned his or her "special words," the experimenter would leave the lighted room, close the door, and play four prerecorded sentences for the child who was to say his or her special words after each sentence. This procedure was repeated for a second trail. The sentences were different for each group and represented elaborations of the key content of the self-statements. Thus, one of the sentences heard by the children in the competence group was, "when you are in the dark you know that you can turn on the light when you feel like it," while the stimulus group heard, "the dark is the best place to go to sleep and have good dreams." The neutral group, on the other hand, heard sentences that elaborated on Mary's interactions with her lamb.

Directly after completion of the training phase, each child was again tested for dark tolerance. This posttest consisted of three trials. In the first two the conditions of the pretest were repeated in that the child was left in the dark for a maximum of 3 minutes (180 seconds) or until the child turned the light back on. For the third posttest trial, the experimenter turned the dial of the rheostat to its highest position and, before leaving the room, instructed the child to turn the dial down so as "to make the room as dark as you can stay in it for a long time" (sic) (Kanfer et al., 1975, p. 254). This trial was terminated after 90 seconds or earlier if the child increased the illumination or called for the experimenter over the intercom. The number of seconds the child was able to tolerate the darkness and the intensity reflected in the voltage setting of the rheostat were the dependent variables for the pretest and all posttests.

The analysis of the time data revealed that the children in both the competence group ("I am a brave boy") and in the stimulus group ("the dark is a fun place to be'') were able to tolerate the dark for a significantly longer time than did the children in the neutral control condition (''Mary had a little lamb''). As shown in Figure 18, the competence group did somewhat better than the stimulus group, but the difference between them was not significant. As Figure 18 also reflects, all groups improved their performance from the first to the second posttest trial. The rate of this change was not different for the three groups. On the third posttest trial during which the children had been asked to turn the illumination down to their own level of tolerance, the time they were able to remain in the room did not differ for the three groups. (The data for this third trial are not shown in the accompanying figures.) The analysis of the light-intensity data revealed similar results (see Fig. 19). Here all groups set somewhat lower levels on the first posttest trial than on the pretest trial but the means of the three groups did not differ significantly. Only on the second post-test trial did the competence group reveal that they had been able to tolerate a lower level of light intensity than either of the other groups, which again did not differ from each other. The data for the light-intensity setting during the third posttest trial showed that the children in the competence and stimulus groups, which did not differ from each other, had selected significantly lower settings than the children in the control group.

As Kanfer, Karoly, and Newman (1975) concluded from their study, the content of the sentences the children had learned during the training phase differentially affected their tolerance of exposure to darkness, phrases having to do with competence being the most effective. As these authors pointed out, the exact process by which the verbal statements affected the children's behavior is not entirely clear. The relevant sentences had been rehearsed only while the children were in the brightly lit room and they had not been instructed to say these words to themselves while in the dark nor was there any indication that they were saying them aloud while they were alone in the room.

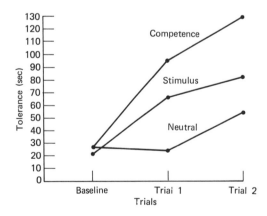

Figure 18. Mean time for tolerance of the dark for the competence, stimulus, and neutral verbalization groups during pretest, baseline, and the two test trials. (Kanfer, Karoly, & Newman, 1975. Copyright by the American Psychological Association. Reprinted by permission.)

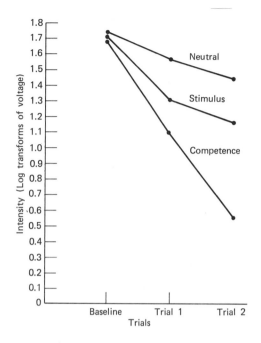

Figure 19. Mean light intensity settings for the competence, stimulus, and neutral verbalization groups during pretest, baseline, and the two test trials. (Kanfer, Karoly, & Newman, 1975. Copyright by the American Psychological Association. Reprinted by permission.)

In view of the fact that all groups, including the one of the children who had been trained on the neutral words, showed an increased tolerance from the first to the second posttest trial, it would appear, as the authors recognize, that some adaptation effect may have resulted from the nonpunished exposure to the feared situation. In other words, some degree of *in vivo* desensitization seems to have entered into this procedure. Whether this meant, as Kanfer et al. (1975) put it, that "the children who remained in the dark room for longer than usual . . . experienced some satisfaction with their achievement" (p. 257) is of course open to question. Inferences about cognitions are easy to draw but difficult to substantiate.

Another point to keep in mind when considering the experiment by Kanfer et al. (1975) is that the children were at all times in direct control of the source of light. With or without self-statements about competence, the recognition of being in control of the source of one's fear may, in itself, help one to tolerate the feared situation. It certainly presents quite a different situation from one where a person perceives himself or herself as helpless in the face of potential danger. Lastly, it should be noted that the children who participated in this study may or may not have been fearful of the dark under conditions other than being left alone in the testing room at their school. Nothing is known about their behavior at home so that it is not possible to tell whether the experimental manipulation in any way affected their fear of the dark in other situations, if it indeed existed.

A clinical application of a procedure based, in part, on the work of Kanfer et al. (1975) was reported by Graziano, Mooney, Huber, and Ignasiak (1979). These investigators worked with seven children between the ages of 8 years, 7 months, and 12 years, 8 months who had highly disruptive nighttime fears of long standing. The behavior of these children included severe panic about going to bed, crawling into the bed of other family members, or insisting on having a bright light in the room, all of which resulted in highly emotional and disruptive nightly scenes that had been taking place during the past three to six years.

The children and their parents were seen once a week for five weeks, the children in one group and the parents in another group. The children were taught a self-control exercise that they were to practice every night before going to bed. This consisted of muscle relaxation, the imagining of a pleasant scene, and the reciting of a "brave" self-statement, similar to the one used by Kanfer et al. (1975). In coordination with their parents, a token reward system was also instituted whereby the child could earn tokens toward a special treat for doing the self-control exercise and for being "brave" about going to bed and remaining so through the night. With this mixture of procedures Graziano et al. (1979) succeeded in having all of the children reach the criterion of 10 consecutive fearless nights within a mean of 8.7 weeks. When they were followed up a year later, all but one of the children were completely free of nighttime fears and none had developed new fears or other problems.

While the study by Graziano et al. (1979) is encouraging from a clinical point of view, it failed to demonstrate the clinical effectiveness of self-control statements *per se* because, as the investigators recognized, the relative contributions to the outcome by the various components of the treatment package had not been ascertained. On the whole, neither the work by Kanfer et al. (1975) nor the report by Graziano and his colleagues (1979) can dispel the skepticism of those who hold the view that so-called cognitive behavior therapy has little empirical support and that it may, in fact, be "a step in the wrong direction" (Ledwidge, 1978) as far as progress in the field of behavior therapy is concerned.

Recapitulation

Fears and phobias were construed as excess avoidance responses and the therapeutic task was seen as reducing these while concurrently increasing adaptive approach responses. Although most treatment procedures combine a variety of methods and principles, investigators have, by and large, focused their studies on one method at a time. Systematic desensitization and its variations were reviewed and it was recognized that while these approaches seem effective in reducing avoidance and increasing approach responses, the theoretical principles underlying them are not always readily apparent. Moreover, it is probably a mistake to assume homogeneity among children who manifest the avoidance behavior from which one draws inferences about the presence of fear. In the context of discussing the various treatment methods based on observational learning we pointed out that what appears to be a fear may reflect a skill deficit, an avoidance response that is actually maintained by the reduction of a conditioned emotional reaction, or a combination of the two. Whenever the treatment of fears succeeds in helping a child approach the previously avoided situation an opportunity for receiving reinforcement presents itself. It may thus be possible to structure treatment in such a way that reinforcement for approach responses becomes the focus of the intervention. Various procedures based on operant principles follow this logic. In practice, however, it is again likely that both operant and respondent processes enter into these treatment approaches. In fact, it has been assumed that certain cognitions may be taking place while a child participates in a treatment designed to increase his or her approach responses. The possibility that by merely inducing such cognitions a therapist might succeed in helping a fearful child has been explored but the result of such research has thus far remained ambiguous.

12

Somatic Disorders

GENERAL CONSIDERATIONS

This chapter deals with topics that have traditionally been viewed as falling within the realm of medicine and although the psychological aspects of physical illness have long been recognized, behavior therapists have entered this area only relatively recently through efforts that have come to be called *behavioral medicine*. Before beginning a discussion of this approach as it applies to the treatment of children it is necessary to consider a number of important points.

First of all, it must be stressed once again that no intervention should ever be undertaken unless it is preceded by a careful assessment of the problem and of the antecedents and consequences that surround it. In the case of somatic disorders it is vital that such an assessment include a thorough medical examination. In fact, it is in the area of behavioral medicine that one finds a welcome collegial collaboration between the medical and the psychological specialists who, approaching the problem from their distinct perspectives, work together on behalf of their patient, the physician dealing with the physical, the psychologist with the behavioral aspects of a case. It should not be assumed that psychological approaches are applied only when biological approaches have been tried to no avail although this has been the case in a number of instances, cited in this chapter, where behavioral methods were only brought to bear when all else seemed to have failed. This, however, seems more often the result of the physician's skepticism about the efficacy of psychological approaches than of any explicit treatment plan.

There are historical reasons for both the physician's skepticism and the relatively recent arrival of the behavioral approach on the medical scene and a recognition of these may facilitate the further development of behavioral medicine. The treatment of physical illness by what might loosely be viewed as psychological methods dates from the tribal shaman, through faith healing, to the exaggerated and unfounded claims of those who came to view a wide range of physical disorders as falling into the realm of psychosomatic illnesses which they proposed to treat by insight therapy. Little wonder that physicians have their doubts when the behavior therapist offers to help on a case by the systematic application of the principles of conditioning and learning. Moreover, it did not take long before exaggerated claims were also made for behavioral approaches, particularly for those based on providing the patient with information of his or her physiological responses, the so-called biofeedback method. As Shapiro and Surwit (1976) have pointed out, much research will be necessary before biofeedback can be advocated as a viable treatment although there is now tentative evidence that this approach can help in the remediation of some physical problems that once could be treated only by such somatic approaches as medication or surgery. The acceptability and respectability of biofeedback methods were unfortunately not furthered by the appearance and promotion on the consumer market of devices of questionable quality and doubtful efficacy, nor by notices in the advertising pages of the public press through which unscrupulous purveyors with uncertain qualifications hawk biofeedback as the nostrum for a wide variety of problems.

Another reason for the slow development of the promising field of behavioral medicine can be found in the psychologist's hesitation to participate in the treatment of individuals whom the physician has identified as suffering from a physical illness. In reaction to traditional approaches, early behavior therapists had found it necessary to stress that the disease analogy is not applicable to psychological disorders; that the behavior they set out to treat is not a symptom of an underlying illness; that psychological principles, not metaphors from medicine must guide the treatment of their clients. Their rejection of the "medical model" became a hallmark of behavior therapists and, in their struggle to establish themselves in the field of behavior disorders, the issue at times found expression in statements that were little short of polemics (Ross, 1964). It seems that only when behavior therapy had become firmly established as an accepted approach to the treatment of psychological disorders that its practitioners were willing to venture forth and become involved in the treatment of medical patients with somatic disorders.

A final point to be stressed is that behavioral treatment and medical treatment should not be seen as competing approaches where one must be proven to be superior to the other. Whether one or the other or a combination of both approaches are to be used in a given case should be based on considerations of effectiveness, side effects, cost, permanence, efficiency in terms of time, and—last, not least—on the informed choice of the patient or, in the case of children, their parents.

Unlike previous chapters which were organized around various psychological approaches to the changing of deficient or excessive behavior, this chapter will be divided according to some of the diagnostic categories of medicine, subordinating the various behavioral treatment approaches to these well-established labels. It will soon be noticed that in every one of the medical disorders here discussed, one is dealing with a difficulty that must be reduced in frequency or intensity, thus justifying the placement of this chapter under the overall heading of the treatment of behavior excesses.

ANOREXIA NERVOSA

This somewhat archaic term which translates as "nervous loss of appetite" identifies a condition in which the individual, usually an adolescent female, voluntarily reduces her food intake to the extent that she suffers such drastic loss of weight, often accompanied by such symptoms as amenorrhea or bradycardia, that she presents a bona fide medical problem that may endanger her survival. As Stunkard and Mahoney (1976) have observed, the term "anorexia" is probably a misnomer in that these patients do not lose their appetite until they reach a fairly advanced stage of the disorder. The suggestion, advanced by these investigators, that the central problem of this disorder may be more accurately reflected by speaking of it as a weight phobia has much merit. The term "weight phobia" not only relates this disorder to such psychological problems as were discussed in the previous chapter but it also provides the basis for treating it as an excessive avoidance behavior.

The disorders we are examining in this chapter inevitably raise the question whether they are physiological aberrations that find expression in disturbed behavior or whether they are psychological problems that affect physiological functions. Anorexia nervosa is no exception. The name implies that the problem is psychological ("nervous") but the question of etiology is far from answered. However, as Bemis (1978) was led to conclude on the basis of his extensive review of the existing literature, "there is still no consensus as to whether organic factors in anorexia nervosa are primary or secondary to the disorder, [but that] it is clear that they form part of a vicious circle in which abnormal physiology further affects emotional state" (p. 611). It is well to keep this point in mind as we review the behavioral approaches that have been used in treating patients with anorexia nervosa. Furthermore, it should be recalled that it is a fallacy to assume that the effectiveness of a treatment permits one to draw conclusions about the origin of the treated disorder. Thus, if psychological principles can be effectively applied in the treatment of anorexia nervosa it does not prove that these principles were involved when the disorder first developed.

It is one of the diagnostic criteria of anorexia nervosa that the patient denies having a problem, enjoys losing weight, and thus sees no need for treatment (Bemis, 1978). This often results in situations where therapeutic intervention only becomes feasible when the patient has had to be hospitalized because her malnutrition has taken on crisis proportions. At that point the obvious treatment priority is to restore the patient's body weight and it is here that behavioral methods aimed at increased food intake have found their most frequent application. Unfortunately, once the patient has regained an approximation of normal body weight and is therefore discharged from the hospital, treatment is usually discontinued even though the number of pounds gained during the crisis management may not be a good criterion of therapeutic success.

If the food refusal of anorexia nervosa is construed as weight phobia, it would seem logical to treat it by one of the methods that have been found to be successful in the treatment of other phobias, such as systematic desensitization. It is therefore surprising to find that this approach has been used only rarely. In an uncontrolled case report Hallsten (1965) described treating a 12-year-old anorectic girl by systematic desensitization. This girl was able to verbalize an explicit fear of "getting fat." She had been overweight some three years earlier. At that time she had been placed on a diet and strongly reinforced for weight loss. Following this she unfortunately had continued to limit her food intake until her drastically low body weight compelled hospitalization. Inasmuch as this girl also had a profound fear of storms, the therapist decided to begin treatment by focusing on that fear. She was taught muscle relaxation and, while thus relaxed, presented with a hierarchy of images regarding storms. Neither her eating pattern nor her weight changed during the three sessions devoted to this procedure. The focus of treatment was then shifted to her fear of gaining weight. The girl was instructed to relax and to imagine a series of scenes where she was comfortably at home, being called to dinner, sitting at the table, eating, eating particularly fattening foods and enjoying them and, having eaten, going to look at herself in a mirror and noting signs of gaining weight. Hallsten (1965) reports that this child was able to receive these instructions without giving any indication of becoming anxious. On the evening of the day when this treatment session had taken place she was reported to have eaten her entire hospital meal. She also ate at subsequent meals and began a steady gain in weight as treatment was continued for a total of 12 intermittently scheduled sessions. It is not clear to what extent the change in this child's eating behavior had been influenced by a threatened (though never implemented) procedure under which hospital visits by her family were to be contingent on her gaining weight. A follow-up five months later showed this girl to be at normal weight for her age and height and to have made an uneventful adjustment to her home and school situation. It may be that this maintenance of improvement had been aided by family group therapy, instituted after the girl's discharge from the hospital.

Making visits from relatives and other privileges contingent on weight gain is a procedure based on operant formulations that has been the focus of several reports dealing with the treatment of anorexia nervosa. Among the earliest of such reports is one by Leitenberg, Agras, and Thomson (1968) who treated two adolescent girls, hospitalized because of their drastic weight loss. In order to test the hypothesis that food refusal was maintained by the reinforcing consequences of the social attention this elicited from hospital staff and others, these investigators introduced a nonreinforcement phase after having taken baseline measures for 10 days. In this phase the staff was instructed to ignore all comments the girls would make about eating or such physical complaints as headaches, nausea, or cramps. While this extinction procedure resulted in a drastic reduction of these verbal statements, it failed to increase food intake or body weight, suggesting that food refusal was not being maintained by contingent social attention.

At this point Leitenberg et al. (1968) instituted a reinforcement phase during which the girls were praised for food intake. Weight gain was to be rewarded by permission to engage in such pleasurable activities as watching television or going on walks in the hospital grounds. While this regimen resulted in very rapid weight gain for both girls, it was not possible to attribute it to the reinforcement procedures since the intervention had also included instructions to the girls that they count and record the mouthfuls of food they consumed during each meal. They were also given feedback on how many calories they had eaten and how much weight they had gained. These confounding features and the puzzling failure of the girls' food intake to decrease when the reinforcement contingencies were experimentally withdrawn, led the investigators to undertake another study (Agras, Barlow, Chapin, Abel & Leitenberg, 1974) in which they sought to isolate some of the variables that had not been controlled in the earlier work.

In a series of studies with nine girls who had been hospitalized with anorexia nervosa Agras et al. (1974) examined which of four variables was primarily responsible for the improvement that had been noted in the earlier study. The variables were size of meal, information feedback, positive reinforcement, and negative reinforcement. These were systematically varied by providing the patients with daily meals of either 3,000 or 6,000 calories and by giving or withholding information about the number of mouthfuls eaten, the number of calories consumed, and the weight gained. Positive reinforcement was similarly manipulated by either giving or withholding praise contingent on weight gain. Since being in the hospital can be construed as an aversive state of affairs, discharge from there contingent on reaching a specified weight goal represents a negative reinforcement. In the earlier study (Leitenberg et al., 1968) positive and negative reinforcement had been confounded since the patients had been praised and given hospital discharge contingent on weight gain. Agras et al. (1974) separated these two kinds of reinforcement by arranging an experimental condition in which discharge from the hospital was not contingent on how much weight the patient had gained. Having controlled these four variables, the investigators were able to conclude that each of them contributed to increased food intake and weight gain but that their relative effectiveness varied considerably. It emerged that information feedback was more potent than positive reinforcement and that positive reinforcement in the absence of feedback was relatively ineffective. In terms of its contribution to weight gain, size of meal eaten was the least significant of the four factors.

The importance of combining positive reinforcement with information about food consumption and weight gain is highlighted by the rather unsatisfactory results reported by Bhanji and Thompson (1974) who did not use this combination in their treatment procedure. These investigators worked with eleven females who ranged in age from 13 to 21 years and who had been hospitalized with anorexia nervosa. The patients were able to receive reinforcement from a self-selected list of rewards if they consumed eight consecutive meals within 60 minutes of their being served. This criterion was subsequently lowered by reducing the time limit in 5-minute steps. It is noteworthy that contact with the hospital staff had been deliberately minimized and that no mention was ever made of the patient's weight. Furthermore, as the investigators recognized in their report, it had been possible for patients to dispose of food surreptitiously since they were expected to eat their meals without supervision. It thus appears that the reinforcement contingency was based on making food disappear from the plate within a set time limit. Any weight gain achieved was thus quite incidental and could, in fact, have been partly due to the fact that all but four of the patients had, in addition to the behavioral treatment, also been on various forms of medication. Under these conditions, it may not be unexpected that one of the patients failed to gain weight while three others required readmission after discharge, one of them on four separate occasions. On a mail follow-up, conducted between 2 and 72 months later (mean = 32 months), but returned by only 7 of the 11 cases, four patients were reported to be of normal weight but only one was rated as having "good" overall adjustment.

Bhanji and Thompson (1974) concluded on the basis of their study that an operant approach is effective for producing rapid weight gain in a crisis but that "more is needed" to assure maintenance of the improvement. Others too have concluded (Agras et al., 1974; Bemis, 1978) that therapists must take steps to see that the discharged patient's natural environment operates under contingencies that support maintenance of appropriate eating behavior.

Since one can sometimes learn as much from failure as from success, it may be instructive to examine just what Bhanji and Thompson (1974) had done with their patients. When one seeks to conduct treatment based on the operant paradigm one must ask just what responses one wishes to strengthen by introducing reinforcement contingencies. One must then have a reliable source of information that indicates when the desired response has taken place and one needs a means of informing the client when reinforcement has been earned and for what behavior. The patients in the study under discussion had been given to understand that the behavior for which they could earn reinforcement was emptying their plate as quickly as possible so that they could ring a bell to notify the nurse that they were finished. Nobody watched them eat the meal and nobody told them whether they were gaining weight which, after all, is the ultimate criterion of success in the treatment of anorexia nervosa, particularly if it is viewed as a weight phobia. Unsound from the point of view of operant procedures, this approach was even questionable from a medical perspective since teaching an anorectic girl to bolt down her food seems contraindicated with a group of patients whose history often includes periods of overeating (bulimia) and whose emaciated state may result in complications with the sudden onset of rapid eating (Bemis, 1978).

A treatment program based on operant principles that set a moderate standard of gradual weight gain and made weight gain, not rapid eating, the criterion for reinforcement was reported by Halmi, Powers, and Cunningham (1975) whose eight patients included four adolescents between the ages of 14 and 17. Here the reinforcement (in the form of social and physical activity and visiting privileges) was based on the youngster having gained at least 1.1 lbs. during each 5-day period. A follow-up, conducted from 3 to 13 months after discharge, revealed that all four of these young people had maintained at least 92 percent of their normal body weight. Unfortunately, this study shares with most that deal with the behavioral treatment of anorexia nervosa such inadequacies as small size, mixing of various treatment modalities, limited follow-up at varying intervals, and questionable measures, such as a questionnaire mailed to the adolescent's parents. With these limitations on our knowledge about the effectiveness of behavioral treatment procedures with cases of anorexia nervosa, the best that can be said at this time is that in the hands of qualified therapists such treatment seems to have a high potential for short-term success in life-threatening crisis situations. Considerably more work will be required before we can be confident about the long-range effectiveness of behavioral treatment for this condition and about its applicability with non-hospitalized persons whose weight phobia has not yet reached crisis proportions.

PERSISTENT VOMITING

The food refusal that characterizes anorexia nervosa is, in some instances, accompanied by vomiting but regurgitating what has been eaten, so-called *ruminative vomiting*, is also found in the absence of direct food refusal. While this problem is more often encountered with infants, there are cases on record where mentally retarded adults (Kohlenberg, 1970) or intellectually normal adolescents manifest that difficulty which, like anorexia nervosa, will ultimately lead to severe loss of weight. A case reported by Ingersoll and Curry (1977) was that of a 14-year-old girl whom they successfully treated by making social, monetary, and activity reinforcers contingent on food retention, while combining this with a time-out contingency for vomiting. With this approach they were able to eliminate the girl's vomiting within one day and her improvement had been maintained when she was contacted for follow-up a year later.

If the patient is carefully observed during and after eating, the reverse peristalsis that leads to vomiting can be detected before the stomach contents reach the mouth. This makes it possible to anticipate the actual vomiting and to interrupt the response chain in its incipient stage either by substituting an incompatible response or by delivering an aversive stimulus. Morgan and O'Brien (1972) employed the former procedure by pairing the incipient signs of the vomiting response with sips of ginger ale. Sajwaj, Libet, and Agras (1974), on the other hand, treated a 6-month-old infant with an aversive stimulus in what they called "lemon-juice therapy." Though the latter is a study of a single case, the investigators employed sufficiently reliable measures and experimental controls to warrant more detailed examination.

When the infant, Sandra, was admitted to the hospital she was about six months old but weighed less than she had at birth. Born with a harelip and cleft palate, for which she had been hospitalized once before, she was now suffering from malnutrition and dehydration. She was emaciated and unresponsive to her environment, displayed very little grasping of objects, no smiling, no babbling, no gross movements, and some crying (Sajwaj, Libet, & Agras, 1974). After each feeding with a commercially prepared formula she would begin her ruminative vomiting, opening her mouth, raising and folding her tongue, and then thrusting her tongue vigorously forward and back until, a few seconds later, milk would appear at the back of her mouth and slowly begin to flow out. This behavior would continue for 20 to 40 minutes until she had apparently brought up all of the milk she had previously consumed. Throughout this sequence, which was repeated after each feeding every four hours, Sandra neither cried nor showed other evidence of pain or discomfort. Thorough medical examinations failed to reveal an organic cause for this behavior which, like other cases of chronic rumination in infants, appeared self-induced.

While others (e.g., Lang & Melamed, 1969) had treated ruminative vomiting by administering contingent shock to the thigh which is a rapid, but also very drastic form of intervention, Sajwaj and his colleagues chose a less controversial aversive consequence for their treatment of Sandra. It consisted of squirting about 5 to 10 cc of lemon juice into the girl's mouth as soon as the vigorous tongue movements were detected. A simple and relatively benign treatment, this could be applied not only by the investigators (who could not be present for every feeding) but also by the ward staff and, if necessary, by the foster parents to whom the infant was discharged some 2½ months later.

The data reported by Sajwaj et. al. (1974) are based on the infant's weight and on observers' records of the number of tongue-thrust movements per 10-second interval during 20-minute observation periods following a feeding. During baseline, tongue-thrust rumination was observed in 40 to 70 percent of the intervals and the girl's weight continued to fall rapidly to below 8 pounds. At the first feeding under the lemon-juice regimen 12 applications were required, a number never again reached after that. During the next 15 feedings, the number of ruminations and tongue movements fell to below 10 percent of observation intervals. At that point an experimental reversal, during which the lemon juice was omitted for two feedings, revealed a dramatic increase of rumination with some 65 percent of the observation intervals reflecting that activity. Treatment was then resumed, quickly resulting in a decreased rate of the target behavior. After the twelfth day no regurgitated milk was ever observed in the infant's mouth and the tongue thrusts were replaced by what the investigators deemed normal mouth and tongue movements. Concurrently, the infant's weight began to increase and continued to do so until she was discharged from the hospital weighing 12 pounds, 5 ounces, an increase of 54 percent since the start of treatment two months earlier. About a month before discharge and after the rumination had essentially ceased the congenital harelip was surgically repaired but while this interrupted the weight gain for a few days it did not affect the rumination. It is also of interest that this infant who had been so lethargic and unresponsive at the time of admission was noticed to become more attentive to the adults about her, to begin smiling and grasping at objects, and to start babbling during the course of her hospitalization. This development continued after discharge and at follow-up 10 months later testing revealed only a slight developmental delay.

Sajwaj, Libet, and Agras (1974) recognize that although their reversal design permitted them to demonstrate the critical role of the lemon-juice application in the treatment of this infant, factors other than the presumably aversive quality of this acidic substance may have played a role in the child's improvement. As these authors point out, the interruption of the ruminative behavior, the forceful injection of a fluid into the mouth, the difference between the room-temperature lemon juice and the temperature of the mouth fluids, or the attention entailed in the administration of the lemon juice might, alone or in combination, have contributed to the effectiveness of the treatment and the contribution of these factors remains to be assessed. Lastly, two cautions voiced by Sajwaj and his associates are worthy of note. The acidity of the lemon juice, they point out, results in mild irritation to the interior and immediate exterior of the mouth and represents a minor negative side effect. More important is the possibility that careless administration of the procedure may result in the infant's aspirating the lemon juice into the lungs. This risk can be minimized by keeping the child's head upright when injecting the juice, by reducing the quantity of juice used, and by minimizing the force with which the juice strikes the inside of the mouth. Sandra, they report, was never observed to aspirate or even gag when the lemon juice was injected into her mouth. These risks and the relatively slow effect of lemon-juice therapy notwithstanding, it is in many ways preferable to the use of contingent shock which may so easily be abused and is unacceptable to many people. Nonetheless, when the alternative may be the infant's death even this drastic procedure has its place.

It was as a last resort and after several other procedures had failed to bring relief that Lang and Melamed (1969) used avoidance conditioning with a nine-month-old boy. This infant's ruminative vomiting had begun when he was five months old and had increased in severity until he would vomit within 10 to 15 minutes after every meal. At the time the conditioning procedure was decided upon, this child weighed only 12 pounds and was being fed through a nose tube. An electrode was attached to the child's calf and a brief, repeated shock, paired with a loud tone, was administered as soon as electromyographic monitoring confirmed the observing nurse's report that vomiting was about to take place.

Treatment sessions of less than one hour each were held following feedings and after only two such sessions shock was rarely required. By the third session only one or two brief presentations of the aversive stimuli were necessary to cause cessation of any vomiting sequence. After the first day of treatment only a few shocks were administered and both the time spent vomiting and the average length of each episode were abruptly reduced. By the sixth session the infant no longer vomited during the testing procedures and the nursing staff reported a progressive decrease in the child's ruminating and vomiting behavior during the rest of the day and that they were able to block these by loudly clapping their hands, indicating that the pairing of tone and shock had led to higher-order conditioning and stimulus generalization. Following three sessions during which there was no vomiting at all the procedure was discontinued. As conditioning theory predicts there was some spontaneous recovery of a mild version of the response two days later but three additional therapy sessions reinstated the treatment effect. Concurrent with the treatment and beginning on the day it was instituted the boy gained weight. Five days after the last conditioning trial he was discharged from the hospital and he continued to eat well without further vomiting. A month later he weighed 21 pounds and was described as alert, active, and attentive to his social environment. There seemed to have been no adverse consequence to the treatment which may well have served to save the boy's life.

OBSESITY

The food refusal and food rejection of anorexia nervosa and chronic ruminative vomiting are relatively rare disorders that demand therapeutic intervention because of their life-threatening aspects. Obesity, when based on excessive consumption of food, though rarely life-threatening, is nonetheless one of the nation's major health problems (Stunkard & Mahoney, 1976) because of its high incidence and its indirect contribution to poor health and reduced life expectancy. When one realizes that, in addition, today's society tends to take a highly negative view of people who are overweight so that this condition becomes a social handicap it is clear that overeating, no less than food refusal, calls for therapeutic intervention. We shall here examine some behavioral approaches to attaining weight reduction in obese children, recalling that obesity can only be defined in terms of a person's weight so that the cut-off point between normal and excessive weight is necessarily arbitrary. It must also be recognized that obesity may be due to one of several causes. These may include metabolic disorders and genetic factors. Here, as in other forms of somatic problems, close collaboration between behavioral and medical specialists is therefore essential.

The Parent's Role

Particularly with young children, eating is largely a behavior that occurs in the context of the family. It is therefore not surprising that the more effective treatment programs have been those where at least one of the parents was intimately involved in the procedure. In fact, Kingsley and Shapiro (1977) demonstrated that mothers who had been in a child-focused treatment group without their obese children were able not only to lose weight themselves but also to affect their children's weight reduction. This study was conducted with 40 children (24 girls and 16 boys), aged 10 or 11, whose initial weight was above the 90th percentile for their age. They were assigned to one of three treatment, and one no-treatment control condition. In one condition, the child-only group, the children attended eight weekly, one-hour group meetings that were built around a modification of the weight-reduction program developed by Stuart and Davis (1972). In line with this program, the children were provided with factual information regarding obesity and nutrition, taught the concept that weight loss can best be obtained by a combination of reduced food consumption and increased exercise, and asked to reduce their caloric intake. To aid them in this effort, the children were given small pocket calorie counting booklets and pocket diaries in which to record their daily food intake. Written instructions were handed out at the beginning of each session and the children were asked to show these to their parents. One of these handouts recommended that the parents institute a token reinforcement program in which the children could earn tokens and back-up reinforcers for following the program instructions and procedures. The authors do not report that any attempt was made to ascertain whether the parents did, in fact carry out these instructions.

In a second treatment group mother–child pairs attended the group sessions together, the program being the same as the one just described. In the third, mother-only group, the mothers attended alone and the program focused on having them help their children to overcome their weight problems by teaching them the necessary behavioral techniques. The analysis of the results revealed that the children's weight loss did not differ among the three treatment groups but that for each it was significantly greater than for the no-treatment control group. The children in the three treatment groups had lost a combined mean of 3.5 pounds over the eight weeks while those in the control group had gained a mean of 2 pounds during the same period. The weight of the mothers had not been a focus of treatment in any of the groups so that any change in their weight was incidental to that of their children. Interestingly enough, the women in the mother-only group lost an average of 6.25 pounds, significantly more than those in the mother–child, child-only, and no-treatment control groups.

On follow-up 6 and 20 weeks later Kingsley and Shapiro (1977) report that the three child-treatment groups did not differ from each other and that the weight gain of the children was age-appropriate in terms of norms for this age group. No comparison with the no-treatment control group was possible at follow-up because that group had been taken into treatment at the end of the 8-week waiting period. As for the mothers, those who had been in the mother-only group continued to weigh significantly less at 6-week follow-up than the women in the other groups, but at the 20-week follow-up intergroup differences were no longer in evidence.

The work by Kingsley and Shapiro (1977) suggests that mothers can succeed in helping their children lose weight and maintain that weight reduction even when the children themselves are not seen in treatment. It is of interest, however, that some of the mothers in the mother-only group expressed dissatisfaction at the exclusion of their children from treatment and that they doubted that the program could be effective. Conversely, some of the mothers in the child-only group resented being excluded from treatment while some of the children in the mother-only group were dissatisfied at not being allowed to take part. Judging by comments made on the posttreatment questionnaires, the participants in the mother–child group seemed most satisfied with the arrangement. While we do not know whether these reactions affected the outcome of treatment, it is not unusual for both parents and children in child behavior therapy to be at least surprised if one or the other does not have contact with the therapist. Parents, in particular, often have difficulty understanding how one can conduct child therapy without working directly with the child which tends to be the practice when treatment of young children is conducted by focusing on the reinforcement contingencies prevailing in the home. Clinicians often find it simpler to "see" the child from time to time than to explain to the parents that they can be the agents of therapy through their contingency management without the child ever being brought to the clinic.

Contingency Contracting. In a weight-reduction program for children conducted and evaluated by Aragona, Cassady, and Drabman (1975) all the work was done through the parents. The children, after being weighed, were sent to a playroom while the therapist discussed the program with and trained the parents. The focus of the treatment was on showing the parents how to teach their children to eat more slowly, to delay meals, to leave food on the plate, and to follow an exercise program. The youngsters were 15 girls, ranging in age from 5 to 10 years, whose physicians had recommended that they participate in a weight-reduction program. The 15 mother–child pairs were divided into three groups, two of whom received treatment while the third served as a no-treatment control.

The 12-week treatment program evaluated by Aragona et al. (1975) was based on a *response-cost contingency contract* between the therapist and the parents. The contingency contract operated as follows. Each mother was asked to decide on a weight-loss goal for her child, ranging anywhere between one and two pounds per week. She was then asked to deposit with the therapist an amount of money that, based on a sliding scale determined by family income and number of dependents, ranged between $12 and $30. This deposit could be redeemed in 12 weekly installments as a function of attendance at weekly group meetings (25% refund), bringing in the required graphs and charts reflecting the child's weight, eating, and exercise behavior (25% refund), and the child's reaching the agreed-upon amount of weight loss (50% refund). Conversely, proportional amounts of money were to be forfeited when any aspect of the contract was not met. This fine represented the response-cost. Every six weeks any deposit money that had not been earned back was divided as a bonus among the successful parents, the amount being determined by how often during the preceding periods their child had met the weight-loss criterion.

The contingency contract with its response-cost provision was in effect for both treatment groups which differed only in terms of the use of reinforcement. The mothers in the response-cost-plus-reinforcement group had been instructed in how to employ reinforcement principles to change their child's eating behavior. The children were to earn points and receive negotiated monetary reinforcements and praise for reducing their daily caloric intake, exercising, and following such stimulus control techniques as eating more slowly and only in one designated area. The mothers in the response-cost-only group had received no such instructions although, as it later emerged, some of them did reward their child for weight loss, one by sharing her redeemed deposit and bonus money with the child, and another by giving her daughter new clothes for losing weight.

When the baseline weights of the children were recorded before treatment began the three groups showed no statistical difference in their mean weights. When weighed again at the end of treatment, the four children remaining in the response-cost-plus-reinforcement group had lost an average of 11.3 pounds, the three who were still in the response-cost-only group averaged a loss of 9.5 pounds, while the five in the control group had gained an average of 0.9 pounds. The difference between the two treatment groups was not statistically significant but both groups did differ significantly from the control group. Given the fact that attrition had reduced the five children in the response-cost-only group to three and that the mothers of two of these had used a reinforcement system of their own, this lack of difference between the two treatment groups cannot be interpreted in terms of the effectiveness of reinforcement techniques in children's weight-control programs.

At a follow-up eight weeks after the end of treatment the children in the response-cost-plus-reinforcement group had maintained a mean weight loss of 7.9 pounds below baseline; those in the response-cost-only group were at an average of 5.0 pounds below their baseline weight, while the four children still in the control group had gained an average of 3.6 pounds over their weight at the start of the study. Statistical analysis showed that the response-cost-plus-reinforcement group had gained back significantly less weight than the controls while the difference between the other treatment group and the controls just missed reaching the conventional level of statistical significance. Another follow-up weight was obtained 31 weeks after treatment. By now only two children remained from the original control group. These had gained an average of 10.2 pounds but the small number precludes statistical comparison. The four children from the response-cost-plus-reinforcement group had maintained an average weight loss of 0.7 pounds while those from the response-cost-only group showed an average net gain of 7.3 pounds. Although the group that had been under explicit reinforcement contingencies thus seems to have done better than the other group, the difference between these two treatment groups is not statistically significant.

In evaluating the results of this study one must of course keep in mind that the participants were children aged 10 years and younger so that one would expect them to gain some weight as part of their normal physical development. Since Aragona et. al. (1975) report their data in terms of net change from baseline, a gradual reduction of this figure over a period of almost a year was to be expected. Unfortunately they do not relate these changes to the weight increase normally to be expected for children of a given age and height, nor did their design include a group of children with normal body weight whose weight increase could have served as a maturational control. In discussing their results, these authors point out that while both treatment groups had regained some weight after the termination of the program, the children in the response-cost-plus-reinforcement group regained weight more slowly than those in the response-cost-only group. Maybe, they say, the mothers in the former group continued to use reinforcement procedures and perhaps "the addition of a post-treatment contingency contract to ensure the long-range maintenance of weight loss attained during treatment would have been a valuable addition to the procedure" (p. 276).

Probably in part because food intake is such a powerful, primary reinforcer, obesity is a problem that is very difficult to overcome. While various weight-reduction programs are effective with some overweight persons, the maintenance of weight reduction, once achieved, is a problem for many. As with weight reduction programs for adults, it would appear that programs aimed at children must be designed explicitly to assure maintenance of any progress that has been achieved. One important aspect of such a design seems to be the individualization of the approach, something that is not possible when the experimental design of a study, such as the one we have just discussed, demands that individuals be randomly assigned to treatment conditions that are then applied to everyone in the group without consideration of individual differences. It is questionable, for example, whether the same treatment procedure can be expected to be equally effective for both a 7-year, 3-month-old child and a 10-year, 1-month-old child. Two children with these ages were included in the response-cost-plus-reinforcement group of Aragona et al. (1975) and on the last follow-up they were at opposite extremes of the distribution, the older one having gained more, the younger one less than the other children in the group. In the treatment program conducted by Wheeler and Hess (1976) emphasis was placed on individualization. We turn to that study next.

Individualization of Treatment

In examining the work of Wheeler and Hess (1976) one is once again struck by the troublesome dilemma so often found in therapy research that forces a choice between experimental rigor and clinical relevance. Almost inevitably a study either has good experimental controls but relatively little bearing on the issues faced in day-to-day clinical practice or it has high relevance to clinical practice but lacks important experimental controls. The Wheeler and Hess (1976) investigation is an example of the latter.

Working in a health maintenance organization where subscribers to the health plan are entitled to free services, Wheeler and Hess (1976) sought referrals of obese children from the staff pediatricians. The 40 children thus gathered ranged in age from 2 to 11 years and they represented "a reasonably broad range and degree of obesity" (p. 238). Fourteen of these children were assigned to a control group that was never contacted but for whom weight data were available from their routine visits to the health care facility. Of the 26 children who had been randomly assigned to the treatment group, 12 dropped out of treatment after three or fewer sessions; they constituted a "drop-out control." Treatment involved individual half-hour session with each mother–child pair. These sessions were initially scheduled at two-week intervals but they were gradually spaced further apart so that, as treatment was proceeding well, they were often at intervals of three weeks or longer. While this varying schedule served the clinical goal of encouraging the parents to become independent and to make appointments according to their needs, it is the kind of uncontrolled variable that an experimentalist finds most perplexing.

The treatment was predicated on the intention to achieve a reeducation of eating habits. This was to be accomplished by a combination of parent-training and child-management procedures, designed to reach a permanent change through a series of gradual approximations of that goal. Their behavioral orientation led Wheeler and Hess (1976) to emphasize an analysis of the stimuli surrounding and maintaining excess eating so that they might identify and later manipulate the antecedents and consequences that control and support overeating. In order to help identify the relevant aspects surrounding eating, each mother and her child were asked to maintain a "food intake record" on which they were to enter how much of what food was eaten when and in what social and physical surroundings. The information contained in this record was then discussed in the treatment sessions where recommendations for changes were presented. "The focus was upon a constantly evolving situation that was practical for the given patient in his particular environment" (p. 236), a sound clinical procedure but hardly an operational description of an independent experimental variable.

The authors provide a list of the eight most frequent problems together with the interventions they recommended. For example, where the child consumed large quantities of candy, cookies, and ice cream in the house, the recommended intervention was to eliminate such foods from the home and to obtain treats from outside sources, such as the ice cream vendor on the street. The mother would also be instructed to purchase food in portion-controlled packages that permit one to keep a clear record of the amounts consumed, to provide attractive snacks of lower calories, and to reward appropriate eating by selecting one food as a daily treat. Other problems such as a child's eating overly large quantities at mealtime or a child's inadequate exercise were handled in similar "common sense" fashion whereby inappropriate stimulus conditions were eliminated or controlled, appropriate conditions provided, and improvements in behavior rewarded by positive consequences.

The results of this study suggest that this highly individualized but vaguely defined intervention was effective in bringing about a reduction in the overweight condition of the 14 children who had remained in treatment for four or more sessions. The measure used by Wheeler and Hess (1976) is far superior to a simple report of the number of pounds lost or gained. In order to take account of the fact that children are expected to gain weight as the normal consequence of their development, these investigators obtained the average expected weight for each child's height, sex, and age from U.S. government statistical tables and compared that with each child's actual weight both before and after a uniform period of 7.3 months of treatment. The difference between expected and actual weight was expressed as percentage overweight and the comparison of percent overweight before and after treatment (or nontreatment for the controls) served as the measure of outcome. Of the 14 treated children 10 (71 percent) were closer to their appropriate weight at the completion of the study than at the onset, while four (28 percent) were further away from that ideal. Having been an average of 40.4 percent overweight at the beginning, the group as a whole was only an average of 34.9 percent overweight at the end, a mean individual reduction of 4.1 percent. Compared with this, the 12 children who had dropped out of treatment had increased their overweight by 3.0 percent and the 14 children in the control group had increased a mean of 6.3 percent. Statistical analyses showed that the 26 children who had been in treatment for any length of time (including those who had dropped out prematurely) had done significantly better in terms of reduction of their overweight than had those in the no-treatment control group. Apparently even those who dropped out of the program after less than four sessions had derived some benefit from the contact, suggesting that even a relatively modest intervention had been effective for these children whose mothers probably continued to follow some of the suggestions that had been made to them regarding their children's eating and exercise patterns.

The approach to weight reduction taken by Wheeler and Hess (1976) is noteworthy for its focus on the child's eating pattern as opposed to a focus on calories or other dietary considerations. Since the eating of young children largely takes place in close contact with their family, the child's eating pattern often relates to the life-style of the family. Changes in this pattern thus impinge on that life-style, hence the emphasis on working with both mother and child. One of the problems encountered among the families who participated in this study, for example, centered on parents who would eat inappropriate foods between meals and who, in order to be fair, shared these with their obese children. To eliminate the inappropriate foods from the child's world, such parents were advised to limit their own inappropriate eating to occasions when they were outside the home and to use "low risk foods" as special treats for the child. It is these family eating patterns that are often reflected in the high positive correlation between obesity in parents and obesity in children and it is of interest in this connection to note that the children who dropped out of the Wheeler and Hess treatment program tended to be those who had overweight parents. Although this study lacks data from a long-term follow-up, it is likely that a program of weight reduction aimed at a gradual altering of a family's eating pattern has a better chance of achieving long-term success than one where dramatic weight loss is sought by temporary adherence to a prescribed diet. At the same time, it is no doubt more difficult to change the eating pattern of a family than only to put the overweight child on a diet. The preliminary work by Wheeler and Hess (1976) would seem to point in a promising direction for achieving weight control when dealing with preadolescent children.

Obesity in Adolescents

When the participants in a weight-reduction program are not young children but adolescents, treatment can be effective without necessarily involving others in the family. This was demonstrated in a well-controlled study conducted by Weiss (1977) who used a behavioral approach to treat 46 obese adolescents, whose mean age was 13.5 years. Based on their expected weight relative to their age, height, and sex, these young people were overweight by an average of 42 pounds. The clients were assigned to one of five groups, balanced for sex, age, weight, and percent overweight. One group, a no-treatment control, had no contact with the therapist until the 12-week treatment period for the other groups had ended. Weiss (1977) describes the four treatment conditions as follows:

> *Diet-no-reward group*. The individuals in this group were instructed to follow the diet outlined by Stuart and Davis (1972). They could earn points for following this diet. These points, however, could not be exchanged for another reinforcer.
> *Diet-reward group*. This group was given the same diet but here the points could be exchanged for a variety of individually determined, self-administered back-up reinforcers, such as watching television.
> *Stimulus-control group*. The young people in this group were asked to engage in such stimulus control behaviors as eating in only one room of the house, doing

nothing else while eating, and chewing each bite thoroughly. They could earn points for each such behavior and these could be exchanged for self-administered reinforcers.

   Stimulus-control-plus-diet-reward group. This group combined the conditions of the diet-reward and the stimulus-control groups.

In all four treatment groups the responsibility for adhering to the program rested entirely with the adolescents, the parents having been asked to refrain from all interference. Each participant was seen individually for a 12 week period in therapy sessions that, with the exception of the first, lasted from 10 to 15 minutes. Participants were asked to engage in some form of physical exercise and to complete daily report forms that they were to turn in to the therapist at the next session. There was no external check on the extent to which the young people followed their prescribed program nor was the administration of the self-reinforcement controlled by anyone other than the client.

   At the beginning of treatment the individuals in the four treatment groups and in the control group had weighed an average of 154 pounds, representing an average overweight relative to their appropriate weight of 42.6 percent. All participants, including those who had been in the control group, were weighed again at the end of the 12-week treatment period. At this point the members of the control group had gained an average of 4.2 pounds while each of the four treatment groups had registered an average reduction in percent overweight. For all the treatment groups except the diet-no-reward group this change was statistically significant, as was the difference between the change in the control group and the changes in all treatment groups with the exception of the diet-no-reward group. A comparison among the four treatment groups showed the greatest change in percent overweight to have been achieved by the stimulus-control-plus-diet-reward group where the average weight reduction had been 2.9 pounds, representing a negative change in relative overweight of 6.9 percent.

   In order to assess the long-range effectiveness of his treatment program Weiss (1977) conducted a follow-up approximately one year after the start of treatment. Since the members of all groups had grown an average of 1.3 inches, the merit of the percent-overweight measure over a measure based on absolute weight becomes immediately evident. By the time of the follow-up, the control group had increased in percent overweight by 7.4 percent; that is, while they had been an average of 52.1 percent over their ideal weight prior to the treatment phase they were now an average of 59.5 percent above that weight. The young people in the diet-no-reward group who had shown a minor net loss (−3.2 percentage points) at the end of treatment had, a year later, increased their weight, as reflected in a net gain of 2.8 percentage points. The diet-reward group was barely holding its own, having reduced their percent overweight by an insignificant amount (−0.1 percent). The most encouraging follow-up results were shown by the two groups for whom the emphasis in treatment had been on changing their eating habits—the stimulus-control group and the group for whom stimulus control had been combined with diet and reward. These groups had continued to reduce their percent overweight by significant amounts, -9.0 and -10.5, respectively. Statistical comparisons of changes in percent overweight showed that each of these stimulus-control groups had done significantly better than either the no-treatment control group or the diet-no-reward group. Furthermore, when the data for the two stimulus-control groups were combined and compared with those for the combined diet groups (diet-no-reward and diet-reward) it was shown that the former had done significantly better than the latter.

Since only the two groups who had been instructed to practice stimulus control over their eating behavior were able to maintain their weight loss and thereby decrease the degree to which they were overweight, it appears that stimulus control is a more effective means for achieving weight reduction and weight maintenance than merely placing a person on a diet. When added to a stimulus-control regimen a diet does seem to contribute to a more rapid initial weight loss although it seems to have little influence on the maintenance of reduced weight. Weiss (1977) reports that many of the young people who had been assigned to the stimulus-control group wanted to have guidelines on what they should and should not eat, apparently expecting a weight-reduction program to include a diet. Since it is clearly not inappropriate to teach youngsters something about good nutrition, Weiss recommends that stimulus control instructions be combined with diet and self-reward for maximum effectiveness.

Before leaving the topic of obesity it is worth examining why a stimulus-control procedure, such as the one Weiss (1977) had used, is so effective in bringing about weight reduction and weight maintenance for a period of at least one year. What is there about eating in only one room of the house, doing nothing else while eating, chewing each bite thoroughly, using smaller plates, leaving some food on the plate at the end of the meal, and waiting a half hour before eating dessert that accomplishes what elaborate diets seem unable to? One possible answer to this comes from looking at eating in terms of the principles of operant learning. The act of eating is a response that carries its own, immediate reinforcement in terms of the food that is placed in the mouth and consumed. What are the discriminative stimuli in whose presence this response-reinforcement contingency operates and that thus come to control this behavior? For many people who find it difficult to lose weight these discriminative stimuli are many; watching television, sitting in a movie, lying in bed reading, or the sight of the refrigerator may all have acquired control over the eating response by having been paired, at one time or another and often repeatedly, with eating and its reinforcing consequence. What a stimulus-control approach to weight reduction seeks to accomplish is to limit the number of stimuli that control the eating response. When only one room in the house (kitchen or dining room) contains stimuli for eating, the person should no longer "feel hungry" in the living room or the den. When the sight of food on the plate no longer controls eating until it is all gone, the person should find it easier to stop eating. Since, as in the study by Weiss, the individuals seeking weight reduction are themselves rearranging these stimulus conditions, programs of this nature can be construed to be programs in self-control. They are more effective than methods based on what is usually conceived of as self-control (gritting one's teeth and thinking, "I must not eat, I must not eat") because, by changing one's external environment, one no longer exposes oneself to the stimuli that have gained the power to seduce one into eating.

ASTHMA

The breathing difficulties associated with asthma have long been viewed as a classical example of a so-called psychosomatic disorder, one involving psychological as well as biological factors. The physical symptoms of asthma can be found in a variety of conditions, not all of which are appropriately classified as asthma. These symptoms are difficulty in inspiring and, particularly, expiring air, accompanied by sensations of chest tightening and a characteristic wheezing during the expiratory phase of breathing. The restriction of air flow is due to a swelling of the mucous membranes of the trachea, the bronchi, or both. Such swelling can be the result of exposure to any of a variety of allergens, such as pollens, dust, or animal fur and it is often precipitated or exacerbated by psychological or physical stress. The relative contribution psychological and biological factors make to this disorder seems to vary from individual to individual.

An oft-cited study by Purcell, Brady, Chai, Muser, Molk, Gordon, and Means (1969) demonstrated that among a group of asthmatic children one can identify at least two subgroups. In one of these the asthmatic attacks are usually preceded by emotional arousal, such as anger, sadness, excitement, or anxiety while in the other group children will manifest asthma attacks in the absence of identifiable emotional antecedents. More children in the former group than in the latter responded favorably to a temporary absence of their family, suggesting that some aspects of interpersonal relationships contribute to both the frequency and the intensity of the asthmatic episodes of these children. Given this information it stands to reason that therapeutic intervention based on psychological principles will be more effective with those children whose asthma has psychological antecedents than with those where such precipitating factors cannot be demonstrated. There is therefore a great need for assessment instruments that can reliably differentiate between subtypes of asthmatic children (Knapp & Wells. 1978). Even the simple dimension of severity of asthma appears to be a factor in whether a psychological approach to treatment will lead to improvement, because while milder cases seem to benefit (Alexander, 1972), the more severe cases appear adamant to such intervention (Alexander, Cropp, & Chai, 1979).

A number of studies that were reviewed by Knapp and Wells (1978) had suggested that teaching progressive relaxation to asthmatic children might be an effective means of improving their respiratory function (Alexander, Miklich, & Hershkoff, 1972; Davis, Saunders, Creer, & Chai, 1973). This conclusion had been based on findings of statistically significant changes on a laboratory measure, the peak forced expiratory flow rate, that records the speed with which the child is able to expel air when instructed to do so with as much force as possible after having inspired to maximum capacity. As Alexander, Cropp, and Chai (1979) have pointed out, statistical significance obtained when measuring a rather atypical kind of breathing is not the same thing as clinical significance in the sense of improvements in the child's asthmatic condition outside the laboratory. When these investigators replicated earlier studies of the effect of progressive relaxation on asthma, using more sophisticated measures of several aspects of pulmonary function, they failed to find a clinically meaningful change for the severely asthmatic children with whom they had conducted their study. Again, the issue of assessment and case selection emerges. For, as these investigators themselves point out, in the discussion of their results, progressive relaxation may well be useful when it is employed in the context of systematic desensitization with children whose fear of asthma has complicated their condition.

A differential effect of relaxation training with asthmatic children was also found by Davis et al. (1973) who report that such training significantly increased the peak expiratory flow rate of children with relatively mild cases of asthma who were not on any medication, while it had no effect on the expiratory rates of cases whose condition was considered so severe that they required ongoing medication. An innovative aspect of the treatment conducted by Davis et al. (1973) was the use of electromyographic (EMG) feedback. In this method the therapist provides the patient with visual and/or auditory signals that indicate the state of relaxation of various muscles by means of electrodes that are sensitive to changes in muscle tension. Such *biofeedback* enhances a person's ability to acquire voluntary control over a variety of bodily functions, such as heart rate or blood pressure, that are difficult to monitor without the information provided by the electronic sensing device.

Learning to control autonomic and other bodily functions by means of a biofeedback device can be construed in terms of the operant conditioning paradigm in that the individual's covert response (e.g., slowing of heart rate) has the consequence of an observable change in the biofeedback signal in the direction therapist and client have agreed as being desirable. For adults and older children, reaching this desired result may serve as a reinforcer but with younger children the procedure can be presented as a game in which points and prizes can be earned for keeping the biofeedback signal at a specified level.

Biofeedback, however, is not the only instance where operant principles can be applied to the treatment of asthma. Creer (1970), for example, succeeded in reducing the frequency and duration of hospitalizations of two 10-year-old asthmatic boys by limiting access to such reinforcers as visitors and toys while the children were in the hospital. A reversal design revealed that having asthmatic attacks severe enough to require hospitalization was indeed under the control of such reinforcers so that time-out from the availability of these reinforcers was an effective treatment method. A somewhat similar approach has been used by Neisworth and Moore (1972) in the case of a 7-year-old asthmatic boy whose asthmatic wheezing was particularly severe at bedtime. A functional analysis of this behavior suggested that the solicitous attention the child's parents gave him during these episodes served as the maintaining consequence. They therefore instructed the parents to ignore the asthmatic responses and to tell the boy that he could earn a monetary reward for decreasing the time he spent coughing at bedtime. This procedure had an immediate effect. After an initial increase in the amount of time the boy spent coughing in the evenings (the spurt so typical of the onset of an extinction procedure), the time spent coughing decreased dramatically. A reversal of procedures, where the parents were instructed to resume attending to the boy's asthmatic responses showed the expected increase, followed again by a decrease when the treatment contingencies were reinstated. Follow-up over a period of 10 months revealed that the improvement was not only maintained but was, in fact, continuing. It is noteworthy that they boy's parents, who had unwittingly reinforced his asthmatic coughing, were able to act as his therapists once they had been given relevant professional advice.

Nonasthmatic Respiratory Distress

As pointed out earlier, the term "asthma" is used rather loosely to label a variety of respiratory difficulties. Sometimes, in fact, the diagnosis may be employed in order to obtain admission to a specialized treatment facility even when the problem does not entail the typical asthmatic wheezing. This seems to have been the case with a 15-year-old boy who was treated by Alexander, Chai, Creer, Miklich, Renne, and Cardoso (1973). Fourteen months earlier, this boy had suddenly developed a severe, hacking cough that had occasioned eight visits to hospital emergency rooms, 25 hospital admissions, and 113 missed school days. Often the coughing bouts had been so severe that the boy lost consciousness. When the problem resisted all treatment except hospitalization 500 miles from home, the boy's physician, "in desperation," diagnosed it as asthma, thereby facilitating his admission to a well-known asthma research institution specializing in children. There it was discovered that the cough had no apparent physical basis, nor was there any evidence that the boy was suffering from asthma. Several specific stimuli, such as the odor of beef grease, shampoo, hair spray, and bath soap were found to be precipitating the cough and the response seemed to be maintained by the consequent concern and attention by all members of the boy's family whose entire life pattern had come to revolve around his coughing. While this information might have suggested a less drastic form of treatment based on manipulating the reinforcing consequences, Alexander et al. (1973) chose to use an avoidance learning procedure, employing what they call "faradic aversive stimulation," which is a euphemism for electric shock.

The presentation of painful stimuli can be justified as a treatment procedure when the alternative is permanent injury or death, as in cases of chronic vomiting or severe self-injurious behavior, and when more benign treatment methods have failed or would be too slow. Although the case presented by Alexander et al. (1973) was surely of considerable severity, their report fails to convince that the use of a punishment procedure was absolutely essential. While their approach is thus not necessarily a model to be readily emulated, the procedure is worth describing since it is one of the few instances in the literature on child behavior therapy involving the use of the avoidance conditioning paradigm.

At first, a simple punishment procedure was tried. This consisted of presenting the boy with the odor of shampoo which would elicit a cough, whereupon a 5-milliampere shock of 1-second's duration was delivered to his right forearm. Under this contingency the coughing response showed a sharp increase over the baseline frequency and the boy (not unreasonably) expressed resentment at being made to cough in order to punish him. The investigators thereupon changed to an avoidance procedure where, instead of being shocked each time he coughed, the boy could avoid the shock by holding off or delaying the cough for a very short interval after presentation of the shampoo odor. He was told that as he learned to suppress his cough, the intervals would be progressively lengthened until he did not cough at all but that, if he coughed prior to the end of the interval for a given trial, he would receive one shock.

As described by Alexander et al. (1973), treatment now proceeded in the following manner. The open jar of shampoo was held directly under the boy's nose for 2 seconds and he was instructed to inhale deeply. During baseline the latency between presentation of stimulus and appearance of the cough was 6 seconds so that this was used as the initial critical delay interval. If the boy could suppress his cough for that length of time, no shock was delivered and a new trial was begun after an interval of about 2 minutes. The delay interval was gradually increased over succeeding trials if the cough had been suppressed but it remained the same if shock had to be delivered because of a failure to delay that response. Using this method, the boy's cough in response to the shampoo was eliminated after 75 trials during 24 of which the shock had to be delivered. The same procedure was then successfully used to shape cough suppression to beef grease, bath soap, and hair spray. Follow-up over a period of approximately 18 months revealed no further coughing despite frequent exposures to the substances that had formerly elicited that response. There were no reports of the appearance of other problems and since the family had been advised to help the boy develop alternatives to the coughing behavior as a means of gaining attention, he was able to resume the active life of a typical adolescent. This boy's cough had apparently been an operant response, maintained by its consequences. Clearly, it was not a case of asthma.

SEIZURE DISORDERS

The seizures associated with epilepsy are generally believed to be due to a sudden and excessive discharge of cerebral neurones. They are often manifested by individuals who have suffered verifiable damage to the brain and whose abnormal brain-wave pattern can be substantiated by electroencephalography. While such seizures thus have a definite neurological basis, they are, in some individuals, precipitated by environmental factors such as stress or fatigue. As we shall see, behavioral interventions have proven effective in bringing about a reduction in the frequency of seizure episodes.

Many seizure-prone individuals experience or display phenomena that reliably precede the onset of a seizure. Such *prodromes* may take the form of headaches, ringing in the ears, excessive thirst, localized spasms, or fixed stares. Zlutnick, Mayville, and Moffat (1975) conceptualized seizures that are preceded by such premonitory episodes as the terminal link in a behavior chain and they reasoned that if such a chain could be interrupted in an early stage, it might be possible to abort the seizure. Working with five children whose pre-seizure behavior could be reliably identified, these investigators found interruption of the behavior chain sufficiently promising to warrant further explorations. With four of these children, the interruption took the form of having another person (attendant, parent, teacher, or even another child) shout "No!" loudly and sharply while, at the same time, grasping the child by the shoulders with both hands and giving him or her a single, vigorous shaking. With the fifth child, the interruption took the form of a differential reinforcement (DRO) procedure.

The shake-and-shout procedure was most effective with a 7-year-old boy who had a history of seizures dating back to when he was 2 years old. Though not diagnosed as epileptic, he was receiving anticonvulsant medication but would still have an average of 12 seizures per day. These seizure episodes had three distinct components. They would begin with a fixed stare at a flat surface, followed by the boy's body becoming rigid, whereupon he would exhibit clonic muscle spasms, violent shaking, and then fall to the floor. Since no seizures were observed that were not preceded by the staring, it was that behavior which Zlutnik et al. (1975) chose as the target for modification.

During a three-week baseline period observers recorded just under 60 seizures per five-day school week, or about 12 per day. With the introduction of the interruption procedure described above, the frequency of seizures initially fell to about one or two per day and dropped to zero after eight weeks of this treatment, which was then continued for another three weeks. At follow-up six months later, the boy was reported to be seizure-free except for one questionable incident where he had fallen on the playground. Concurrent with the treatment, the anticonvulsant medication had been systematically reduced so that the boy was off the drug when the treatment ended. In order to obtain a minimal control that might answer the question whether the interruption procedure had indeed been the critical variable in the reduced seizure frequency, the investigators applied a reversal procedure for half a day, after the seventh week of treatment since they were reluctant to reinstate a behavior as severe as a seizure for longer than that. During the morning of that day the preseizure staring was not followed by the interruption procedure and this resulted in six full seizures during the 3-hour period. When the interruption contingency was reinstated in the afternoon, the seizures again dropped to the prereversal level, providing strong evidence that the procedure was truly the effective independent variable. It is of particular interest that the interruption procedure not only eliminated the seizures but that this boy's preseizure staring had also been removed from his repertoire. With other children, whose rate of preseizure behavior was not affected by the procedure, the reduction of seizure rate was less dramatic.

As stated earlier, one of the children on whose treatment Zlutnik et al. (1975) reported had received differential reinforcement of behavior incompatible with the responses in the early part of the seizure chain. Here, the seizures took the following form. The girl, a mentally retarded, epileptic, 17-year-old, would display rigidity and tensing of her body, a clenching of her fists and a raising of her arms at a 90-degree angle from the body, followed by her head snapping back and a grimace appearing on her face, whereupon a major motor seizure would ensue. Since the arm-raising was the most reliably observable part of the early phases of the chain, it was selected as the target for intervention. As soon as the girl would display this behavior, another person would place her arms back down at her side, wait for 5 seconds, then praise her effusively for having her arms lowered, and present her with a piece of candy. This procedure was at first carried out by one of the investigators or other members of the institution's teaching staff. Eventually, however, other students at the training center were able to assume this responsibility. During baseline, this girl had an average of 16 major motor seizures per day, but with the introduction of the differential-reinforcement procedure, the frequency of seizures very quickly dropped to and remained near zero. After nearly two months the contingency was removed as part of a reversal design whereupon seizures reappeared at the rate of about six per day. Reintroduction of the DRO procedure again reduced seizure frequency to a near-zero level where it remained over a nine-month follow-up period. The only instances of seizure activity took place when no one was able to reach the girl in time to interfere with the arm-raising, which always preceded the seizures.

Not with all of the five children with whom Zlutnick et al. (1975) applied their interruption procedures was the seizure-suppression as successful as with the two whose cases we have here presented. For example, with a 4-year-old, brain-damaged boy whose seizures took the form of mild arm and head spasms or brief episodes of vacant staring, followed by vomiting, the use of the contingent shouting and shaking had only a transitory effect on the frequency of these episodes. The major difference between this child and the two previously discussed was that his motor seizures were preceded some 60 percent of the time by a lowered activity level, a prodrome more difficult to observe than an arm-raising, while the vacant stare–vomiting sequence had no discernible antecedents. As a result, the interruption method could be applied to the motor seizures only intermittently and with the vacant staring it was used not before but during the episode itself. It appears that the effectiveness of the procedures used by Zlutnick et al. (1975) depends on the ability of an observer reliably to predict a seizure so that the behavior chain leading up to it can be consistently interrupted. Such an interruption can either take the form of a punisher, such as the shout-and-shake procedure described, or of the differential reinforcement of an incompatible response alternative, like lowering the raised arms. As these investigators pointed out, their procedures may hold promise in the treatment of some types of epilepsy although further research is required before the mechanisms underlying the effect can be understood.

One of the imponderables in the procedures used by Zlutnick et al. (1975) and recognized by them has to do with the reliability of the seizure-frequency data. In counting the number of seizures per day, it is obvious that only those seizures will be reported that take place while an observer is present. A frequency of zero thus means that no seizures were observed, not that none had taken place. With a problem such as seizures one would have to observe a child 24 hours a day in order to obtain truly reliable data. Lacking this total surveillance, it is conceivable that an interruption procedure, particularly one involving punishment, may succeed in reducing seizure frequency only in the presence of observers who also manage the contingency, but not when the child is alone. In other words, the observer-contingency manager may become a discriminative stimulus for seizure suppression. This hypothesis could be tested by separating the contingency managing from the observing function as might be done if seizure frequency were monitored by a telemetry device that the child would wear throughout the day and, if necessary, at night so as to obtain a 24-hour record of seizure activity.

The same reliability problem encountered by Zlutnick et al. (1975) also plagues the data reported by Balaschak (1976) who instructed the teacher of an 11-year-old epileptic girl how to reinforce seizure-free periods and who succeeded thereby in reducing the frequency of her seizures from three to one per week. The teacher maintained a chart on which she entered check marks reflecting seizure-free time periods that earned the girl a reward at the end of the week. The child's mother introduced an informal contingency management system at home and succeeded to reduce seizure frequency there also. Unfortunately, neither the teacher nor the mother seemed to have become fully convinced of the efficacy of this procedure and when they therefore decided to discontinue it the girl's seizures returned to pretreatment levels. While this provided a certain amount of experimental control that lends support to the assumption that the contingency management had indeed been responsible for the improvement, it regrettably spelled an early end to what appears to have been a promising intervention. This experience is one with which child behavior therapists are not unfamiliar; often there is little that can be done for a child when important adults like parents or teachers are unwilling or unable to cooperate with a treatment plan.

This dependence on the cooperation of others makes procedures that do not rely on such cooperation particularly attractive. If a therapist can help children to manage their own contingencies, thus acquiring control over their own behavior ("self-control"), the need for help from parents or teachers is obviated. Along this line, a case study reported by Ince (1976) points to one of the most promising behavioral methods for the control of epileptic seizures. This therapist based his intervention on relaxation training and succeeded thereby in providing a 12-year-old epileptic boy with a technique for preventing his own seizures. The treatment began with reducing the boy's anxiety that had become associated with his recurrent seizures. To accomplish this, Ince used systematic desensitization and the relaxation training that had been part of this procedure was then employed to eliminate the seizures. Ince taught the boy to associate the word "Relax" with the relaxed body state and to use this cue word as a conditioned stimulus to elicit that state at will. Later, whenever the boy experienced the aura of an approaching seizure, he was to induce relaxation by saying the cue word. This method enabled the child to avoid the onset of seizures and to eliminate completely both the grand mal and petit mal episodes he had previously been experiencing at the rate of 9–10 grand mal and 25–26 petit mal seizures per week. Systematic desensitization had, in this case, served as a self-control procedure much as Goldfried (1971) had conceptualized.

MISCELLANEOUS SOMATIC DISORDERS

Insomnia in a case of an 11-year-old girl was treated by Weil and Goldfried (1973), employing a method of self-relaxation. This child's problem had led her to be so fatigued that the school nurse's concern eventuated in referral for treatment. Partly because of her sensitivity to external noises, it would take this child as long as two hours to fall asleep at night. Along with this, her parents complained about her reluctance to remain at home when they went out in the evening, even when they had engaged a sitter to stay with the child. This suggested that the sleep problem had a strong psychological component.

Weil and Goldfried (1973) decided to focus the treatment of this girl on her insomnia problem, assuming that her fear of being alone would be minimized once she could fall asleep more readily. Accordingly, a therapist visited the home in the evening and, with the girl lying in bed, gave her instructions for relaxation, based on the alternate tensing and relaxing of various muscle groups. The child responded favorably to this and fell asleep one hour later. The therapist's relaxation instructions were now put on a tape recording, 30 minutes in length, and the girl was instructed to listen to this tape at bedtime every evening. After she had done this for two weeks, during which time improvement began to be reported, the tape was changed so as to eliminate the muscle-tensing phase, providing only instructions for relaxation. By now, the girl would fall asleep either during or immediately after the playing of the recording so that, after one week, a 15-minute version of the tape was substituted. She used this version each night for another two weeks when she was given yet another tape that lasted for only five minutes and contained instructions for self-relaxation. The girl used this tape for approximately one week more and had no difficulty falling asleep shortly after the end of the recording. Weil and Goldfried (1973) report that they eliminated the use of external instructions for relaxation at this point. Instead they told the child that she was to concentrate on self-relaxation to the exclusion of all other thoughts as soon as she was in bed and ready to go to sleep. The girl did this for the following few weeks and reported that she was able to sleep almost immediately. As the therapists had hoped, the problem about letting the parents go out in the evening had abated concurrently with this improvement. The girl was generally a more relaxed person. When the family was contacted for a follow-up six months after termination of treatment all previous difficulties had disappeared. It is noteworthy that in the two months taken up by the treatment, direct contact between the therapist and the child and her parents had been limited to seven sessions, including two assessment interviews and a home observation. Nevertheless, by using the tape recordings, the girl had been able to receive some 40 sessions of relaxation training, thus affording a remarkable economy of therapist's time. The method thus not only provides a form of self-management but it also comes close to being a self-help procedure.

Another problem relating to sleep where psychological and biological factors are difficult to separate is presented by *somnambulism*, or sleepwalking. A treatment, based on a rationale similar to that underlying the conditioning procedures used with enuretics, was developed by Clement (1970) who worked with a 7-year-old boy whose somnambulism was associated with nightmares, crying, and talking in his sleep. This child had been averaging four nights of sleepwalking per week when the therapist introduced a regimen that called for waking him up whenever he engaged in this behavior or when he was about to begin it. Assessment had revealed that sleepwalking was always preceded by a recurrent nightmare that involved being chased by "a big black bug." The boy would then begin to sweat heavily, moan, talk in his sleep, and toss about in his bed. He would then get out of bed and begin walking around the house.

Clement (1970) reasoned that if his client could learn to awaken himself whenever he experienced the nightmare, the behavior chain leading to sleepwalking would be interrupted and the somnambulistic episode aborted. The boy's mother was instructed to be alert for such precursors as moaning or tossing in bed and to wake the boy up whenever these occurred or, when she had missed these cues, to awaken him when she found him walking around the house. While this method was anything but systematic and the mother not entirely consistent in her behavior, it nonetheless succeeded in reducing the sleepwalking to less than one per week. The boy reported that he would now wake up whenever he had his nightmare and on follow-up a year later sleepwalking had ceased almost entirely. While Clement (1970) views his procedure as derived from a conditioning model, this case study is at best suggestive. Inasmuch as getting out of bed could easily be monitored by a simple, automated device that might activate a signal awakening the sleeper, a more rigorous application of the conditioning model should be possible for the purpose of the controlled experimental study that this author advocated.

The somnambulistic boy just discussed had reported that he could "wake himself up" when he had his nightmare. In that sense, his treatment, too, was a form of self-management. Another self-management procedure was used by Hutzell, Platzek, and Logue (1974) in working with an 11-year-old boy who manifested a condition called *Gilles de la Tourette's syndrome*. This is a very rare, poorly understood, presumably neurological disorder in which the patient manifests such motor tics as head jerking accompanied by loud noises that sound like barking. The latter sometimes develop into compulsively emitted obscene words or swearing, referred to as *coprolalia*. This bizarre behavior often has its onset with adolescence and it obviously not only interferes with a youngster's social relationships but also disrupts classroom decorum, often leading to disciplinary actions. Lahey, McNees, and McNees (1973) had reported on a case like this in which they helped the classroom teacher control a child's "verbal tic" by a time-out procedure. In contrast, Hutzell et al. (1973) placed control over this behavior directly into the hands of the afflicted child. This boy had developed a skipping motion while walking, a severe head jerk, and an intermittent utterance of a peculiar "barking" sound some six months earlier. Medication and an attempt to use a positive reinforcement procedure had proven unsuccessful. The self-monitoring procedure introduced next and focused on the head movements and barking noises was described as follows.

Treatment took place in two half-hour sessions per week during which one therapist played a simple game with the child while an observer recorded the frequency of the head jerks and barks per 30-second interval. During the first nine sessions, which were used to establish a baseline, the boy displayed a mean rate of 1.20 head jerks and 1.58 barks per minute. The experimental design called for a multiple baseline across responses. Therefore the boy was first taught to monitor his head jerking behavior. This was accomplished by providing him with a hand-held counter, demonstrating the head jerking to him, having him produce this movement intentionally, and instructing him to score one point on the counter each time he jerked his head. It should be pointed out that the boy was highly motivated to cooperate in the treatment program because his bizarre behavior was causing him considerable social embarassment.

After the boy had been instructed in monitoring his head movements he and the therapist again engaged in play sessions during which he was to continue scoring his tics on the hand counter. The accuracy of these counts was checked against those maintained by the observer and the boy received praise when the two counts matched. The accuracy of the self-monitoring gradually increased and with it the rate of head jerks decreased to an average weekly rate of about 0.50 per minute. Meanwhile, the barking noises that had not yet been made a target of the self-monitoring showed a marked increase, reaching an average weekly rate of more than 6.5 barks per minute. With the eighteenth session, when head jerking had been reduced to a moderate rate, self-monitoring of the barking noises was initiated. The boy was told that henceforth, instead of counting the head movements, he was to count the barking behavior. The training for this again included modeling by the therapist, intentional production of the response by the child, and demonstration of the use of the counter. With the introduction of this procedure, the barking behavior immediately decreased in frequency, falling to a rate of 0.21 per minute. By now the boy had no difficulty with accurate monitoring, his count showing a very high level of agreement with that of the observer.

Treatment was discontinued after 27 sessions at which point the boy's mother was instructed how to observe and record the two target behaviors. Follow-up sessions were conducted at the clinic 1½ months, 2½ months, and one year after termination. These showed that the frequency of the target behaviors was still low, though it was not zero. Interestingly enough, at the time of the one-year follow-up when some of the target behavior was observed at the clinic, the boy's parents and teachers reported that he no longer displayed any of it. This discrepancy is difficult to explain. The authors report that the boy had been extremely anxious on his first return to the clinic and they speculate that this may have been responsible for reinstating an occasional barking response for which the clinic setting may well have been a discriminative stimulus. However, as Hutzell et al. (1974) observe, what is of practical importance is not whether a treatment effect can be demonstrated in the clinic but whether it is apparent in a child's natural environment. From that standpoint the self-monitoring they had taught to their patient had clearly been successful.

Recapitulation

Somatic disorders represent an interface between the behavioral and the medical sciences where collaboration between specialists from these fields often serves to enhance the help that can be made available to a patient. As in the case of anorexia nervosa, it is often difficult or impossible to determine whether psychological or organic factors are the principal contributors to the condition, yet, while psychological interventions have often shown to be highly effective, this does not permit one to draw conclusions as to the cause of a disorder.

In problems relating to eating—food refusal, persistent vomiting, and obesity—the manipulation of the consequences of the behavior often succeeds in modifying the problem but attention to the immediate antecedents in the form of discriminative stimuli may well be equally useful. With young children, in particular, eating usually involves an interaction with parents whose collaboration in a treatment plan thus becomes very important. This is also true in the treatment of asthma since the pulmonary distress that is associated with that condition almost inevitably elicits a reaction from the child's family.

Interruption of a behavior chain has been shown capable of reducing the frequency of seizures and of sleepwalking, while self-management procedures have been used effectively with such somatic problems as insomnia and the bizarre, ticlike behavior associated with Gilles de la Tourette's syndrome. These demonstrations of the positive contributions to the treatment of somatic disorders of which the behavioral sciences are capable have, to some extent, reduced the historically based hesitation and skepticism of the medical profession about collaboration with specialists in psychology, resulting in what has come to be known as behavioral medicine.

CHAPTER 13

Self-Stimulation and Self-Injury

GENERAL CONSIDERATIONS

The bizarre and puzzling excess behavior to be discussed in this chapter is exhibited primarily by such profoundly impaired children as those labeled mentally retarded, schizophrenic, or autistic. *Self-stimulatory behavior* takes such forms as stereotyped, repetitive spinning of objects, flapping of fingers or arms, and rhythmic rocking. Such behavior is often very persistent and therefore tends to interfere with therapeutic attempts to teach the child language or other adaptive responses (Koegel & Covert, 1972). For this reason it must be reduced or eliminated in an early stage of treatment so that constructive intervention can become effective. Standing in the way of the child's acquisition of adaptive behavior, self-stimulation is detrimental to the child though it is obviously not as detrimental as self-injury which, as the term implies, represents actual physical damage to the child's body and may, in extreme cases, actually be life-threatening. *Self-injurious behavior* by retarded or psychotic children takes such forms as head-banging, hitting one's eyes, biting parts of one's body, or repeated scratching that creates deep and open wounds. The magnitude of this behavior may be such as to threaten permanent blindness, concussions, large, bleeding, and infection-prone lesions, or the loss of a finger. At lower levels of magnitude self-stimulatory or self-injurious behavior can occasionally be observed in relatively normal children. For example, young children are sometimes reported to rock in their bed or to hit their head on the side of the crib in the process of falling asleep. Excessive scratching has been found in otherwise unimpaired youngsters, and, as we shall see, hair-pulling to the point of creating bald spots is not an unknown clinical phenomenon in otherwise normal children.

A discussion of behavioral treatment of self-stimulatory and self-injurious behaviors is impeded by several factors that reflect the difficulties faced by investigators seeking to do research on this topic. There is, first of all, the fortunate circumstance that, though not unfamiliar to those working with profoundly disturbed or retarded children, the overall prevalence of these behaviors is relatively low. This accounts for the fact that the information available on the treatment of these self-directed behaviors is based largely on studies of individual children or of a very small number of rather dissimilar individuals. Children labeled as autistic or mentally retarded represent quite heterogeneous groups, partly because the diagnostic labels are so nonspecific, and partly because each of these difficulties encompasses a range of impairments along the dimension of severity. Thus, an autistic child who is mute presents a different case from one who possesses some language, and a retarded child at the trainable level is not the same as one who is so profoundly impaired that little more than maintenance care is feasible. On top of this, children who engage in self-stimulatory behavior do so in a variety of ways, from a boy who crosses his eyes to a girl who flaps her arms. Similarly, self-injurious behavior may range from mild face-slapping to violent head-banging. To speak of treating self-stimulatory or self-injurious behavior as if these were circumscribed categories is therefore an overgeneralization. The treatment approaches discussed in this chapter should thus be viewed as suggestions for procedures a therapist may wish to try with a specific child and not as recommendations of proven methods. It should further be stressed that while several of the procedures to be discussed have proven effective under the carefully controlled conditions of highly specialized treatment and research facilities, their transferability to other settings often remains to be demonstrated.

There remains yet another point that must be stressed before we can turn to the substance of this chapter. It derives from the fact that the self-injurious behavior manifested by profoundly impaired children often endangers such a child's health and survival. Faced with problems of such proportions many investigators have reluctantly turned to the use of a punishment procedure as the most effective treatment strategy presently available. This, as Harris and Ersner-Hershfeld (1978), among others, have pointed out, clearly entails major ethical issues, particularly when the procedure involves the infliction of pain. No one should apply punishment as a treatment procedure without full awareness, exploration, and discussion of its ethical implications and never before less drastic measures have been considered. Moreover, as Lovaas and Newsom (1976) have so cogently stated in their discussion of behavior therapy with psychotic children, no one should undertake to punish self-injurious behavior who is not prepared to invest much time and effort in establishing and maintaining adaptive response patterns that can take the place of the suppressed behavior and serve the child as a means of obtaining social reinforcers (p. 319). In the absence of such efforts, procedures employing punishment, especially those that involve the infliction of pain, are totally unacceptable. The elimination of self-directed behavior should not be an end in itself but always a means toward the end of increasing a child's repertoire of adaptive responses.

SELF-STIMULATORY BEHAVIOR

Before examining some of the procedures that have been used for the purpose of reducing or eliminating self-stimulation of profoundly impaired children, it is fitting to ask when it is appropriate to interfere with such behavior. In reading, for example, that Doke and Epstein (1975) sought to reduce the persistent thumb-sucking of two 4-year-old, retarded children one wonders why this behavior was viewed as calling for intervention. Only when one considers that these children's self-stimulation prevented them from effective participation in a language-training program does the investigators' strategy become understandable. Intervention can be justified only when self-stimulation actively interferes with the acquisition of adaptive behavior. There is, however, some controversy whether self-stimulation necessarily prevents a child from learning.

A study by Koegel and Covert (1972) lent support to earlier findings by Lovaas, Litrownik, and Mann (1971) who had shown that the amount of self-stimulation by autistic children varied inversely with their obtaining reinforcement for other behavior. Attempting to teach three autistic children a simple discrimination, Koegel and Covert (1972) found that these children made no progress as long as their self-stimulatory behavior remained unchecked. The children were able to acquire the correct discrimination only when self-stimulation was suppressed by the investigator yelling "No" and, if necessary, slapping the child on the hands when self-stimulation occurred. Self-stimulation also appears to interfere with appropriate play behavior that emerges only once self-stimulation has been suppressed (Koegel, Firestone, Kramme, & Dunlap, 1974) but a more recent study by Klier and Harris (1977) suggests that this statement has to be qualified by taking into account the nature of the self-stimulation, the requirements of the task, and the level of the child's impairment. Profoundly autistic children, as Lovaas et al. (1971) had suggested, may be unable to attend to more than one stimulus at a time so that self-stimulation may functionally interfere with other behavior. Children at somewhat higher developmental levels, on the other hand, may be able, in the metaphor of Koegel and Covert (1972), to have their cake and eat it too. They might, for example, be mouthing their left hand while working on a puzzle with their right or engage in body-rocking while listening to a story. Only when the self-stimulation physically interferes with the demands of a task, as hand-slapping does with placing pieces in a puzzle, would it seem necessary to suppress that behavior in order to enable the child to learn adaptive responses. As always, intervention must be based on careful assessment so that treatment can be individualized. With this proviso, we turn to an examination of available treatment procedures.

The Treatment of Self-Stimulation

If one seeks to reduce the frequency of an excess behavior, an extinction procedure readily comes to mind as a method likely to be successful. It is known that by withholding the reinforcer that maintains a response the frequency of that response will decrease after the typical extinction spurt has subsided. In order to employ extinction, however, it is first necessary that one identify the reinforcer that maintains the behavior. The same is true if one were to contemplate a time-out procedure where access to the reinforcer must be suspended contingent on the response one seeks to weaken. The most obvious consequence of self-stimulation that might serve as a reinforcer is the attention that adults tend to pay to the child who is engaged in self-stimulation. Yet with many children this behavior is known to continue even when adult attention is systematically withdrawn and does, in fact, often take place when such children are alone and observed without their knowledge. Unlike other operant responses, self-stimulatory behavior thus does not seem to produce external consequences. For this reason it has been assumed that the sensory effect that the stimulation creates is, in some fashion, reinforcing in itself. This would mean that the reinforcers are under the child's own control so that another person is not in a position to withhold them, greatly complicating the use of extinction or time-out procedures for the purpose of therapy.

The reinforcing aspects of self-stimulatory behavior were demonstrated by Solnick, Rincover, and Peterson (1977) who had been working with a 6-year-old autistic girl, trying to teach her the discrimination of colors. Frequent tantrums (not self-stimulation) would interfere with the lessons and whenever such a tantrum took place, the teacher would pick up the candy reinforcers being used for the training and leave the room for 10 seconds. This was thought to be a time-out procedure and the investigators assumed that it would reduce the frequency of the tantrums. Tantrums, however, increased dramatically. What had been expected to serve as a punisher (the teacher's leaving the room) seemed to be a reinforcer. Observations of the child during the time-out periods revealed that she would engage in self-stimulatory behavior while alone. In terms of the principle first explicated by Premack (1959), the opportunity to engage in a high-probability behavior (self-stimulation) had been made contingent on a lower probability behavior (tantrums) thereby reinforcing the latter and leading to its increased frequency. When Solnick et al. (1977) now changed their procedure by having the teacher physically restrain the child from self-stimulation for 10 seconds whenever she emitted a tantrum, the tantrums quickly decreased in frequency and did not occur at all during the last four treatment sessions. Self-stimulatory responses appear to have a reinforcing property and if these responses are to be reduced or eliminated, this reinforcing property must be identified so that it can be made available or substantially altered.

Sensory Extinction. An investigation conducted by Rincover (1978) not only identified some of the reinforcing properties of self-stimulatory behavior but also pointed out a direction that therapeutic intervention might conceivably take. The procedure involved the masking or removing of various types of sensory stimulation that were produced by a child's stereotyped, repetitive behavior. One child, for example, would persistently spin objects, such as a plate, on the table. When one does this a number of effects will result. One sees the plate twirling, hears the sound it makes, feels the slight current of air that is set in motion, and gets the kinesthetic feedback from one's fingers and hand as the object is set in motion. If the behavior follows operant principles, one or more of these sensations must be the consequence that maintains the response at such a high frequency. The relevant consequence could be identified if one were to eliminate one of these sources of stimulation at a time until one observed a change in the response frequency. In practice, this might prove rather difficult; how, for example, would one control the kinesthetic feedback?

In the case described by Rincover (1978), the functional analysis of the behavior was facilitated by careful observation of the boy's behavior. This showed that he would cock his head to the side each time he had set the plate spinning, as if he were listening to the sound it made. This led the investigator to cover the table at which the child was sitting with a thick but hard and flat carpet thereby making the spinning inaudible. As soon as this had been done the percentage of time this boy spent on plate-spinning dropped from a high of 72 percent to near zero. When, as part of a reversal design, the carpeting was removed from the table, the spinning again increased, taking up some 83 percent of the time devoted to the testing session. Since a different intervention, blocking visual feedback by placing a blindfold over the boy's eyes, had little effect on the self-stimulatory behavior, it was concluded that the auditory effect had indeed been the reinforcing consequence. This conclusion was confirmed in a different study (Rincover, Cook, Peoples, & Packard, 1979) which showed that contingent access to such auditory stimulation as the sound of a music box could serve as a reinforcer for appropriate toy play on the part of this child.

Two other severely psychotic children whose self-stimulatory behavior was also studied by Rincover (1978) seemed to be controlled by different reinforcers. One boy engaged in excessive finger-flapping, placing one or both hands in front of his face and vigorously moving the fingers back and forth. The other child, a girl, would twirl such objects as a feather or a string of beads in front of her eyes. In these cases, the visual and proprioceptive components of the behavior were experimentally manipulated. Visual feedback was easily blocked by means of a blindfold but proprioceptive sensations could only be masked and not removed. Masking was attempted by placing a small vibratory mechanism on the back of a child's hand that generated a repetitive, low-intensity, high-frequency pulsation. The finger-flapping of the boy did not seem to be a function of the visual sensation because the blindfolding had little effect, but when the proprioceptive sensations were masked by means of the vibrator, his self-stimulation decreased from an average of 83 percent to an average of 5 percent. With the girl, removal of the visual effect of the object-twirling also had little effect and while the reduction in her behavior under the condition of proprioceptive masking was less dramatic than it had been with the boy, she nonetheless reduced her response rate from an average of 95 percent to an average of 49 percent.

The function of the vibrator in this experiment is unfortunately somewhat ambiguous. Taping such a mechanism to the back of a child's hand will *change* the sensations created by finger-flapping, but it does not remove the proprioceptive consequence. Conceivably, flapping one's fingers while one has a vibrator taped to the back of one's hand serves to make finger-flapping unpleasant so that the reduction in that response under the masking condition might have been the result of the introduction of a punisher and not of the removal of a reinforcer. This comment, however, is not meant to detract from the value of Rincover's (1978) pioneering study because it does permit one to view the reinforcement functions of self-stimulatory behavior in a new light. It further opens possibilities for the therapeutic use of sensory extinction with children where the sensory feedback of self-stimulation is easily controlled.

As we pointed out earlier, the elimination of self-stimulatory behavior should never be an end in itself for unless children who engage in such behavior are helped to replace it with other, more adaptive responses they might as well be permitted to obtain whatever positive consequences behavior like finger-flapping seems to provide. In fact, under certain circumstances, the reinforcing potential of self-stimulatory behavior might be used for strengthening other, more adaptive behaviors. Rincover (1978) suggested that a child who is reinforced by the auditory consequences provided by a spinning object might be taught a new response if one made the opportunity to listen to the recorded noise of a spinning plate contingent on the emission of that response.

Hung (1978) reported the use of self-stimulation in just such a fashion and Devany and Rincover (1978) studied whether this had any adverse consequences. If one permits a child to engage in self-stimulation contingent on some other behavior one desires to reinforce, the questions arise whether this will increase the amount of self-stimulation that children will engage in during other times of the day and whether once having used self-stimulation as a reinforcer, such self-stimulation will be more difficult to treat at a later time. If either of these consequences were to occur, it would clearly be a questionable, if not unethical practice to use self-stimulation as a reinforcer. In what they considered an experimental analysis of an ethical issue, Devany and Rincover (1978) found neither of these undesirable consequences; children so reinforced did not engage in more self-directed behavior during extratherapy time and when sensory extinction was later applied to that behavior it was readily eliminated.

Time-out Procedures. In its technical meaning time-out entails the response-contingent withdrawal of the opportunity to obtain positive reinforcement and since this procedure reduces the frequency of the response it had followed, time-out is a form of punishment, punishment by removal. In order to use time-out correctly, it is necessary to ascertain the positive reinforcer that is maintaining the behavior so that access to this reinforcer can be contingently withheld (Solnick, Rincover, & Peterson, 1977). In certain respects, the sensory extinction procedure used by Rincover (1978) contains an element of time-out in that he sought to prevent the child's self-stimulatory response from having the reinforcing consequence that had presumably been identified. Thus, when the child spun the plate and this failed to produce the sound that seemed to have maintained that response in the past, the frequency of the plate-spinning behavior began to decrease. That is to say, the child had been placed under a time-out contingency. There is only a very subtle difference between therapy in which padding is placed on a table so that subsequent plate-spinning will fail to produce a noise and therapy that actively prevents a child from obtaining a reinforcer *after* the response has been emitted. In either case one is dealing with punishment by removal, in other words, time-out.

Some investigators have made the assumption that the consequence that maintains self-stimulatory behavior is not the sensory stimulation that Rincover (1978) sought to remove, but the response-contingent attention that others in the child's environment provide when the behavior is observed. Some support for this assumption comes from a report by Risley and Wolf (1967) who had been working on the development of speech in echolalic children whose self-stimulatory behavior interfered with the training efforts. They found that they were able to bring mildly disruptive behavior under control by having the teacher simply look away until the child would once again sit quietly in the chair. For more severe forms of self-stimulatory behavior they used a procedure whereby the teacher left the room for a brief period whenever such behavior occurred, returning only when the child had not engaged in self-stimulation for a few moments.

Although their approach enabled Risley and Wolf (1967) to reduce self-stimulatory behavior sufficiently to permit them to teach the children some communicative speech, the function of the manipulated teacher attention is not entirely clear. It may be that the teacher's watching the child engage in self-stimulation and commenting on it with words like, "Don't do that," had indeed served as a social reinforcer so that looking away or leaving the room introduced a time-out contingency. On the other hand, it is possible that the teacher's leaving the child alone in the room introduced an aversive state of affairs that was terminated contingent on the child's not engaging in self-stimulation, thereby delivering negative reinforcement contingent on the omission of that response. As MacDonough and Forehand (1973) have pointed out, many parameters of the time-out procedure are yet to be studied and many therapists use that term rather loosely and practice the procedure a bit haphazardly. As is always the case when one seeks to use a time-out procedure in hopes of reducing the frequency of a given behavior, one must have established what consequence is maintaining the behavior before one can arrange a response-contingent withdrawal of that consequence. This was cogently pointed out by Plummer, Baer, and LeBlanc (1977). When, in order to withdraw attention contingent on misbehavior, a teacher suspends a child's instructions this may serve to strengthen the misbehavior through negative reinforcement if receiving instructions happens to be an aversive experience for that child. Plummer et al. (1977) recommend the use of paced instruction, wherein the lesson continues regardless of the child's behavior, and they demonstrated that when misbehavior no longer led to interruption of the lesson it could be reduced to zero.

If the withdrawal of another person's attention contingent on a self-stimulatory response can serve to reduce such responses, as one interpretation of the Risley and Wolf (1967) data would suggest, then the self-stimulatory behavior of at least some children might conceivably be maintained by two sources of reinforcement. One of these sources would be extrinsic in the form of social reinforcement so that a reduction of the behavior would have to be brought about by withdrawing attention from the child whenever self-stimulation takes place. The other source would be intrinsic, stemming from the sensory consequences produced by the response itself and here a reduction would have to be accomplished by preventing the child from experiencing the consequences, as Rincover (1978) had done. The answer to whether a given child's self-stimulatory behavior is best reduced by sensory extinction procedures or by withdrawing social attention or by a combination of the two lies, of course, in a careful functional analysis of the objectionable behavior. Such assessment may also reveal whether yet a third form of intervention, *response prevention*, might be the treatment of choice. Here a child is kept from obtaining reinforcement from self-stimulation by physically interfering with that response, as in grasping the hands of a child whose self-stimulation takes the form of finger-flapping. Inasmuch as doing that is inevitably linked with the therapist attending to the child whenever self-stimulation takes place, that form is obviously contraindicated if the assessment has shown that adult attention serves as a reinforcer for self-stimulation.

Overcorrection. A method that has shown some promise for reducing the self-stimulatory behavior of profoundly disturbed or retarded children is *positive practice overcorrection* which we previously examined in connection with the treatment of certain control deficits (Chapter 7). As conceptualized by Foxx and Azrin (1973b) self-stimulation reflects a gross imbalance in reinforcement for self-directed versus outward-directed activities. Profoundly impaired children such as the severely retarded or the autistic have few responses in their repertoire that might result in their receiving reinforcement from the external, social, or physical environment. What responses they do emit toward that environment are often so inadequate or maladaptive that they are more likely to be ignored or punished than rewarded so that even these responses are likely to drop out of the repertoire. Self-directed behaviors, on the other hand, regularly result in direct and immediate consequences which, to judge by the fact that once begun they are maintained for long periods of time, appear to be positively reinforcing. When self-stimulation is thus reinforced, it attains progressively greater strength and frequency, consequently reducing still further the likelihood that the child will engage in reinforced, outward-directed activities. To be successful, a therapeutic intervention would therefore have to be capable of reversing the balance of reinforcement for self-directed as opposed to outer-directed responses, self-directed responses being made less, and outer-directed responses more reinforcing. Overcorrection is successful, Foxx and Azrin (1973b) believe, because it is capable of doing just that.

Basically, overcorrection for self-stimulation consists of having another person (attendant, teacher, therapist, or parent) immediately interrupt every episode of such behavior and manually guide the child in *functional movement training,* that is, in an activity where the body parts involved in the self-stimulation are employed in an incompatible, socially adaptive form. Since this intervention has been shown to reduce the frequency of the self-stimulation which it follows, overcorrection is technically a form of punishment, probably because being held and required to engage in a physical activity have aversive aspects for a child. However, as will be seen when we examine the cases of children with whom Foxx and Azrin (1973b) used this procedure, the punishment involved is so mild that most people would probably not view it as such.

One of the four children with whom Foxx and Azrin (1973b) demonstrated the effectiveness of overcorrection in eliminating self-stimulation was a 7-year-old boy, Mike, who had been diagnosed as autistic by three different treatment facilities. Among other autistic behaviors, he engaged almost continuously in clapping his hands and this was chosen as the target for intervention. Before describing the procedure that was used, it is important to note the setting where it was applied since the use of overcorrection presupposes that the child's environment provides the continuing availability of positive reinforcement for outward-directed activities that can take the place of self-stimulation once that has been reduced or eliminated. Mike was enrolled in a behaviorally oriented day-care program with a high (1 to 3) ratio of teachers to children where the teachers had ample time to focus on instructing the children in constructive behaviors and in providing frequent reinforcement for appropriate, outward-directed responses.

After 11 days during which baseline observations on Mike's hand-clapping behavior were gathered, Foxx and Azrin (1973b) introduced the overcorrection procedure that in his case, took the form of "functional movement training," which they describe as follows. Any time the boy began clapping his hands, a teacher would immediately tell him to stop and then instruct him to move his hands in one of five positions: held above his head, held straight out in front of him, placed in his pockets, or held together and placed behind his back. The teacher would manually guide the boy's hands whenever he failed to follow one of these instructions. Each of the required positions was to be maintained for 15 seconds and then another instruction would be given until all five had been carried out. The sequence in which these instructions were given was kept random in order to assure that the child learned each individual instruction rather than a set sequence. Manual guidance was faded out as the boy began following the verbal directions but the teacher remained ready to provide the guidance, if needed, by "shadowing" the boy's hands with her own.

The overcorrection condition remained in effect for 20 days after which a procedure of verbal warning was instituted. This was intended to approximate the conditions that might exist in the child's natural environment and entailed merely saying something like "Stop that!" when self-stimulation was observed. If the child failed to cease self-stimulating or repeated that behavior during the remainder of that day's school session, overcorrection was used again but, as Figure 20 shows, there was no need for that in the case of Mike who had not engaged in the hand-clapping since the eleventh treatment day. However, while his hand-clapping had been eliminated during the entire school day, he was almost continuously doing so at home. One of the day-care teachers therefore went to instruct the boy's parents in the functional movement training

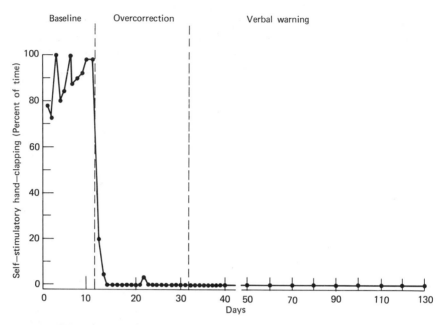

Figure 20. The effect of Overcorrective Functional Movement Training and Verbal Warning procedures on the self-stimulatory hand-clapping of an autistic boy. The ordinate is labeled in terms of the percent of time samples in which hand-clapping was observed. During the baseline period, no contingencies were in effect for hand-clapping. (Foxx & Azrin, 1973. Copyright by the Society for the Experimental Analysis of Behavior, Inc.)

procedure that had been used so successfully at school. Two days after the parents had instituted that procedure at home, Mike's hand-clapping ceased to occur and on the very rare occasions when he did display it, a verbal warning was sufficient to stop him.

The experimental design used with Mike did not include a reversal procedure so that this case provides only presumptive proof that the overcorrection was indeed the effective independent variable. However, with the three other children, who were severely retarded and whose self-stimulatory behavior took the forms of object-mouthing, hand-mouthing, and head-weaving and with whom overcorrective procedures had also been used, reversal to baseline condition resulted in an immediate increase in the frequency of the target behavior with a similarly dramatic decrease when the treatment was reinstituted. The self-stimulation of all of these children was essentially eliminated by the end of 10 days of treatment and sometimes even sooner.

Again, it should be recalled that the setting in which this study had taken place provided many opportunities for having a child's outward-directed activities earn immediate positive reinforcement. It is unlikely that similar success would be possible in a relatively impoverished setting, such as an overcrowded institution, where a child's self-stimulation might be one of the few sources of gratification. As previously noted, Foxx and Azrin (1973b) base their treatment procedure on the rationale that self-stimulation reflects a gross imbalance in reinforcement for self-directed, versus outward-directed activities and consider overcorrection a method for reversing this imbalance in favor of the latter. A summary of this rationale and of the treatment procedures derived from it are shown in Table 2.

Table 2   Summary of Rationale for Treating Self-stimulation by Overcorrection (after Foxx & Azrin, 1973b)

Treatment Aim	Treatment Effect
Decrease the duration of reinforcement intrinsically provided by any given instance of stimulation.	Teacher immediately interrupts each instance of self-stimulation that is observed.
Prevent further instances of self-stimulation and the consequent strengthening of that behavior.	Self-stimulation is physically prevented while the teacher manually guides the child through the overcorrection.
Arrange annoying (aversive) consequences for each instance of self-stimulation so as to reduce its frequency.	Annoying consequences for self-stimulation result from the physical effort required by overcorrection and from being manually guided.
Teach outward-directed activities that can take the place of the self-stimulation.	Outward-directed activities are taught by manual guidance and instruction.
Provide an environment that will assure a high frequency of positive reinforcement for continuing outward-directed activities.	Provides an enriched school or home environment where positive reinforcement for outward-directed activities is continuously available.
Qualitatively alter the tactile, proprioceptive, visual, gustatory, or other sensations resulting from self-stimulation since these presumably account for its reinforcing value.	Requiring movements, postures, and gustatory experiences* that are opposite or different from those naturally resulting from self-stimulation, qualitatively changes the physical sensations naturally associated therewith.
Provide negative reinforcement (relief from annoyance) in addition to positive reinforcement for outward-directed behaviors since positive reinforcement alone seems insufficient.	Provides negative reinforcement for outward-directed behavior when the child moves spontaneously or attends to the teacher, thus eliminating the annoyance of being manually guided.

*The reference to gustatory experiences refers to work with children whose self-stimulation takes the form of mouthing objects or body parts and for whom overcorrection involves the use of a mouthwash, introduced as part of an oral hygiene procedure.

An overcorrection procedure was also used by Epstein, Doke, Sajwaj, Sorrell, and Rimmer (1974) with two profoundly disturbed children who displayed inappropriate hand and foot movements and other self-stimulatory behavior. The results of these treatment efforts were as positive as those reported by Foxx and Azrin (1973b) but Epstein et al. also discovered some additional effects of this procedure. With one of the children with whom they worked, overcorrection was introduced to reduce inappropriate hand movements and involved the arm and hand exercises that had been employed in the case of Mike, described above. When the same exercises were then used contingent on that child's self-stimulating foot movements, these too underwent a reduction in frequency. This seems to support the assumption that the overcorrective exercises function largely as a negative consequence (punishment) for the behavior they follow regardless of the topographic similarity of the exercises and the self-stimulation.

With the other boy about whom Epstein et al. (1974) reported, the overcorrection applied to reduce inappropriate hand movements also proved effective when used contingent on the child's inappropriate vocalizations during naptime that disrupted other children's sleep. In the case of this child it was also observed that as the frequency of inappropriate hand movements decreased that of appropriate play increased. It seemed that the self-stimulation had interfered with more appropriate behavior. There was, however, a negative side effect in that at naptime when the boy's inappropriate vocalizations were reduced by overcorrective hand exercises, inappropriate foot movements became more frequent. Epstein et al. (1974) speculate that this paradox might be explained by the fact that during play periods teachers would attend to and thus reinforce manifestations of appropriate play, while at naptime the appropriate alternative to the undesirable vocalizations, namely taking a nap, is not likely to receive explicit reinforcement.

When Doke and Epstein (1975) investigated the effects of overcorrection further, they again found that the procedure can be used to reduce behavior that is not topographically similar to the overcorrection. Here a so-called oral overcorrection that involved the response-contingent application of a strong mouthwash was effectively used to reduce hand- and object-mouthing. When the same consequence was then made contingent on inappropriate behavior that did not involve the mouth, that too underwent a reduction in frequency. Overcorrection appears to serve as a generalized punisher but when used in this fashion it no longer includes the aspect of positive practice that had led Foxx and Azrin (1973b) to introduce this procedure because it not only entails aversive qualities that might suppress the undesirable behavior but also, and at the same time, provides the child with adaptive alternate responses that can take the place of the suppressed behavior.

There is a natural relationship between having to undergo an oral hygiene procedure involving the use of a strong mouthwash in consequence of having placed "dirty" objects in one's mouth. But when that procedure is used as a consequence of not lying quietly at naptime it becomes an arbitrary and illogical punishment that does not contribute to the child's learning a socially adaptive behavior. The punishing quality of their use of oral overcorrection is also suggested by the observations reported by Doke and Epstein (1975) to the effect that verbal warnings ("If you don't lie quietly I'll have to use the toothbrush") were capable of maintaining the reduction of self-stimulation and that, in one instance, a child, having observed another receiving oral overcorrection thereupon showed a reduction in his own self-stimulation.

The side effects of overcorrection that had been reported by earlier investigators induced Wells, Forehand, Hickey, and Green (1977) to conduct a study explicitly aimed at exploring this aspect of the procedure. They also noted that while Foxx and Azrin (1973b) had indicated that overcorrection was aimed at teaching the child "outward-directed activities," the overcorrection procedures, such as the hand exercises that have been described, are outward-directed only in the sense that they are made in response to instructions received from another but that they can hardly be viewed as constructive or socially useful alternatives to self-stimulation. Furthermore, as Wells et al. (1977) point out, no one had ever demonstrated an increase in the frequency of the behaviors actually practiced during overcorrection although other constructive activities, when available and likely to be reinforced, seemed to increase. These investigators thus reasoned that the activities required during overcorrection ought to be something like appropriate toy play which, once practiced under instructions and guidance in consequence of self-stimulation, might become the constructive and desirable alternative to that undesirable behavior. This formulation represents an intriguing challenge to the assumption that overcorrection is a form of punishment for if the activity required during overcorrection were aversive, the child should be expected to avoid that activity at other times so that, if toy play were required during overcorrection, such play should not be something the child would later engage in on his or her own. As we shall see, the results presented by Wells et al. (1977) leave this paradox essentially unresolved.

The two boys with whom Wells et al. (1977) conducted their study were 10-year-old fraternal twins with intelligence test scores in the severely retarded range who engaged in a variety of inappropriate, self-stimulatory behaviors such as flipping toys in front of their eyes, placing fingers, toys, or other objects in their mouths, flapping hands or fingers, body-rocking, and masturbating. The investigators established a time-sampling observation procedure for these behaviors and also for such appropriate toy play as working on a puzzle, stacking wooden blocks, or playing with a log-construction game. Their experimental design called for multiple baselines across subjects and across behaviors such that after an initial baseline period that differed in length for the two boys, overcorrection was introduced in a sequential order for the four classes of targeted inappropriate behaviors: object manipulation, mouthing, hand movements, and other inappropriate behaviors.

The aim of the overcorrection procedure was to engage the boys in appropriate toy play whenever they emitted one of the targeted behaviors. The procedure involved a verbal command to stop the behavior, followed by manual guidance in appropriate toy play. To do so, an investigator would approach the boy after issuing the verbal command, physically stop the inappropriate response, and then guide him through 2½ minutes of appropriate play either with the toy that had been used inappropriately or, where the target behavior had not involved a toy, with one arbitrarily chosen. Manual guidance was faded out when the child spontaneously engaged in appropriate play but the investigator would continue to "shadow" the child's hand until the end of the 2½-minute period. All parts of this investigation took place in a small playroom containing only the toys with which the overcorrection was to be conducted. The two boys and two investigators spent a 30-minute free play period together in this room four days a week for a total of 53 sessions. The rest of these days the boys spent with other children in the day school for developmentally handicapped children in which they were enrolled. It is worth noting that the effects of the intervention were reported only for the 30-minute treatment periods for as long as the investigation lasted. Nothing is known about any generalization to the rest of the children's school day or about maintenance of the treatment effect over time.

Given the limitations just mentioned, the results reported by Wells et al. (1977) are quite impressive. With both boys, every one of the four classes of inappropriate behavior that had been targeted for intervention by the overcorrection procedure showed an abrupt reduction in frequency the moment the procedure was made contingent on a particular class of self-stimulation. Moreover, with one of the twins (John) it was evident that as overcorrection was introduced first for one, and then, one at a time, for additional inappropriate behaviors, fewer overcorrections were needed in order to obtain the desired effect. The percentage of time this boy spent in appropriate toy play increased spontaneously as his self-stimulatory behavior decreased. The other twin (Tim), however, not only failed to show the generalization of the treatment effect across target classes but he also did not engage in spontaneous toy play despite the fact that his self-stimulation was markedly reduced when overcorrection was applied to a given class of these inappropriate behaviors. Even when explicit reinforcement for appropriate play was made available Tim's play failed to increase. Only when Tim was given verbal prompts ("Tim, play with _____ '') in addition to the reinforcement did he begin to play with the toys in an appropriate manner during a high proportion of the available time.

The study conducted by Wells et al. (1977) dramatically underscores the phenomenon of individual differences in response to treatment procedures, differences that manifest themselves even in twins who lived in the same home, attended the same school, and were treated in the same room by the same two therapists. It is well to keep this observation in mind when one examines the findings of treatment research based on the single-subject design or where group data are reported in terms of means or other measures of central tendency which inevitably mask the individual differences among the cases treated. Research that shows a particular treatment to be effective can never provide assurance that the treatment will have the desired results with another individual, in a different setting, treated by a different therapist. All too often careless statements are made that imply that disorders, treatments, therapists, and clients are standardized, homogeneous entities about which one can make glib generalizations. Wells et al. recognize this problem when they conclude that for some children overcorrection may be sufficient to teach and motivate the appropriate behaviors practiced during manual guidance but that for other children caregivers may have to provide an environment that assures a high frequency of positive reinforcement for outward-directed behavior. That is exactly what Foxx and Azrin (1973b) had suggested.

Earlier, we had raised the question why an overcorrective activity that is required of a child as a form of contingent punishment should later become an activity to which the child will spontaneously turn. Should toy play, when used as the overcorrection, not become aversive? At least in the case of John who did spontaneously engage in the very activity that had been used to punish him for self-stimulation, the results reported by Wells et al. (1977) suggest that there is something amiss with this formulation. The answer lies in the manner in which overcorrection was applied.

It will be recalled that whenever a child engaged in self-stimulation an investigator would physically intervene by stopping the inappropriate response and then manually guiding the child through appropriate toy play. Physical intervention and manual guidance entail being held and restrained in one's voluntary movements and that experience is very likely to be aversive. In fact, since Wells et. al. (1977) mention that as much as possible they ignored kicking, crying, or fighting during the 2½ minutes of overcorrection, such reactions to the coercive measure must have taken place, reflecting the aversive nature of the procedure. There is then the following key phrase in their report, "only by engaging in positive practice of appropriate toy play could the child avoid forced manual guidance" (p. 683). In other words, in the context of the overcorrection, appropriate play resulted in immediate negative reinforcement in the form of release from the aversive manual guidance. This then strengthened the desirable play, resulting in its being emitted in what seemed like a spontaneous manner. It is here particularly revealing to note the investigators' report that John's appropriate play responses "resembled those that had been guided by the experimenter during forced manual guidance, suggesting that these behaviors had been learned during overcorrection episodes" (p. 687). It appears that what these investigators called "appropriate toy play" may have been no more than a stereotyped avoidance response that had been learned under conditions of negative reinforcement. The other twin, Tim, who had been described as functioning in school at a less advanced level than his brother, as less attentive, and less quick to learn, might also have acquired that behavior, had he been given more training trials, when in fact (due to the requirements of the multiple baseline design) he had received only 75 overcorrections to John's 109.

Given the above formulation, the question arises why the children in studies like those of Foxx and Azrin (1973b) or Epstein et al. (1974), whose overcorrection had taken the form of various arm and hand exercises, did not also engage in avoidance behavior that took the form of the exercises they had been made to practice before they could return to other activities. Here the answer seems to lie in the fact that these children had been treated in the open setting of the day-care facility where many different activities and toys were available by means of which they could receive positive reinforcement and from which the restraint associated with the overcorrection might have constituted a time-out. The children in the Wells et al. (1977) investigation, on the other hand, had been treated and observed in a small (5 by 4.2 m) playroom where the number of toys was intentionally limited to those used in the study. As Foxx and Azrin (1973b) stressed, a child's caregivers should provide an environment that will make it possible for that child to encounter a high frequency of positive reinforcement for outward-directed activity. Such activity should not be constrained by limiting its range to four types of toys. Under artificial conditions one is likely to observe artificial behavior and that may well have been what Wells et al. (1977) saw in the case of John.

When Ollendick and Matson (1978) reviewed the published studies dealing with the use of overcorrection they concluded that it is a highly effective procedure for the immediate reduction of self-stimulatory behavior in children and that there is evidence that it results in durable response suppression over periods extending up to one year. While questions about the effective components of that procedure must await further research, Ollendick and Matson point out that the most effective way of using overcorrection seems to be one that incorporates the aspects originally recommended by Foxx and Azrin (1972). These are that the procedure should be directly related to the behavior one seeks to suppress, that it should be applied immediately following that behavior, that each instance of overcorrection should last for longer than a few moments, and that the exercises should be actively and vigorously performed by the child. Though, as we have seen, overcorrection has also been shown to be effective when one or another of these characteristics are omitted, Ollendick and Matson (1978) believe that they are nonetheless desirable if one wishes to maximize the effectiveness of the procedure.

On the whole, overcorrection is, at present, the most effective and the most practical technique available for the suppression of the self-stimulatory behavior of profoundly impaired children. As Foxx and Azrin (1973b) had demonstrated with two severely retarded children, overcorrection is far more effective in eliminating self-stimulation then merely providing more frequent but noncontingent positive reinforcement, delivering reinforcement contingent on the omission of self-stimulation (DRO), or punishing self-stimulation either by giving the child a severe slap on the thigh or (in the case of hand-mouthing) painting the hand with a distasteful solution. Needless to say, overcorrection, though it also is a punishment procedure, is far less objectionable than the infliction of pain which, as we shall see in the following section, should be used only as a method of last resort.

SELF-INJURIOUS BEHAVIOR

When one observes a child who time and again emits presumably painful responses that result in physical injury, one is faced with one of the most paradoxical phenomena involving human behavior. Self-injurious behavior seems to be an exception to the Law of Effect which states that a response that is consistently followed by an aversive stimulus will cease to be emitted. Here, however, is an instance in which a response is maintained despite its aversive consequences. Various hypotheses have been advanced in attempts to resolve this paradox. As Carr (1977) has pointed out in reviewing these attempts, the hypotheses have ranged from inferences about guilt that the child presumably tries to reduce by seeking pain, to notions about aberrant physiological processes, and formulations about a high sensory threshold that leads such a child to seek high levels of stimulation. Two of these hypotheses view self-injurious behavior as a learned operant and they are not mutually exclusive. One postulates that these responses are maintained by positive social reinforcement in the form of the adult attention that self-injurious behavior almost inevitably elicits. The other hypothesis conceives of that behavior as maintained by negative reinforcement in that it serves to terminate or avoid another aversive stimulus. Though he rejects the psychodynamic hypothesis about guilt because, as it is stated, it is incapable of an empirical test, Carr (1977) concludes that self-injury may be multiply determined. He urges continued research into the motivation of that behavior because truly effective treatment may depend on a recognition of its motivational sources. Clinicians, meanwhile, find themselves in a so-called clinical bind. Faced with children who bang their heads to the point where sutures are required to close the resulting gashes, they cannot wait until the needed research is concluded but must seek to intervene in as effective and humane a way as possible, even in the absence of definitive knowledge.

As described by Bachman (1972), self-injurious behavior "often consists of a series of repetitive, sometimes rhythmical responses that include forceful head-banging (against walls, floors, sharp corners, furniture, or other parts of the body), banging and hitting other parts of the body against inanimate objects, face-slapping, and scratching, pinching, and biting body parts. The physical damage sustained by such behavior varies; some individuals . . . produce only minor lesions with few permanent consequences. Others, however, produce serious, permanent damage to themselves, such as blindness, loss of limb, severe bleeding, concussions, etc." (p. 212). The demand characteristics of this behavior call forth a variety of responses on the part of the adults responsible for these children; all are designed to prevent that behavior in order, as it were, to protect these boys and girls from themselves. Institutions with self-injurious children among their charges often resort to keeping them physically restrained by tying their feet and arms to the bed, putting their arms in splints, or placing them in straitjackets. Deep sedation with powerful drugs are also used to keep such children from injuring themselves. It should be readily apparent, however, that these methods prevent the undesired response only for as long as they are being used; as soon as the restraints are removed or the medication suspended, the child will resume the self-injurious behavior. What is more, while under restraint or medication these children can engage in little or no behavior and prolonged "treatment" of this kind has been known to result in arrested motor development and in physical changes of the limbs due to disuse.

This dismal picture has been presented for several reasons. One is to underscore the urgency of finding a therapeutic alternative to the measures of desperation that are now so widely used; another is to set the stage for a discussion of the drastic intervention to which some behavior therapists have turned. A third reason is to highlight the most immediate environmental consequence of self-injurious responses since an explanation for the paradoxical persistence of these responses may well lie in that consequence which is the inevitably immediate attention by caretakers who will regularly rush in to stop the self-injurious behavior in which a child is engaged.

The Treatment of Self-Injury

Given the fact of immediate adult attention and ministration that Lovaas, Freitag, Gold, and Kassorla (1965) have shown to be a reinforcing consequence, the most obvious form of treatment suggesting itself is to place the behavior on an extinction schedule by the simple expedient of ignoring it. While this does indeed work (Lovaas & Simmons, 1969) it is unfortunately not a readily feasible method because, like any other response at the beginning of an extinction procedure, the self-injurious response will first increase in magnitude before it undergoes extinction (the extinction spurt). In the case of life-threatening behavior that is obviously unacceptable. Moreover, as Carr, Newsom, and Binkoff (1976) have demonstrated, self-injurious behavior may, in some instances, be maintained not by positive but by negative reinforcement in that its appearance interrupts an activity, such as a training session, that is aversive to the child. These investigators present a case of a mildly retarded boy who would hit his head with his fist to the extent of bruising and cutting his face, immediately after a tutor had issued a request that he do something, like pointing to the window. Having been trained to use time-out procedures, this tutor would thereupon interrupt the lesson and momentarily turn away from the boy, only to find that the self-injurious behavior during these lessons would increase rather than decrease in frequency, a result not dissimilar to that reported by Plummer, Baer, and LeBlanc (1977) in the case of milder forms of disruptive behavior. When Carr et al. (1976) changed the nature of the tutoring sessions, making them less aversive by having the teacher present her requests in the context of an animated, entertaining story, the frequency of the child's self-hitting decreased dramatically.

Differential Reinforcement. When one approaches self-injurious behavior from the point of view of a functional analysis of behavior that inquires into the consequences of a given response because it is that consequence that is likely to be maintaining the behavior, one finds that one of the consequences that follow self-injury with a good deal of regularity is that these children are placed in physical restraints, aimed at preventing their dangerous behavior. It may seem a paradox to state that the very restraint that is supposed to prevent self-injury actually serves a reinforcing function that maintains such behavior. But paradox or no, this seems to be exactly what physical restraint is doing, at least in some cases. Favell, McGimsey, and Jones (1978) had informally observed that some profoundly retarded residents in an institution seemed to enjoy being physically restrained. They therefore reasoned that if such restraint has the function of a positive reinforcer, it ought to be possible to use it to strengthen a desirable alternative to self-injurious behavior. Indeed, when these investigators reversed the contingencies so that an 8-year-old retarded boy could "earn" brief (3½ minutes) periods of being restrained on his bed, contingent on increasingly longer periods during which he did not engage in self-injurious behavior, that behavior showed a dramatic decrease in frequency as soon as this change in contingency was introduced. From a near-zero level, self-injury again rose to occur in 100 percent of the observation intervals when the original, baseline contingency was experimentally reinstated in the service of a reversal design, falling again to near-zero when the treatment contingency was once more put in place.

Favell et al. (1978) speak of their procedure as a "treatment package" because their intervention was not limited to using physical restraint as a positive reinforcer for periods during which no self-injury was emitted; they also engaged the boy in alternative activities while he was not restrained. The observed reduction in self-injurious behavior may thus have been due to more than the mere reversal of the restraint contingency. Support for the reinforcing function of constraint was adduced, however, in that these investigators demonstrated that a retarded, self-injurious adult learned a new, arbitrary marble-dropping response when the only contingent consequence was that each correct response led to her having her arms placed in rigid splints for a period of 30 seconds. The self-injurious behavior of that woman had also been drastically reduced by reinforcing periods during which no self-injury had taken place by brief moments of restraint. This work thus not only permits one to view the function of physical restraint in a different light but it also suggests a means whereby the self-injurious behavior of some individuals might be reduced.

It is important to note that Favell, McGimsey, and Jones (1978) had not merely reduced self-injurious behavior by reinforcing the absence of such behavior. There can be no such thing as the absence of behavior for some behavior must be present when another behavior is absent; a child who is not engaging in self-injury is doing something. What that something is to be, what is to replace self-injury once that has been reduced or eliminated is the responsibility of the therapist. Explicit plans for establishing response alternative must be an integral part of any treatment strategy aimed at the removal of an undesirable response. Favell et al. had initially engaged the eight-year-old in primitive play with pieces of string; later they encouraged him to join group activities on the ward. In that respect, their procedure falls under the rubric of differential reinforcement of other behavior (DRO), where the "other" behavior was the play activity.

Another instance in which a DRO procedure was used to treat the self-injurious behavior of a retarded child was reported by Weiher and Harman (1975) who viewed their approach as *omission training* because they explicitly reinforced only the absence of a head-banging response. By so doing, they succeeded in reducing head banging from a baseline mean of 14.34 instances per minute to a near-zero rate within fewer than 50 training sessions. Fortunately, in the sense that these investigators had apparently not made explicit plans for strengthening alternate behaviors, they observed the emergence of such socially desirable behaviors as smiling, laughing, and vocalizing which, occurring during self-injury-free periods, had received adventitious reinforcement. The establishment of alternative behaviors should, however, not be left to chance but built into the treatment procedure.

From the standpoint of failing to build constructive alternatives to the behavior being reduced in frequency the work reported by Repp and Deitz (1974) can also be faulted. These investigators employed a DRO technique to treat the severe face-scratching of a profoundly retarded, 10-year-old girl whose self-injury required that she regularly wear elbow splints that prevented her from reaching her face. In order to obtain a baseline measure, the splints were removed for ten 15-minute sessions during which the teacher's saying "No" was the only consequence for scratching. Under these conditions the girl was observed to scratch her face an average of 17.2 times per minute. The treatment plan consisted of reinforcing the child with bits of candy for increasingly longer intervals without the splints during which no face-scratching took place. When such a self-injurious response was observed during these sessions, the teacher would say, "No" and pull the girl's hand down to her side. Treatment began with the child and the teacher alone in a room and each session lasted 25 minutes. At first the scratch-free intervals for which reinforcement was earned were only 1 second long but gradually they were increased so that after 45 days of treatment the girl had to go 2 hours without scratching in order to earn a reinforcer. After 20 sessions, child and teacher moved into the activity room where other teachers and children were also present and with that, the length of the sessions was gradually lengthened so that by the end of the study the entire 2-hour session was taking place in the presence of others.

Repp and Deitz (1974) report that within seven days after the DRO-verbal reprimand procedure had been introduced the rate of face-scratching had fallen to zero and that it remained at or close to that level for the remaining 50 days of the study. They point out that a comparison of the last 43 sessions of the treatment phase with the 10 baseline sessions revealed a reduction by 1/1000 in the self-injurious scratching.

One hesitates to find fault with such an impressive result but two points should be made. As suggested earlier, Repp and Deitz (1974) had viewed the target of their intervention as increasing the periods of time during which this girl would not scratch her face. At least as far as their report reveals, they had made no attempt to teach this child a constructive response that might have taken the place of the face-scratching during the increasingly longer periods of time when she did not emit that response. She seems to have been reinforced for merely sitting with her hands in her lap, doing nothing. Though this child was severely retarded and functioned at the 9- to 12-month level on motor activity and language expression, it would seem that she should have been explicitly taught to engage in some form of activity once she and the teacher had moved their sessions into the activity room and her elbows no longer had to be in the splints. Maybe some simple activity was inadvertently reinforced in the context of the DRO procedure but building constructive alternatives to self-injurious behavior should be an explicit part of the treatment plan. The mere absence of self-injury is not a sufficient treatment goal.

The other comment on the Repp and Deitz (1974) study is not a criticism but an observation. Their record shows that for three 5-minute segments during the 10 baseline sessions when the girl's elbow splints had been removed she manifested a very high rate of self-injurious responses. With the advantage of having the results of the subsequent study by Favell, McGimsey, and Jones (1978) available it is now possible to wonder whether this frequency really represented the "normal" rate at which this child scratched her face. Could it be that the elbow splints served as a reinforcer for scratching so that their removal represented an extinction procedure? The high rate of scratching might then be an extinction spurt and the subsequent reapplication of the splints a reinforcer for that high rate. This would have inflated the baseline rate. Nonetheless, there is little doubt that this child was indeed highly self-injurious, and the results Repp and Deitz (1974) obtained with her were indeed remarkable.

When people are working with profoundly retarded or severely impaired children who engage in self-injurious behavior it may seem unreasonable to expect them to combine the elimination of that dangerous behavior with the explicit teaching of alternative, constructive response patterns. Such children have such a limited response repertoire that it is difficult to think of a constructive response that they might be taught. Saposnek and Watson (1974) point the way in their report of the case of a 10-year-old, nonverbal, profoundly retarded boy who had been diagnosed as autistic. This child had been institutionalized largely because his parents had been unable to cope with his severely self-injurious behavior which consisted of a rapid and vigorous slapping of the sides of his head with both hands that inflicted bruises and abrasions. Because he was thought to be in imminent danger of detaching his retinas and causing serious damage to his middle ear, his arms were kept in restraints during both day and night. He spent his waking hours sitting on his bed rocking and although he was able to walk he was not toilet trained.

Treatment involved having the therapist hold the boy in a horizontal position on his lap with the child's neck and knees loosely cradled in the therapist's arms. The boy responded to being held in this position by flailing, kicking, squirming, and screaming loudly. When he began slapping the sides of his head, the therapist blocked the child's arms and encouraged him to hit the therapist's hand both by verbal instruction ("Hit my hand") and by physically guiding the boy's arm through the appropriate motions. Based on the rationale of the somewhat obscure rage-reduction method of treating autistic children (Zaslow & Breger, 1969), each session lasted until the child ceased the struggling and squirming and his body became relaxed. We need not here be concerned with the question whether the rage-reduction method is effective; what is important is that the child treated by Saposnek and Watson (1974) soon began hitting the therapist's hand instead of his own head and that by the end of this study, when his head-slapping had virtually disappeared, he would playfully and lightly slap the hands of various adults or the flat armrests of ward furniture. This then is an instance where treatment not only essentially eliminated self-injurious behavior but succeeded in establishing a play behavior that could take its place. What is more, during the early phases of this study, Saposnek and Watson would use the periods when the child was not engaging in self-injurious behavior to train him in dressing and playing with toys, reinforcing him with food, praise, and pats on the shoulder when he engaged in these socially appropriate competing responses.

The approach followed by Saposnek and Watson (1974) is clearly a constructive, clinically appropriate method that would permit a child to move from sitting on the bed and rocking back and forth with his arms tied to his side, to free participation in the regular institutional habilitation program. It is again a reflection of the inverse relationship between experimental rigor and clinical relevance that these investigators felt the need to apologize for confounding several procedures in the early parts of their study, thus being unable to ascertain which aspect of their approach was the critical independent variable. They therefore introduced a series of sessions in later phases of their work with this boy where no incompatible activities or responses, and no food or praise reinforcements were used and only the treatment procedure described earlier was applied. They were thus able to demonstrate that, at this point at least, this procedure alone was capable of controlling the boy's face-slapping. That having been established to their satisfaction, the boy was again introduced into the habilitation program and the report ends with the encouraging statement that the boy had become an active participant in recreation, concept formation, and language training programs.

Overcorrection. In the case reported by Saposnek and Watson (1974) one of the procedures used entailed guiding the boy's hand so that he would slap the therapist's hand as an alternative to his hitting his own head. That procedure thus contained an aspect of overcorrection and serves to introduce an examination of a study by Harris and Romanczyk (1976) who explicitly used overcorrection in treating the self-injurious behavior of a moderately retarded, 8-year-old child. This boy had been born with multiple defects that had required several instances of corrective surgery, leaving him with a profound hearing impairment and very poor eyesight. Though he possessed no speech, he communicated in a rudimentary fashion by means of about a dozen hand signs. He was adept at handling mechanical objects and physically quite agile. Though he displayed several characteristics of autistic children, such as an indifference to other people and self-stimulatory behavior, this boy was in many respects less profoundly impaired than the self-injurious children we have discussed thus far. Even his self-injury, consisting of banging his head or chin against solid objects, had a different quality in that he would engage in it primarily when he was unable to get his own way or in order to communicate his needs. Furthermore, his head-banging had never drawn blood although it was so intense that he had shattered automobile windshields on two separate occasions and had dented the walls of the rooms in his foster parents' house. During a 14-day baseline period this violent behavior was recorded on an average of 32 times per day.

The overcorrection procedure that was implemented at the end of the baseline period took the following form: Contingent upon each instance of head- or chin-banging, the boy's head was guided in an up–down, left–right movement pattern. This was repeated every 5 seconds and continued for 5 minutes. Following this, the boy's arms were guided to his side, in front, over his head, out to the side at shoulder height, and back to his side. This cycle was also repeated every 5 seconds and continued for 5 minutes. If any self-injurious behavior took place during overcorrection, timing began anew. At the end of the overcorrection, the task that had been interrupted was resumed and continued until the boy had made at least one correct response related to the goals of the individual tutoring program in which he was enrolled. This program emphasized attending, discrimination skills, and reading.

During the first week in which the overcorrection contingency was in effect, the boy's self-injurious behavior decreased to a mean of five episodes per day and during the second week it fell to two per day. Following this, the behavior remained at or near zero for the remaining 4½ months of observations. Apparently, however, the improvement was specific to the day-treatment program where the treatment had taken place. At home the boy continued to bang his head at the average rate of 15.44 times per day. When overcorrection was initiated at home, following a 29-day baseline period and 20 days after it had been introduced at the treatment center, the self-injurious behavior dropped to two episodes on the first day and to zero on the second. Nine months later, self-injury had remained at or near zero both at home and at the center. Meanwhile, the boy's appropriate behaviors had increased; he had acquired a sight reading vocabulary of 25 words, was able to attend to a learning task for 30 minutes of concentrated attention, and was described by his family as increasingly responsive and affectionate.

All this progress should obviously not be attributed to the overcorrection itself for that had been aimed merely at eliminating the self-injurious behavior. The overall improvement in adaptive behavior had apparently been the result of intensive efforts by tutors who were working with the boy in the day-treatment center but these could not have taken place had he continued to respond with head-banging whenever a task-oriented demand was made of him or when he was prevented from some other activity, as had been the case at the start of the intervention.

It appears that overcorrection is an effective means of suppressing self-injurious behavior of moderate severity, such as had been manifested by the boy

whom Harris and Romanczyk (1976) had treated or had been displayed in the
eye-poking of a visually handicapped 3-year-old on whose treatment Kelly and
Drabman (1977) reported. Whether this procedure alone would be effective
with the extreme forms of uncontrolled self-injury that results in bleeding lesions or concussions remains to be seen. In combination with other behavioral
procedures, overcorrection may well be capable of accomplishing that end.
This was shown by Azrin, Gottlieb, Hughart, Wesolowski, and Rahn (1975)
who worked with a group of 11 institutionalized patients, five of whom were
18 years old or younger. These investigators employed what they called "educative procedures" with which they quickly eliminated severe self-injurious behavior of long standing. The procedures involved required relaxation, hand
control, and hand-awareness training that were administered by the ward at-
tendants in the context of everyday ward activity.

As described by Azrin et al. (1975), required relaxation involves having
the patient go to his bed and lie there for 10 minutes with his arms at his sides
after self-injurious behavior had been emitted. For patients with whom this
procedure was ineffective or inappropriate, the hand-control procedure was
applied. Hand control is based on the overcorrection principle and involves
arm and hand movements that are incompatible with self-injury on the occurrence of which it was contingent. Hand-awareness training was not used as a
consequence for self-injury but consisted of ongoing efforts during the rest of
the day to give the patient feedback and positive reinforcement for keeping his
hands away from his head or other parts of the body that had been the target
of the self-injurious behavior.

Azrin et al. (1975) report fairly rapid success with the 11 individuals with
whom they used this combination of procedures. There was an average reduction of about 90 percent of self-injurious behavior on the first day of treatment
and of about 96 percent by the seventh day. Three months after treatment the
self-injurious behavior was down by an average of 99 percent compared with
its rate during baseline observations. These impressive results are all the more
remarkable because the investigators had made no attempt to select the individuals with whom they used the procedure. They had simply approached several
institutions with the offer to assist in treating residents who repeatedly inflicted
self-injury that resulted in evident tissue damage. All individuals, referred to
them on that basis, were accepted for treatment. This included an 18-year-old,
profoundly retarded female who had been exhibiting self-injurious behavior
since birth and who, when not restrained, had been slapping her face, ears,
and head at the rate of 3,500 times per day.

Given the demonstrated effectiveness of methods such as the one just described that provide a constructive and readily acceptable alternative to physical restraint, heavy sedation, seclusion, and punishment by the infliction of
pain, there would seem to be little reason why institutions persist in routinely
using these methods for the control of self-injurious behavior. Yet there may

be instances where none of these alternatives are effective or where very rapid response-suppression is absolutely essential and it is here that a punishment procedure based on the application of pain may be the method of last resort. It is from that perspective that we turn to the final segment of this chapter.

Punishment. In a technical sense, any contingent response consequence that results in reducing the magnitude of that response is a punisher so that, as we pointed out earlier, such interventions as time-out and overcorrection represent forms of punishment. Here, however, we are concerned with punishment that involves the response contingent application of pain. It is rightfully a highly controversial procedure which inevitably raises ethical and moral questions when it is discussed. The various procedures that we considered earlier were almost always developed by investigators who sought alternatives to physical punishment because, like others in our society, they found its use aversive. Responsible therapists who have used physical punishment to suppress self-injurious behavior invariably mention the ethical and moral issues in their reports and take pains to point out that they turned to it only because it was the less objectionable of two undesirable alternatives, where the choice was between permanent injury or even death or, as Lovaas and Newsom (1976) put it, where the use of a relatively small pain in the present prevented a relatively large pain in the future.

The pain of which we are here speaking is usually applied by means of a hand-held, battery-operated rod that, when brought in contact with an exposed part of a person's body, such as the legs, delivers between 4 and 5 milliamperes of current. This is experienced as a shock which, though painful, is entirely safe and harmless. What is more, the pain is localized at the point of contact and terminates immediately when the current is turned off a moment later. Though usually referred to as "electric shock" it should not be confused with the shock used in electroconvulsive therapy that many psychiatrists apply in the treatment of their patients and that, incidentally, has also been tried (though unsuccessfully) with children who engage in self-injurious behavior.

The aversive faradic stimulus (a euphemism for electric shock), has repeatedly been shown to be a highly effective means for the rapid suppression of self-injurious responses when it is delivered immediately following the emission of such a response (Lovaas, Freitag, Gold, & Kassorla, 1965; Lovaas, Schaeffer, & Simmons, 1965; Lovaas & Simmons, 1969; Risley, 1968; Tate & Baroff, 1966). All of these investigators combined the response suppression thus achieved with the positive reinforcement of constructive alternative responses, thereby adhering to the requirement voiced by Lovaas and Newsom (1976) and mentioned at the beginning of this chapter that no one undertake to punish self-injurious behavior who is not prepared "to invest considerable time and effort in explicitly building and maintaining adaptive behaviors which will have a chance of displacing [the self-injurious responses] as a means of obtaining social reinforcers'' (p. 319).

Corte, Wolf, and Locke (1971) compared three procedures for reducing the self-injurious behavior of four institutionalized, profoundly retarded adolescents who engaged in such activities as face-slapping, face-banging, hair-pulling, face-scratching, and finger-biting. With two of these individuals they attempted to use an extinction procedure by eliminating all social consequences of the self-injurious behavior but they found this to be ineffective. They then sought to reduce the self-injury by systematically reinforcing non-self-injurious behavior by the contingent delivery of food. This worked only with one of these two individuals and then only when he was made mildly hungry by depriving him of food. Only when response-contingent electric shock was introduced did the self-injury of all four residents decrease rapidly and fall to zero or near-zero frequency.

The use of pain to suppress a response that in itself is presumably painful for the person who engages in self-injurious behavior raises not only the ethical and moral issue we have already touched on but also the more theoretical question why someone who is hurting himself can be kept from doing so by hurting him further. Particularly those who view behavior as being motivated by inner needs have difficulty fitting such treatment into their conceptual scheme. Lovaas and Newsom (1976) suggest two related explanations for the effectiveness of punishment in the suppression of self-injurious responses. One is that these responses have, in the past, almost invariably had the consequence of adult sympathy and attention, thus becoming associated with reinforcement. Such social reinforcement is absent or greatly reduced in the application of shock. The other possible explanation is that the magnitude of self-injurious behavior usually increases gradually over a period of months or years, growing from relatively mild slaps to blows of full intensity. This progression would enable a child to adapt to the pain associated with these blows. The shock, however, being introduced suddenly and at full strength, does not permit such adaptation so that it is indeed an effective punisher, at least at the beginning of its use. It is conceivable that if shock were to continue to be used over a long period of time it too might lead to adaptation so that it would lose its effectiveness. On this point, however, we have only suggestive evidence, some of which comes from the following case report.

A Case Study

Most reports on the use of electric shock as a punisher for self-injurious behavior are based on relatively time-limited, largely experimental interventions, lacking long-term follow-up and failing to report on the behavior of the children so treated in settings other than those where the intervention was con-

ducted. An exception to this is the detailed case report presented by Romanczyk and Goren (1975) who describe a treatment program they conducted with
a severely self-injurious boy that exceeded 1,000 therapy hours, extending over
a period of 10 months. The child, identified as Peter, was 6½ years old when
he came to the attention of these investigators. Diagnosed as a case of "infantile autism with functional retardation without evidence of organic involvement", his repertoire consisted almost exclusively of self-stimulatory and self-
injurious behavior, the latter taking the form of scratching and head-banging.
This was so bad that he had to be kept in total restraint because when either his
legs or his hands were released, he would immediately bang his head either
against his limbs or any available object, often with such intensity that it was
"bone jarring or flesh tearing." Despite this problem and the fact that this boy
had no functional speech or self-help skills, and had to be force-fed because he
would otherwise spit out all food placed in his mouth, he was being cared for
at home by his parents. This is where Romanczyk and Goren (1975) began
their intervention.

    With the consent of Peter's parents, Romanczyk and Goren decided to in-
troduce response-contingent electric shock for self-injurious behavior because
it was clear that the boy was in severe physical danger from his self-inflicted
blows that even constant adult attention could not always prevent. The treatment can be viewed as having taken place in four distinct phases that represent
sequential changes in the approach, based on conclusions drawn from observations during the previous phase. In the first phase, the boy's right arm was
freed from restraint whereupon he immediately began hitting his head at the
rate of one hit every 2 seconds. Converted to an hourly rate to permit later
comparisons, this would represent a rate of approximately 5,400 hits per hour.
Because Peter hit himself so severely and frequently that he began bleeding
after 10–15 seconds, baseline observations were limited to two sessions each
lasting only 1 minute. Intervention consisted of delivering a shock to the boy's
free forearm each time he hit himself. The instrument used for this purpose
was a hand-held inductorium capable of delivering an extremely painful
shock, localized to the point of contact, and lasting approximately three-tenths
of a second. During the first of six treatment sessions, each lasting for 20 minutes, the frequency of the boy's self-injurious responses showed a decrease
which, though dramatic relative to the baseline frequency of 5,400 per hour,
was still unacceptably high since, converted to an hourly rate, it would have
amounted to 300.

    In order to increase its effectiveness, the treatment was then shifted to the
psychological clinic where the punishment procedure was combined with the
teaching of socially adaptive, alternative behaviors. Self-feeding, self-toilet-
ing, and the use of appropriate speech were shaped by prompting and reinforcement, the boy's echolalia was reduced by fading and ignoring, his spitting

was eliminated by overcorrection, and he was taught to fold his hands and hold them in his lap by shaping and reinforcement procedures. Meanwhile, the boy's mother was phased into the therapy sessions and taught some of these treatment methods, including the use of a modified shock device with which the suppression of the self-injurious behavior that had been accomplished at the clinic could be generalized to the home. During this, the second phase of treatment, the following distinct procedures were used to deal with the self-injurious responses. At the beginning, each such response was followed by a brief shock and the reapplication of the constraint for a period of 5 minutes. Since shock was now delivered via an electrode attached to the boy's wrist, more immediate application of the punisher was made possible because the therapist no longer had to reach over to contact the boy's arm. Combined with this procedure was an attempt to provide differential reinforcement for acceptable alternatives to self-injury. As the boy's self-hitting decreased in both frequency and intensity, the restraints were gradually removed and shock came to be delivered each time he raised his hand, thus *before* he would hit himself. This did not prove feasible, however, and punishment after the self-injurious response was again instituted.

By the 39th treatment session all restraints had been removed, hitting was at near-zero level, and the boy was eating solid foods. He had begun to ask for certain foods, using language. At home, Peter spent most of his waking hours without restraint, playing, or following his mother about, only occasionally hitting himself. The mother, however, continued to be in a position to administer shock, when needed. This was done by having the wrist electrode attached to a long cable, thus giving both mother and boy a certain amount of freedom of movement. Most interesting, from the point of view of understanding the function of the shock apparatus, is the fact that Peter could not tolerate the removal of the wrist electrode. As soon as this was attempted, he appeared to panic and would engage in self-injurious behavior. This of course is reminiscent of the report by Favell, McGimsey, and Jones (1978) who hinted at self-injurious individuals' responding to restraint as if it were reinforcing. One is tempted to raise the (unanswerable) question whether self-injurious individuals seek to be prevented from hurting themselves.

At any rate, as Romanczyk and Goren (1975) point out, it is usually at the point when self-injurious behavior of a child has been brought under almost complete control that reports of the treatment of such children are prepared for publication. The literature thus gives the impression that electric shock is a highly effective mode of treating self-injury. What is often ignored, however, is that the response suppression has been achieved only in the highly controlled and easily discriminated environment of the laboratory and treatment facility. It is to the credit of these authors and the fact that makes their report so unique that they carried their work beyond the point of apparent success so that one can learn not only of the experimental effectiveness but also of the clinical utility of shock in the treatment of self-injurious behavior.

The third phase of this study follows Peter into a day-treatment school for severely impaired children which the boy was now able to attend due to the remarkable improvement he had made in the 10 months of treatment that had entailed more than 1,000 therapy hours. In the highly individualized program provided in the treatment school setting, Peter was given training in preacademic and academic skills and encouraged to interact with the other children. For about two months all went well. His self-injurious behavior was almost totally suppressed both at home and in school, there was little or none of the screaming, scratching, spitting, or throwing that had been a part of his behavior pattern. He was making rapid progress in acquiring appropriate speech, self-help, academic, and social skills.

About this time the records of the frequency of Peter's various behaviors, which had been continuously maintained, began to show a gradual increase in the unacceptable behaviors. First the spitting slowly reappeared, then the throwing, followed by scratching and screaming, and finally self-injurious behavior showed up with increasing frequency. In order to increase the potency of the food reinforcers used in school for strengthening desired behaviors, Peter was deprived of his breakfast but this succeeded only temporarily in reversing the trend of deterioration. After a week, the unacceptable behaviors appeared again, with their rate increasing at a quickly accelerating pace so that on one day the frequency of Peter's self-injurious responses reached over 200. This happened to be a day when the shock equipment had malfunctioned at home the night before so that the boy's parents had been unable to apply the shock contingency on a systematic basis. Romanczyk and Goren (1975) speculate that this intermittent punishment, the necessary resort to full physical restraints, and the parents' excitement surrounding it all might have been responsible for the sudden breakdown of the acquired control over the self-injury but, as they recognize, the trend toward increased self-injury had been reflected in the record for some weeks before that day.

In order to obtain some leads on what might have gone wrong and on how they should proceed, Romanczyk and Goren (1975) conducted a brief functional analysis of the shock contingency in a controlled setting. This suggested to them that the social consequences always associated with the application of shock, that is, the therapist's observing the child's self-injurious response and reacting to it, might be serving as a reinforcer. They therefore tried to apply an extinction procedure by totally ignoring all self-injurious responses. The only way this could be done was to place heavy padding on the boy and on all objects in the room and to observe him over a TV monitoring system while he was left alone. Although the self-injurious responses decreased under this condition, Peter was still able to hurt himself by extricating himself from the padding so that the observer had to rush into the room to prevent serious injury, thereby providing social reinforcement for high-intensity responses and vitiating the extinction procedure. Furthermore, since there were unexplainable daily variation in response frequency and no significant reduction of self-injury could be obtained by this extinction approach, this phase was terminated after 19 days.

The investigators ultimately assumed that unspecified variables were controlling the self-injurious behavior and that these had probably contributed to the eventual deterioration of the gains that had been achieved during treatment. To speak of "unspecified variables" that are controlling a behavior is to admit that assessment procedures are not sufficiently refined to permit a thorough functional analysis of that behavior. Where that behavior takes the form of self-injury carrying out such an analysis is of course severely constrained by the reality that one cannot manipulate the many potential variables while permitting the response one is studying to be emitted at a high, baseline rate.

Under the circumstances, Romanczyk and Goren (1975) reviewed Peter's status with his parents and advised them to consider institutionalizing the boy since continuing to keep him at home and in outpatient care seemed no longer practicable. The parents reluctantly agreed and Peter was placed on a small children's ward of a state hospital where a low staff-to-patient ratio permitted sufficient supervision so that the boy did not have to be kept in constant restraint. With only partial restraints, he was able to attend school at the institution for approximately 5 hours a day and to participate in some simple tasks. On visits to his home, where unlike at the institution the use of the portable shock apparatus was permitted, Peter was seen during occasional follow-up visits by the investigators. They report that approximately a year later, the rate of his self-injurious responses never exceeded 15 per hour and that it was usually less than 5 per hour. Compared to the 5,400 per hour at the beginning of the intervention this is a remarkable change, all the more so since Peter was never observed during these visits to administer a blow sufficiently intense to cause injury or bleeding. Nonetheless, Romanczyk and Goren (1975) are suitably conservative in concluding that "the degree of suppression achieved was not sufficient to justify evaluating the outcome as clinically effective" (p. 738) because Peter required institutional care for his continued well-being. They correctly believe that the only acceptable criterion for the effectiveness of a procedure aimed at the treatment of self-injurious behavior is the complete suppression of that behavior for extended periods of time and in the child's natural environment.

At the present time, as Bachman (1972) has pointed out, the contingent application of electric shock is the treatment of choice for severely self-injurious behavior but, thus far, it is capable only of response-suppression under fairly circumscribed, quasilaboratory conditions. One source of this limitation, as Romanczyk and Goren (1975) reason, seems to lie in the fact that all currently available devices for the administration of shock have a highly discriminative quality so that their presence or absence is readily noticed, thereby complicating or precluding a gradual fading of their presence and eventual removal. Lovaas and Newsom (1976) also speak of the high degree of discriminability of the shock effect that seems to result in a child's learning to suppress self-injurious behavior under specific stimulus conditions without generalizing this to other conditions. There is no reason, however, why further research, improved technology, and more sophisticated clinical use of response-contingent punishment should not succeed in making this promising technique more effective so that it can be available as a last resort when other forms of treatment have failed and when, as Romanczyk and Goren (1975) put it, the consequences of *not* employing contingent electric shock for the punishment of self-injurious behavior are unacceptable.

Other Forms of Self-injury

While self-injurious behavior is generally associated with children who are classified as autistic, retarded, or brain damaged, some milder forms of this behavior are also encountered among less profoundly disturbed individuals. In a sense, nail-biting, eyelash-picking, and excessive scratching are forms of self-injury and the hair-pulling, technically known as trichotillomania, that results in large bald areas on the child's head should also be viewed as falling into this category.

Effective treatment methods for these so-called habits have been reported in the form of self-monitoring (Anthony, 1978), behavioral contracting (Stabler & Warren, 1974), differential reinforcement (Allen & Harris, 1966; Evans, 1976; Lowitz & Suib, 1978; Mulick, Hoyt, Rojahn, & Schroeder, 1978), response cost (McLaughlin & Nay, 1975), and the delivery of aromatic ammonia as an aversive stimulus (Altman, Haavik, & Cook, 1978). Azrin and Nunn (1973) reported success with the use of competing response practice that, quite similar to overcorrection, involves having the child engage in a movement pattern that is either the opposite of or incompatible with the self-injurious response.

In the reports just cited one is dealing almost exclusively with uncontrolled studies on single cases. Because of this and in view of the fact that, compared with life-threatening self-injury, nail-biting and hair-pulling are minor irritants, we have concentrated in this chapter on the more profound and alarming behavior found among the severely impaired.

Recapitulation

Profoundly disturbed children often engage in self-stimulation that precludes their acquiring more adaptive responses or in self-injury that endangers their health and, in some instances, their very lives. For these reasons, such self-directed behavior calls for intervention designed to suppress these responses and to replace them with constructive alternatives. Self-stimulation appears to be maintained by the reinforcing qualities inherent in the stimulation itself. One means of reducing such behavior should therefore be to remove or mask this reinforcing quality and some success has been achieved with sensory extinction and time-out procedures. The response-contingent introduction of the negative consequences entailed in overcorrection, particularly when combined with positive practice of response-alternatives, has also been shown capable of reducing self-stimulation and this appears to be the most promising method presently available for this purpose.

Any discussion of the treatment of self-injurious behavior must take cognizance of the fact that the function of these responses is, as yet, unknown. The immediate social attention that this behavior invariably calls to itself may well be among the reinforcing consequences, but it is obvious that this attention cannot be withheld because of the dangerous nature of much of this behavior. Those charged with caring for these children have often had to resort to extreme measures to prevent self-injury, raising ethical and moral issues that must be taken into consideration when one is contemplating such intervention. For some milder forms of self-injury, differential reinforcement or overcorrection have been used with some success. In the more virulent forms of this behavior procedures based on the punishment paradigm and involving the delivery of a brief but painful stimulus have been the method of last resort. Given such choices as permanent, self-inflicted physical damage, deep sedation, or total restraint, that method may well be the most humane of the presently available forms of intervention, *provided* it is used in the context of an explicitly planned, systematic program that is designed to teach such a child alternative responses with which to obtain social reinforcement.

CHAPTER 14

Noncompliant Behavior

The topic to which this chapter is devoted takes us to the indistinct border between behavior therapy, child-rearing practices, and what has sometimes been called behavior modification because we shall examine the changing of behavior that is not necessarily deviant, but which someone nonetheless wishes to see changed. We are here talking about children who may be variously referred to as disobedient, rude, ill-mannered, negativistic, oppositional, uncooperative, undisciplined, rebellious, defiant, or just plain brats. Each of these terms has found its way into the literature on child behavior disorders, as has a term that reflects the interpersonal nature of this problem, parent-child conflict.

ETHICS, VALUES, AND THE RIGHTS OF CHILDREN

When therapists are asked to intervene with a child to whose behavior we shall here refer as *noncompliant*, they encounter issues of values and ethics that, in this form, enter only rarely into therapeutic considerations. Few would question, for example, whether a child with deficits in social skills, academic performance, language acquisition, or toileting functions should be helped to overcome these. Nor is there ordinarily a question whether children whose excessive fear, aggression, norm-violations, or disruptions interfere with their social relations ought to be given treatment designed to reduce these problems. Surely, no one would quarrel with a therapist's decision to reduce a child's excessive self-stimulation or self-injury even though, as we pointed out in the previous chapter, the methods used to accomplish the latter often raise questions of social acceptability and ethics. Yet, when a parent comes to a therapist and complains about a child's misconduct, disobedience, or defiance and wants help in "disciplining" the child, the therapist must proceed with great care. Here, more than in any other problem area, an intervention may entail an unwarranted intrusion into a child's rights in that treatment may serve to support a parent's distorted values or unrealistic expectations that may be the core of the problem. Matters of ethics, values, and the rights of children in the context of child therapy have received extensive discussion elsewhere (Ross, 1980) but before presenting material related to the treatment of noncompliance we must take another look at these issues so as to be alert to their implications. Issues related to ethical considerations in therapeutic relationships have been examined by Van Hoose and Kottler (1977), and those dealing more specifically with behavioral interventions were scrutinized by Stolz and associates (1978). The question of children's rights in this context was explored in a work by Koocher (1976), while Rosen, Rekers, and Bentler (1978) addressed the more specific issue of the ethical implications involved in treating children with gender identification problems.

When one person undertakes to intervene in the life of another, whether under the rubric of training, teaching, correction, or therapy, there is always an element of intrusion. The question must therefore be asked whether the person on the receiving end of these ministrations wishes to have this happen. When adults enter treatment, it is they who go to a therapist seeking help, unless they have been institutionalized involuntarily, in which case, the courts have lately come to protect their interests. In the case of children, on the other hand, it is hardly ever they who go to a therapist seeking help. They are almost always brought by their parents or guardians who seek help on behalf of the child. The ethical implications of intervening in a person's life increase in magnitude as an inverse function of that individual's freedom of choice and a child's choice regarding treatment is extremely limited. Not only do children have little say about going to a therapist for help but, unlike adults who have entered treatment, they are also rarely able to terminate treatment when they no longer wish to continue.

Does a child have the right to refuse therapy? Do parents have the right to decide what the child needs or do they, on the contrary, have a responsibility to make that decision? Is a child therapist the agent of the parents? Whose judgment of what is needed should take precedence, the parents' or the therapist's? These are questions that must be asked but there are no clear-cut answers. Our society is remarkably ambivalent about the rights of children vis à vis their parents. "Father (or mother) knows best" is still a generally accepted maxim that is set aside only in cases of obvious neglect or severe abuse. Given this state of affairs, the child therapist has a special responsibility to consider whether the intervention sought by a child's parents is really in the child's best interest; if it is not, the therapist is ethically bound to refuse undertaking that intervention.

Unfortunately, it is not always readily apparent what is in a child's best interest. Let us take the case of a 7-year-old boy who is brought to a therapist by his mother who complains that "he won't ever obey; refuses to hang up his clothes; keeps his room in a mess, and has terrible table manners." He is "sassy" when she asks him to do a chore or run an errand and always insists on an explanation or justification for her demands. All of this has led to a highly charged interaction between mother and child and this, in turn, has resulted in marital discord because when her husband comes home, mother is "on edge," yet he wants to hear nothing about her troubles. During initial assessment, the therapist asks the boy whether he has any problems with which he wants help. Predictably, the boy answers in the negative, saying that as far as he is concerned "everything is o.k. at home." Tentative attempts at helping the mother to be more accepting of the child's behavior, less concerned about messy rooms and scattered clothes, show her to be unyielding. She knows what is right and the boy had better learn to obey. "Children," she asserts, citing the teachings of her church, "are meant to obey their parents."

What is the therapist to do with such a case of noncompliant behavior? Should the therapist recognize the boy's right to self-determination and, respecting it, withdraw from the case or does a 7-year-old not have such a right? Should the adult override the child's wishes to be left alone? Are not the parents, who are going to pay for the treatment, entitled to a service the therapist is holding out to the public? What really is in the child's best interest in such a case? Is it in his best interest to let him struggle through a stressful childhood because one wants to respect his right to refuse help? One might say that in this way he will develop into an adult who is able to assert his rights in the face or irrational authority. That, however, is an uncertain prediction and for that matter, whether it is good to be assertive in this manner is another issue that might be challenged as an idiosyncratic value judgment. On the other hand, it might be in the child's best interest to learn to live in his home with a minimum of stress and conflict; a goal that might be reached if one undertook treatment aimed at helping him to adapt to the existing reality. Yet it is again a value judgment to maintain that stress and conflict are bad, while harmony and serenity are good. Obviously, there are no easy answers to any of these questions, yet it behooves every therapist to explore them and to reconcile the issues they raise with his or her own values and to make these values explicit.

Because of the ambiguity that exists in this realm, it may be useful from the standpoint of making us more aware of these issues, to explicate some specific rights of the children who are clients in therapy (Ross, 1974; 1980). These rights are here presented as absolutes although it will quickly be apparent that they may at times have to be compromised because of overriding considerations, such as a child's safety. Stating them as absolutes, however, should help one recognize when these rights are being violated so that this is done only after due consideration and with the clear awareness that the child's rights are being infringed by one's actions.

The rights cover four basic principles: the right to be told the truth, the right to be treated as a person, the right to be taken seriously, and the right to meaningful participation in decisions that involve the child's life. The first of these rights, the right to be told the truth, should be foremost in any interaction between people, whether in therapy or elsewhere. There is rarely an excuse for lying, particularly to a child. Similarly, the right to be treated as a person is a universal that must be extended to the child. Every human being, no matter how young, how impaired, or how disturbed, is entitled to being treated with respect. Probably the most frequently violated right is a child's right to be taken seriously. Adults have the tendency to view children as inconsequential or insignificant; they are often shrugged off or ignored. "Too young to understand; doesn't know what she is talking about" are heard not infrequently. The fourth right, the right to participate in decision-making, derives from the other three. If one is honest with children, treats them as persons, and takes them seriously, one cannot help involving them in the making of decisions that affect their lives. Participation in decision-making obviously does not mean that the child's wishes or desires must necessarily prevail once the options have been explored, but honesty demands that the child should have been informed of that condition ahead of time, not asked for an opinion only to have it later ignored.

Values and the Methods of Behavior Change

As we shall see, most of the treatment of noncompliant behavior takes the form of teaching a child's parents to apply the principles of operant learning so that they can decrease the child's noncompliance and increase his or her compliance with their requests, demands, commands, and orders. The very use of words like commands gives one pause. What is the content of these commands? What are the parental values and expectations with which the child is to comply? Who are the parents to whom methods of behavior change are to be taught? To what ends will they use them?

Operant methods for behavior change are particularly effective in situations where the person seeking to change another's behavior has control over the reinforcers. In circumstances where access to such basic necessities as food, clothing, shelter, and contact with other people is under the control of any one person or group who choose to make such access contingent on the performance of specified responses, these responses can usually be obtained. Although much of our everday behavior is under the control of contingencies that are managed by others, the amount of control that can be exerted is limited by the fact that as adults we usually have access to alternate sources of reinforcement. If we object to the things someone is trying to make us do, we can usually change our job, move to a different town, transfer to another college, or separate from our spouse. The young child has none of these options available. If his or her parents decide to withhold food, to use social isolation, or to apply physical punishment contingent on the emission of a given response, there is very little the child can do other than to comply. It might be argued that some parents do such things even without knowing about operant principles but the point is that once they have been taught how to use food reinforcers, time-out, or differential reinforcement in a systematic fashion their control over the child will be even more effective. A heavy responsibility is thus placed on the therapist who teaches behavior principles to parents or others who are in charge of children. Before making parents one's auxiliary therapist one must be certain that they will not misuse the techniques that are to be handed to them.

Psychology is in a dilemma, a dilemma not unlike that in which other sciences find themselves when they develop the techniques that can be used for constructive or nefarious ends. The individual psychologist may refuse to teach behavioral principles to parents whose aims and values he or she does not share but such parents can easily obtain that very knowledge at the nearest bookstore where a number of manuals are now available that teach these principles and their application to child-rearing in readily understood form. A recent survey of such parent-training manuals (Bernal & North, 1978) listed no fewer than 20 publications, some written at the seventh-grade reading level. It would, of course, be futile for psychologists to try keeping their knowledge to themselves; knowledge cannot be locked up nor, once available, destroyed. We must recognize that we are faced with an ethical dilemma, that values have become inextricably intertwined with our therapeutic activities, that psychology has lost its innocence, and that, as Krasner (1965) recognized in the early days of behavior therapy, we have "no place to hide." There is no answer to this dilemma; all we can do is to be aware of it as we explore the work that has been done with noncompliant children and look at the procedures that have been used in training parents to be the agents of change for the behavior of their children.

THE MODIFICATION OF NONCOMPLIANCE

Early investigations of the problem presented by noncompliant children had demonstrated that effective intervention was possible if one or both of the child's parents were trained to apply the principles of operant learning. Bernal, Duryee, Pruett, and Burns (1968), for example, reported such an approach with a mother of an 8½-year-old boy who had been quite unmanageable prior to the intervention. The mother was taught to ignore the boy's abusive behavior unless it was excessive, in which case she was to express anger or to spank the child. At the same time, she was to provide positive reinforcement for acceptable behavior. This combination of extinction, punishment, and DRO procedures served to reduce the boy's unacceptable behavior and to increase acceptable alternatives within three weeks, the progress being maintained over a 23-week follow-up period.

A similarly uncontrolled case report was presented by Hawkins, Peterson, Schweid, and Bijou (1966). Here, a 4-year-old boy who had been extremely difficult to manage due to his disobedience, tantrums, and demands for attention, was treated by providing the mother with training in the use of reinforcement principles. Unlike the procedure employed by Bernal et al. (1968) who had relied on instruction and videotape feedback, Hawkins et al. (1966) sent an observer to the child's home so that the mother could be given training in the natural environment where she was interacting with her child. The observer arranged to give the mother three different signals to instruct her in the appropriate consequence to bring to bear on the child's behavior. One signal indicated that the mother was to tell the boy to stop whatever he was doing; another indicated to her that she was to put him in his room and lock the door; and the third cued her to give the boy praise, attention, or affectionate physical contact. After a while the mother learned to discriminate appropriate and inappropriate behavior quite easily and acquired the skill to apply the relevant consequences on her own. Some mothers, it seems, have difficulty discriminating the early stages of unacceptable behavior so that they miss the point where intervention would be most effective. They only intervene, and then often in an inappropriate fashion, when the child's behavior has reached a high level of intensity at which point intervention tends to be ineffective. What such a mother needs is not merely to learn how to apply behavior-change methods but also when to apply them.

A replication of the study by Hawkins et al. (1966) was reported by Zeilberger, Sampen, and Sloane (1968) who describe a 4-year, 8-month old boy whose objectionable behavior included screaming, fighting, bossing, and disobedience. When observed with his peers he continually told them what to do and how to play, enforcing his demands with punches, kicks, and slaps. He had been expelled from two nursery schools because of this behavior and the family's physician had told the parents that the boy had a severe emotional problem. Home observations of mother–child interactions suggested that the mother reinforced undesirable behavior with excessive attention. Her use of consequences was inconsistent and ambiguous since she would often get involved in long verbal explanations before instituting aversive consequences for undesirable behavior.

The boy's physical aggression against other children while playing in his own house or yard was selected as one target for intervention. The other was compliance with his mother's instructions. Observational records were also kept on the frequency of two other classes of behavior; yelling at and bossing other children. After 10 daily one-hour sessions during which baseline observations were conducted, Zeilberger et al. (1968) instructed both of the boy's parents in the use of a combination of time-out, extinction, and positive reinforcement procedures. These were to be employed contingent on aggression and disobedience or on such desirable alternatives as cooperative play and compliance with instructions. One of the family bedrooms was modified for use as a time-out room by removing all toys and any other items that might be of interest to a child, and by installing a hook to keep the door shut. The boy was to be placed in this room for 2 minutes immediately after he had engaged in an aggressive act or disobeyed an instruction. He was not to be let out of this time-out room if at the end of the 2-minute period he was crying or throwing a tantrum (so as not to provide negative reinforcement for that behavior). This meant that the 2-minute period was timed from the end of the last tantrum or cry.

While taking the boy to the time-out room, the parents were to make no comment other than, "You cannot stay here if you fight" or, "You cannot stay here if you do not do what you are told." At the end of the time-out period, they were to take him back to his regular activity in a matter-of-fact manner and without further comment. Any discussion of the program or of the boy's behavior was to be separated from the time-out procedure itself, held at times when no undesirable behavior had occurred, and kept to a minimum. This was in line with the therapists' plan to employ extinction by withholding positive attention from the undesirable behavior. In line with this plan they also had instructed the parents to ignore any aggressive or disobedient behavior that they learned about only some time after it had taken place. On the other hand, the parents were to reward the boy when he obeyed their instructions, to give reinforcement for desirable, cooperative play with frequent comments, such as "My, you are having a good time," that did not interrupt the ongoing play. After periods of such play, the parents were to provide special treats in the form of refreshments or new toys and activities.

In the course of the 10 sessions during which these contingencies were in effect, the boy's behavior showed a distinct change. Whereas he had followed parental instructions an average of only 30 percent of the time during baseline, he now averaged 78 percent. Aggressive behavior reflected similar improvement for while this had been taking place an average of 7.6 percent of the time during baseline, it dropped to zero by the third day of the treatment phase and occurred only rarely thereafter. After the 10 sessions during which the treatment program was in effect, the investigators instructed the boy's parents to resume interacting with him as they had done during the baseline phase. This reversal, carried on for six sessions, demonstrated the effectiveness of the treatment procedure in that the boy's disobedience and aggression quickly reverted to baseline levels, improving once more when the treatment procedures were reinstated as the final phase of this ABAB experimental design.

The investigation by Zeilberger, Sampen, and Sloane (1968) had demonstrated that the manipulation of the contingencies controlled by parents effects significant changes in their child's behavior and that parents can learn to change these contingencies. In that particular case, however, the mother seems to have been more adept at reducing the attention with which she had been inadvertently reinforcing undesirable responses than at increasing the amount of reinforcing attention that she gave to the child's appropriate behavior. Zeilberger et al. also report that this mother gave her boy fewer instructions while the time-out contingency of the treatment phase was in effect. It may of course be that for some reason fewer instructions were required during that phase. On the other hand, it could be that the mother found it aversive to place the boy in the time-out room and reduced the occasions for this procedure by issuing fewer instructions. Clearly, the parent's behavior is as important a topic of study as the child's behavior when the focus is on parent–child interaction. We shall return to this issue after reviewing an investigation where tokens were employed to improve children's compliance with family rules.

A demonstration that it is possible to use a reinforcement program based on a token economy when there are several children in a family was presented by Christopherson, Arnold, Hill, and Quilitich (1972) who worked with two separate families, one with three, the other with two preadolescent children. Points that were exchangeable for specified privileges (like going to a drive-in movie) could be earned for taking care of certain household chores, but they could also be lost for bickering, teasing, or whining. In both families these investigators worked solely through the parents who received the instructions, which they then communicated to their children. Both sets of parents were able to implement the program successfully for, as Christopherson et al. point out, they were interested and cooperative. Furthermore, as Christopherson and his colleagues recognized, none of the children in these families had been exhibiting severely inappropriate behavior and the parents' complaints had been about problems of noncooperation that are not unusual for families with young children.

One might object to the introduction of a token economy into the relationship between parents and their children. Obviously it is preferable that families interact on the basis of such intangible social reinforcers as praise, approval, and affection. Only when these reinforcers fail to maintain desirable behavior should it become necessary to resort to such artificial consequences as tokens and their back-ups. At that point, the mechanical aspects of a token system to which some people object may be a distinct advantage. A parent who might neglect to acknowledge a child's desirable behavior with praise or approval may be more likely to remember to hand out a token or to make a check mark on a chart. In fact, the children may remind the parent that they are due a reinforcer. This makes a token system more systematic and regular, thus more effective than a more haphazard and informal procedure based on social reinforcement.

In the token system that Christopherson et al. (1972) had employed in one of the families with whom they worked, punishment for undesirable behavior was administered by a response-cost system that involved taking away tokens the child had previously earned. While it might have been preferable to have two distinct token currencies, one for use in positive reinforcement and one for use in punishment, because expecting to lose what one has earned may deflate the value of the currency, imposing an effective fine may be preferable to the social isolation entailed in the use of a time-out room. It will be recalled that the mother in the case reported by Zeilberger et al. (1968) seemed loath to impose time-out on her child. She might have found a response-cost system within a token program more palatable.

There is yet another reason why a token program has advantages over other methods of intervention, such as the delivery of treats, snacks, or other tangible rewards contingent on desirable behavior. While a snack may or may not be reinforcing for a child every time it is made available, a token is far more likely to be a potent reinforcer at all times. As a generalized reinforcer, a token is more certain to serve the function of strengthening desirable behavior because the child will later exchange the token for whatever back-up reinforcer is, at that moment, the most attractive, that is, the most reinforcing. The delivery of a token must of course always be paired with such potential social reinforcers as praise which, through such pairing, should acquire reinforcing properties in their own right. A related advantage of a token is that it is always readily available so that it can be dispensed immediately after the desirable response has occurred and, unlike a snack for example, does not require any preparation. Yet, despite these advantages, a treatment program that employs tokens should do so only until the desired behavior has been established and must include a plan for having this behavior maintained over time by more natural, largely social consequences. This is particularly important because, as Christopherson et al. observed, parents often tend to discontinue the token economy once contact with the therapist is terminated.

Variables in Parental Behavior

It will be recalled that in the study reported by Zeilberger et al. (1968) the mother seems to have reduced the number of requests she issued to her child thereby reducing the potential instances of noncompliance and making it less often necessary for her to impose the time-out condition that she appeared to find aversive. Clearly, noncompliance on the part of a child is related to the frequency of parental requests. What is more, whether a child does or does not comply seems a function not only of the consequences that ensue when a request is or is not met, but also of the manner in which that request is delivered. The variables surrounding the delivery of parental instructions have been the subject of a series of studies conducted by Forehand and his colleagues at the University of Georgia (Forehand, 1977). These investigators have chosen a rather unfortunate terminology in reporting many of their studies and lest the following discussion lead the reader to view them in the wrong light it should be pointed out that Forehand (1977) is well aware of the moral and ethical implications of teaching parents the use of effective methods for influencing the behavior of their children. Nonetheless his use of such terms as "commands" and "disciplinary procedures" may be ill-advised, since "requests" or "instructions" and "management procedures" would communicate the same meaning without the rather harsh, drill-sergeant connotations. As Krasner (1976) has pointed out, the methods of behavior change must be not only effective, they must also be socially acceptable and social acceptability is not enhanced by the use of infelicitous terminology that arouses negative reactions.

In order to conduct their studies, the University of Georgia investigators usually advertise in local newspapers, specifying the ages of the children whose behavior they wish to investigate, and offering mothers a nominal fee for their participation. They then ask mother and child to interact in a specially prepared playroom where they can be observed while the mother gives the child instructions to engage in specified activities, to move from one activity to another, or to cease a given activity. Many of their studies thus involve samples of a population that is not typical of the people who seek professional help because their child's noncompliance presents a problem. Moreover, the situations they observe are laboratory analogs of the parent–child interactions that occur in natural settings. The research of these investigators is thus well controlled but its relationship to the clinical treatment of noncompliant children may be somewhat tenuous. Again, the dilemma of research on clinical problems: experimental rigor and clinical relevance stand in an inverse relationship to one another.

In one such analog study, Forehand, Roberts, Doleys, Hobbs, and Resick (1976) investigated the effectiveness of various "disciplinary procedures" in reducing the noncompliant behavior of children between the ages of 4 and 6½. The procedures were negative attention, repeated "commands," ignoring, and isolation. Negative attention entailed the mother's standing up quickly, crossing her arms, firmly saying, "You did not do what I said right away: I do not like it when you disobey me!" and retaining that position for 56 seconds while glaring intently at the child. Repeated commands meant that the mother would repeat her initial command in slightly altered form at 8-second intervals up to three times. Ignoring was implemented by having the mother read a magazine for one minute and not responding to the child after having announced, "You did not do what I said, so I am not going to watch you for a while." The isolation condition entailed having the mother say, "You did not do what I said, so I am going to leave the room for a while" and depart for one minute. The commands consisted of instructions to play with one of five different toys in the room and they were to be issued in "a calm, but authoritative tone" at the rate of one every 30 seconds. In order to maximize the number of trials for meaningful data analysis, children in one experimental condition were given 40 commands. The results showed that in this rather unnatural situation repeated commands (probably the most frequent form of parental behavior when a child "does not listen") failed to reduce noncompliance. On the other hand, negative attention, isolation, and ignoring did have the desired effect of increasing compliance, defined as the child's moving toward the specified toy within five seconds of the mother issuing a command.

In one of the two experiments conducted in the context of their study, Forehand et al. (1976) had the mothers continue to issue commands for four additional sessions during which they were not to invoke any consequences for noncompliance. This revealed that only those mothers were able to obtain continued compliance from their child who had used a combination of negative attention, isolation, and ignoring (in random order) during the preceding three treatment sessions. While this varied use of different discipline techniques thus seems to be the procedure of choice, Forehand and his colleagues point out that negative attention is, on the whole, to be preferred. They base this conclusion on the consideration that the best index of the immediate effect of a consequence used by a mother is whether the child plays with the required toy while the consequence for previous noncompliance is in effect. By this criterion the mother's glaring disapproval ("negative attention") seemed to be the most effective of the four procedures that had been compared. It remains for future research to ascertain whether this procedure would also be effective in the natural setting of the home where compliance with demands entails something other than having the child jump from toy to toy every 30 seconds.

In a study by Roberts, McMahon, Forehand, and Humphreys (1978) the focus was on the nature of maternal commands. These investigators distinguish between two ways in which parents issue commands to a child: The so-called alpha command takes the form of an essentially straightforward, unitary instruction that entails a specific action the child is to perform and is given the opportunity to perform by the parent waiting at least 5 seconds after issuing the command. The so-called beta command, on the other hand, is either a vague, nonspecific command or an alpha command that the child is not given the opportunity to carry out because the parent does such things as physically or verbally interfering with the child during the 5-second period after the command is issued. Peed, Roberts, and Forehand (1977) had found that beta commands are frequently employed by parents of clinic-referred children and Roberts et al. (1978) sought to investigate in their study whether these commands affect the rate of children's noncompliance. Additionally, they set out to examine the effect of a time-out procedure on noncompliance, in relation to the two kinds of antecedent commands.

Again working with mothers and their children whose participation had been solicited through public announcements, Roberts et al. (1978) first observed each mother–child pair for 10 minutes in order to obtain a baseline measure of the mother's ability to "control and direct" her child's behavior. Following this, each of the 27 mothers who were participating in the study was assigned to one of three training conditions. In one condition the mothers received explicit, individual training in issuing alpha commands. In the second condition this command training was combined with training in the use of a time-out procedure. This entailed four steps: Labeling the contingency ("You did not do what you were told, so you must stay in the corner for a while"); guiding the child to the time-out area and saying, "You must not leave this area until I tell you to"; ignoring the child for 2 minutes; and, if the child left the time-out area before the 2 minutes were up, instituting an "escape contingency". For the first escape, this consisted of a warning ("If you leave the corner again before I tell you to, I will take all the toys from this room and leave you by yourself"); this was put into effect for 2 minutes following the second escape. A third group of mothers were given training in a well-known (nonbehavioral) parenting skill called "active listening" in order to provide a placebo control. In each condition the training was conducted individually and lasted a maximum of 30 minutes.

Following their respective training sessions, all mother–child pairs were again observed for 10 minutes in a situation where the mother was to direct her child toward a different play activity every minute. During this posttest and for reasons that are not entirely clear, the experimenters provided feedback to the mothers regarding their appropriate use of commands, praising them for giving alpha commands and pointing out errors in the case of beta commands. Since the mothers in the so-called placebo group did not receive that feedback, which amounts to additional training, comparisons with that group are confounded. The results presented by Roberts et al. (1978) show that from pretest to posttest the number of alpha commands and the compliance ratio of the children increased significantly but there is no support for their conclusion that these changes were due to their training procedures. What they did establish, because the interpretation of these data does not depend on a comparison with the placebo group, was that the combination of alpha commands with time-out for noncompliance was significantly more effective in eliciting child compliance than was alpha command alone. Noteworthy too is their statement that one must attend to both the antecedents and the consequences of child compliance if one seeks to increase it.

That the manner in which a mother issues requests and instructions and what she does after the child emits or fails to emit a response are important variables in child compliance was also demonstrated in a study by Forehand, Wells, and Sturgis (1978). Working with parent–child pairs who had been referred to a clinic, these investigators observed each mother–child dyad in 20 minutes of playroom activity. The observation focused on the mother's issuing beta commands and providing reinforcement for desirable behavior. Forehand et al. (1978) report that these observations were better predictors of the child's noncompliance in the home than were parents' responses to questionnaires about their child's behavior. Given the importance of the nature of parental instructions, it is appropriate to take a closer look at the different forms in which such instructions can be issued. Green, Forehand, and McMahon (1979) provide categories that represent a refinement on their earlier dichotomy of alpha and beta commands, as follows:

> *Labeled commands.* These have a clearly specified objective, are explicitly stated, leaving no doubt as to what the child is supposed to do, such as instructions to the child to start doing a certain thing or to go to a specified place.
>
> *Question commands.* These are prefaced by a question ("Why don't you . . . ?") and involve a motoric response.
>
> *Stop commands.* Here the child is instructed to cease an ongoing behavior or not to begin a behavior that is about to take place. Included here are generalized restrictive rules.
>
> *Vague commands.* These are commands to which compliance is difficult if not impossible; they are the opposite of labeled commands in that they lack an operational referent in behavior.
>
> *Interrupted commands.* These commands also make compliance impossible because the parent issues a new command within 5 seconds and before the child has had a chance to comply. Such interruption can of course take the form of any of the other four commands.

It will be noted that vague and interrupted commands are what had previously been classified as beta commands, while the other three commands had been labeled alpha commands.

The Consequence of Noncompliance. The research by the Georgia group has demonstrated that both the nature of the stimulus and the characteristic of the consequence a mother presents in seeking to obtain a response from her child have a bearing on the child's compliance. Some of their research has focused specifically on the effectiveness of different consequences for noncompliance. In a study cited earlier, Forehand et al. (1976) had mothers impose time-out as a consequence of their child's failure to follow an instruction and this procedure entailed either having the mother ignore the child or having her leave the room for 2 minutes. The differential effectiveness of these two time-out procedures had been investigated by Scarboro and Forehand (1975). They compared a within-room and an out-of-room time-out contingency when imposed on 5-year-old children following failure to comply with a maternal instruction. For within-room time-out, the mother merely stopped playing with the child while for out-of-room time-out, she would leave the room, taking the toys with her. Here as elsewhere, the term *time-out* is used somewhat loosely because in its technical meaning it refers to time-out-from-positive-reinforcement. Not having established whether the mother's attention or her presence in the room were indeed functioning as positive reinforcers for child responses, withdrawing attention or leaving the room may or may not have represented time-out although, since the effect of this procedure was to reduce the behavior (noncompliance) on which it had been contingent, it clearly served as a punisher.

The results of the Scarboro and Forehand (1975) study revealed that both forms of time-out were effective. They significantly reduced oppositional behavior (noncompliance) below the rate the children had displayed during baseline observations. There the mother had been told to instruct her child to play with specified toys, to have the child change from one toy to another, and "to handle any problems in her usual manner" (p. 256). A group of mothers in a control condition who had not been given training in the use of a time-out procedure and who had continued to interact with their children as they had during baseline failed to elicit more compliance, differing in this regard significantly from the mothers in the two training groups. Since there was no statistically significant difference between the two time-out groups in terms of increased compliance and reduced noncompliance they were considered equally effective. In terms of efficiency, however, out-of-room time-out was superior to the other method for the within-room group required significantly more impositions of this consequence than did the out-of-room group. Apparently, having the mother leave the room, taking all toys with her, was a more potent form of punishment than merely having her withdraw her attention for a brief period.

What is the optimal length for a time-out period? This question was investigated by Hobbs, Forehand, and Murray (1978). Again using mother–child pairs solicited by means of newspaper advertisements and the playroom situation in which the mother is instructed to get her child to do a different thing every 20 seconds, the experimenters varied the length of the time-out consequence, using 4-minute, 1-minute, and 10-second periods. In this study the time-out procedure in consequence of noncompliance entailed confining the child to a marked-off corner of the room. In a control group, the mothers merely said to the child, "You did not do what I told you right away" but brought no other consequence to bear. The results revealed that, compared with the control group and with respect to a pretraining baseline, each of the time-out conditions led to a significantly lower level of noncompliance, with the 4-minute period showing the greatest effectiveness. At the end of the treatment phase, all mothers were asked to issue 12 more commands and to behave as they had during baseline. They were given no instructions as to the use of a time-out consequence. Under these conditions, the mothers were able to maintain the significantly higher level of compliance they had achieved during the treatment-training sessions. The study thus suggests that with a nonclinic population subjected to a highly artificial command–compliance regimen, relatively brief within-room periods of time-out can be an effective means of establishing child compliance. We now need to turn to the question whether similar procedures will be effective with children whose mothers bring them to a clinic with the complaint that they are noncompliant and, what is more, whether training given at the clinic will carry over (generalize) to the home.

Clinical Applications

In early work by Wahler (1969a, b) it had been demonstrated that when parents of young boys, aged 5 to 8, were taught to use time-out and differential attention contingent on oppositional behavior, the cooperative behavior of these children showed a dramatic and stable increase. In these cases time-out consisted of isolating the child in his bedroom for approximately 5 minutes contingent on the occurrence of oppositional behavior. This procedure had been taught to the parents by having the therapist visit them in their home where direct observations of parent and child behavior were also carried out. In the cases of two boys (Wahler, 1969b) the oppositional, noncompliant behavior was emitted not only at home but also in school, permitting an investigation of the question whether the treatment-related improvements obtained in the child's home would generalize to the school. This revealed that the home and school settings were functionally independent with respect to the problem behavior because the boys' school behavior did not change when the contingencies were manipulated at home. Only when the teachers also implemented time-out and differential attention in the case of one child and differential attention alone, in the case of the other, did the boys' behavior in school show an improvement.

The studies just mentioned and later work by Wahler (1975) have lent further support to the assumption derived from the principles of operant learning that behavior is specific to situations so that changes in behavior established in one situation should not be expected to generalize to other situations until the reinforcement contingencies there are also changed.

While behavior appears to be situation specific, a report by Bucher and Reaume (1979) suggests that *within* a setting, changes may generalize across behaviors. That is to say that when parents introduce explicit contingencies for one behavior, changes can also be observed in other behaviors within the same response class. In the case presented by Bucher and Reaume a girl was able to earn tokens contingent on her picking up the toys in her room. As this behavior improved, concurrent improvements were also observed in her hanging up her clothes, tidying her bed, and putting her dirty clothes in the laundry in response to her mother's general request that she clean up her room.

In order to conduct well-controlled research it is necessary that behavior observations be carried out in the child's home by trained, independent observers. Treatment effectiveness is probably maximized if the therapist visits the home to instruct the parents in behavior management techniques in their own setting. Such practices are obviously uneconomical from a practical point of view and we therefore turn to an examination of the treatment of noncompliance under conditions that are clinically feasible but where experimental rigor is necessarily compromised. Forehand and King (1974) reported on work they had conducted with five male and three female preschool children whose parents had come to a clinic for help with the noncompliant behavior of their children. Each mother–child pair was seen in a therapy room equipped with a table, chairs, and some toys where observations could be conducted from an adjacent room via a one-way mirror. As in the other work by Forehand and his group that was discussed earlier, the therapist was able to communicate with the mother from the observation room by a device known as a "bug in the ear." When this device is used, the mother wears a small, wireless FM receiver that fits into the ear like a hearing aid and through which she can hear instructions that the therapist delivers into a microphone in the adjoining room.

Treatment began with baseline observations during which each mother was instructed to play with her child, first with any toy selected by the child and then with a game and under rules determined by her. Following this, each mother was instructed in the appropriate use of positive reinforcement of desirable, cooperative child behavior. This was done by means of discussion, modeling, role playing, and direct practice while instructions and feedback were delivered through the bug-in-the-ear device. In subsequent training sessions each mother was taught to use a time-out procedure, contingent on the child's failure to follow her requests. Time-out entailed the use of a chair placed in a corner of the room in which the child was made to sit for approximately two minutes if, following a warning about this consequence for noncompliance, the child had failed to carry out the mother's instruction. If the child left the chair prematurely, a warning was issued that repetition of this would result in a spanking and, when necessary, the child received "two quick spanks on the rear" before being placed again in the chair. (This is the only instance that we have encountered in the behavior therapy literature where spanking is recommended as a formal part of the treatment procedure. The fact that it is here presented is not to be construed as an endorsement of this controversial approach to child-rearing. Some parents may be all too quick to seize on a therapist's recommendation that they spank their child to justify the physical punishment to which they had already been resorting on their own.)

After a mean of 6.2 treatment sessions in which Forehand and King (1974) had taught the mothers the combination of positive social reinforcement and time-out procedures, each mother–child pair was again observed. Comparison between the behaviors of the mothers and their children from baseline to treatment conditions revealed significant changes in a number of categories. The mothers' rate of providing rewards for compliance had increased significantly as had the ratio of child compliance to the commands issued by the mother. During baseline the children had complied with only 43 percent of maternal commands; in treatment this ratio had risen to 81 percent.

From the standpoint of clinical relevance, of course, it is necessary to demonstrate not only that a treatment affects behavior in the laboratory but also that the improvement carries over into the child's own home. To test this, Forehand and King (1974) observed two of the eight mother–child pairs in their own homes and found that in each case the child's compliance was higher at home than it had been in the laboratory, suggesting not only a carryover of the achieved change but, in fact, further improvement. Certain obvious shortcomings in the design of this study unfortunately detract from the confidence with which one can view its results. Among these flaws is the fact that the investigators had not obtained pretreatment observations in the home, that their comparison was between a baseline condition and a treatment (instead of a posttreatment) condition, that they fail to report how they selected the two families on whom posttreatment home observations were obtained, and that there was no control group. Nonetheless, since a somewhat more refined study by the same investigators (Forehand & King, 1977) led to very similar results, there may be some merit to their conclusion that the short-term treatment for noncompliance they have developed has the desired effect. For more substantial support, however, we must turn to a series of studies concerned with the effectiveness of parent-training programs.

Parent-training Programs

The behavioral program for training mothers to increase their children's compliance that Forehand and King (1974, 1977) had described was evaluated by Peed, Roberts, and Forehand (1977) with 12 mother–child pairs, nine of whom had been referred for help by teachers or physicians in the community and three of whom had responded to a newspaper announcement. "Disobedience" was a presenting problem for all of the children; in addition, some were said to have temper tantrums, or to be destructive or hyperactive. Six of these mother–child pairs were assigned to a treatment group while the other six served as a waiting-list control. Direct observations on both groups were gathered before and after treatment, at the home as well as in the clinic. In addition, parental judgments about child behavior were gathered by means of attitude scales and checklists at the beginning and the end of the study. The observations conducted at the clinic took place within the structure described earlier where mother and child spend time interacting around activities selected by the child, followed by a period where the mother issues instructions on what the child should do, based on cues she receives by earphone from a therapist located in the adjoining room. The observations conducted in the home, on the other hand, took place under as natural a condition as possible, the observer having asked the mother to interact with her child according to her daily routine.

The analysis of the results of this study (Peed et al., 1977) revealed that, from pre- to posttest, the children in the treatment group showed a significant increase in compliance to maternal commands both in the clinic and at home. The children in the control group on the other hand decreased their compliance at the clinic and failed to change at home. Furthermore, comparisons between treatment and control groups permitted the conclusion that the treatment had indeed been the effective variable. Not only had the behavior of the children changed in the direction of greater compliance, but the behavior of the mothers had also changed in the predicted direction in that they issued fewer of the ambiguous beta commands, gave more positive reinforcement for compliance, and attended more appropriately to the child's behavior.

While the behavior observations thus supported the conclusion offered by Peed et al. (1977) to the effect that a brief treatment program of approximately 10 hours results in significant improvement in mother–child interaction, the data from the checklists and attitude questionnaires were more difficult to interpret. This was due, in part, to the control parents reporting improvement in the behavior of their children, a result that might raise questions about the validity of such paper-and-pencil instruments if one assumed that the direct observation of behavior by a trained observer can be used as the validity criterion.

The conclusion that training parents in more effective child-rearing methods decreases noncompliant child behavior both at the clinic and in the home received further support from two studies reported by Forehand and his students (Forehand, Sturgis, McMahon, Aguar, Green, Wells, & Breiner, 1979). Here, follow-up assessments were gathered at 6 and 12-month intervals, revealing that the treatment-produced changes were generally maintained over these periods of time. The second study in this series addressed the question whether treatment effects generalize from the home to the school. There is, of course, little reason to expect such generalization if one views behavior to be specific to the situation and if one considers that treatment brought about changed contingencies in the mother–child and not in the teacher–child interaction. In line with this expectation, and confirming Wahler's (1969b) results, the improvement in the child's compliance at home did not have its parallel in the school where the teachers, not having been involved in the treatment, continued to maintain the same contingencies as before.

Issues related to the generalization of treatment effects have been discussed by Forehand and Atkeson (1977), Stokes and Baer (1977), and in a review by Wahler, Berland, and Coe (1979). All of these writers agree that since the behavior of children (as that of adults) is under the control of social reinforcement contingencies, behavior change will be neither generalized nor maintained unless the therapist takes these contingencies into consideration while planning and conducting the treatment.

Group Training. The parent-training discussed thus far involved working with individual parent–child dyads where the parent—usually the mother—was taught behavioral child management methods. We turn now to an examination of studies where several parents gathered in groups to receive training in the use of these methods. One such group program was described by Hall, Axelrod, Tyler, Grief, Jones, and Robertson (1972). The group had met for 16 weeks in weekly 3-hour sessions in the context of a three-credit course, entitled Responsive Teaching. Though the classes varied in size from 40 to above 70 students, meetings in discussion groups of about 10 persons were used to supplement the lectures, films, and quizzes. Hall et al. (1972) report on the successful experience of four of these participants, who applied the child-management skills they had learned in class with the oppositional, noncompliant behavior of their own children. Several investigators have since addressed the question of the most effective means for operating such group-training programs.

A comparison of four instructional techniques for teaching parents to use time-out contingencies was conducted by Flanagan, Adams, and Forehand (1979) who evaluated the relative effectiveness of a lecture format, a printed pamphlet, a videotaped modeling presentation, and a structured role-playing session. Observations conducted in the home by trained observers revealed that the modeling situation was the most effective from the point of view of the mothers' ability to apply what they had learned in the natural environment of the home. While it is worth knowing that mothers can learn to apply a time-out contingency appropriately after only one 70-minute training session, it is necessary to ascertain whether this application will succeed in changing the targeted behavior of the child. Here, a study by Glogower and Sloop (1976) is of relevance. They worked with eight mothers who had sought professional help because of their children's noncompliant behavior. The mothers were assigned to one of two groups that met for 10 weekly 2-hour sessions. In one of the groups the focus was on teaching general principles of behavior during the first four sessions and on changing specific target behaviors during the remaining sessions. The other group spent the entire 10 weeks focusing on specific target behaviors and on how these might be modified by the application of the principles of behavior. The results were evaluated by comparisons between pre- and posttraining administrations of laboratory observations of each mother in interaction with her child, an adjective checklist, and mother's responses to a series of behavioral vignettes depicting problem situations calling for a solution. Five months after conclusion of the training programs all mothers were asked to observe and record again the target behavior they had been taught to monitor during the early part of the training; to respond again to the behavioral vignettes and the adjective checklist, and to repeat a test on operant principles that had been administered at the end of the training program.

The results of the study by Glogower and Sloop (1976) show that combining the teaching of behavioral principles with training in applying these to specific problems was superior on several of the measures to merely dealing with specific problems. While both groups of mothers demonstrated knowledge of the behavioral principles taught and were able to apply these successfully with their children at home, the mothers in the group that had combined general principles with specific applications used these principles with more target behaviors and (unlike the other group) established home projects beyond those dealt with during training. The investigators also report that the mothers in this combination group improved considerably in playing with their children and in their ability to give effective commands.

The efficacy of teaching parents the principles of applied operant learning instead of focusing on helping them solve specific problems and sending them on their way was also borne out in a three-year evaluation of parent-group training conducted by Rinn, Vernon, and Wise (1975). Not only do parents who participated in such programs report improvement in the problem behaviors about which they originally sought help but, as Karoly and Rosenthal (1977) have reported, they also experience improvement in family cohesion; that is, they view their home environments as psychologically less noxious, conceivably because increased compliance on the part of the child reduces the frictions among family members. The observation that a noncompliant child affects the entire family, just as family discord will affect the individual child, was also made by Wahler, Berland, and Coe (1979) who speak of the ecology surrounding child behavior and stress that this ecology must be taken into consideration in planning and conducting the treatment of any member of a family. In fact they suggest that the effect of treatment on child noncompliance and the likelihood of maintaining any improvement may be a function of the social support system in the community that is available to a family and particularly to the mother.

A Methodological Note. In the earlier discussion of the study conducted by Peed, Roberts, and Forehand (1977) we mentioned a discrepancy between results obtained by direct observations of child behavior and those based on parents' questionnaire responses. While in that case the discrepancy lay in the control-group parents perceiving improvements in their children that direct observation could not substantiate, there have also been instances in the literature where parents in the treatment group reported improvements that observers were unable to detect (Eyberg & Johnson, 1974). This, as Atkeson and Forehand (1978) have pointed out, alerts one to the fact that outcome measures furnished by parents may be tapping a source of information regarding child behavior that is different from the one sampled when independent observers collect data in the home. With different measures yielding different conclusions regarding treatment outcome, care must be taken to consider not one, but several sources of data and not to exclude the more rigorous, objective, observational methods that frequently yield the less gratifying results (Forehand & Atkeson, 1977). All of this is of course particularly important when, as in the case of treatment involving the training of parents, auxiliary therapists (the parents) are asked to assess the very treatment in which they themselves have taken an active role. Global ratings may here be particularly subject to distortion and only data based on the recording of objectively defined behaviors permit one to have confidence that the parent is reporting changes that have indeed taken place. When, in addition, some means is available for ascertaining the reliability of the data gathered by the parent, as was the case in the study by Hall, Axelrod, Tyler, Grief, Jones, and Robertson (1972), this confidence is considerably increased.

Effect on Siblings

If a mother is taught child-management techniques designed to increase one child's compliance and if such intervention has implications beyond that mother–child dyad as Karoly and Rosenthal (1977) suggest, it stands to reason that other children in the family may also be affected by the change. Not only would one assume that the mother might apply the newly learned management skills with her other children but, as has been shown in classroom situations (Christy, 1975; Drabman & Lahey, 1974), changes in the behavior of a treated child tend to affect the behavior of other children.

Arnold, Levine, and Patterson (1975) demonstrated changes in the behavior of the siblings of a child whose aggressive behavior had been the target of treatment and Resick, Forehand, and McWhorter (1976) found this to be the case with a sibling of a noncompliant child. Humphreys, Forehand, McMahon, and Roberts (1978) conducted a controlled investigation of this effect with eight cases in which noncompliance had been the target of intervention. Mothers who had sought help from a clinic because of the noncompliant behavior of one of their children were given training in the contingent use of such social reinforcement as positive attention for appropriate child behavior and in employing an in-room time-out procedure contingent on noncompliance to alpha commands. The training procedure was the same Forehand and his students had used in studies we have discussed previously. Prior to the beginning of treatment which took place over a mean of 5.6 sessions, trained observers had visited the family's home four to eight times to obtain a record of the mother's interaction with the boy whom she had referred to the clinic and his untreated, nonreferred sibling. Some of these untreated siblings were younger, some older than the targeted child but all were relatively close in age. The mean age for the targeted children was about 6½ years, that of the untreated siblings about 5 years. The home observations had been explained to the mother as based on the clinicians' interest in typical family interactions but not until the end of the study was it revealed that the actual focus of the observations had been on the untreated sibling.

Criteria for successful completion of the training conducted in the clinic playroom were threefold. The mother had to give an average of at least four rewards and contingent attention per minute during a five-minute observation of child-initiated play, her child had to comply with at least 75 percent of the mother's commands during a five-minute, mother-initiated play period, and the ratio of the mother's contingent reward to the child's compliance during this period had to be at least 60 percent. These are the same criteria of training effectiveness Peed, Roberts, and Forehand (1977) had used in an earlier study. Once a mother's training had reached this criterion of success, Humphreys et al. (1978) conducted four more home observations of the mother's interactions with her nonreferred child while the referred child was also present. A comparison of the pre- and posttreatment observations (see Fig. 21) revealed significant increases in the mothers' use of rewards and contingent attention and a significant decrease in the use of the vague beta commands to which compliance is difficult or impossible. At the same time, the untreated siblings' compliance showed a significant increase, suggesting that the mothers' changed child-management techniques had positively influenced the behavior of children who had neither been the target of, nor participated in the clinic treatment. It is particularly noteworthy that although the mothers had been taught a time-out procedure, this method was used so infrequently that it precluded meaningful statistical analysis. The increased compliance of the untreated children was thus largely accomplished by the mothers using such positive consequences as praise, approval, and positive physical attention for constructive activity and by their practice of stating clearly defined rules, instructions, and requests.

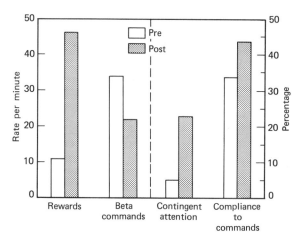

Figure 21. Mean occurrence at pre- and posttreatment of parental rewards, beta commands, and contingent attention addressed to the untreated siblings and mean percent compliance to commands by the untreated siblings. Graphs left of vertical line are expressed in rate per minute; those at right show percentages. (Reprinted with permission from *Journal of Behavior Therapy and Experimental Psychiatry, 9,* Humphreys, Forehand, McMahon, & Roberts, "Parent behavioral training to modify child noncompliance: effects on untreated siblings," Copyright 1978, Pergamon Press, Ltd.)

When parents are taught to act as auxiliary therapists to treat the problem behavior of one of their children, they often express a legitimate concern about what the effect on their other children will be if, as a part of the treatment, they begin to focus their attention on the behavior of the problem child, particularly when that child is to earn tangible reinforcers for desirable behavior. Therapists have found that untoward reactions of siblings can be avoided by permitting them to share in the reinforcers earned by the treated child (as when a family outing is used as a back-up reinforcer) or by seeing to it that everyone can earn explicit rewards for desirable behavior. Lavigueur (1976) reported that involving a sibling as a ''therapeutic aid'' can not only compensate for the parents' increased attention to the treated child but that it also results in positive changes in the sibling's own behavior. In one of the families treated by Lavigueur, a 9-year-old boy, described as ''rude, tense, and demanding'' was treated with the assistance of his 10-year-old brother. Intervention and independent observations of behavior were conducted in the home. After obtaining baseline data, the parents were instructed and cued to reinforce positive verbalizations and either to ignore or follow with time-out any negative verbalizations of the targeted child. After five sessions of this, the sibling was brought into the picture by having the parents instruct him to attend to the positive and to ignore the negative verbalizations of his brother in order to help him overcome his problem. Five sessions later, following a multiple baseline design, the parents (but not the sibling) began imposing appropriate consequences on a new behavior (noncompliance) that had not been targeted before. After yet another five sessions during which these contingencies had been in effect, the sibling was also told to respond differentially to his brother's noncompliance and this phase was continued for a final five treatment sessions.

The data presented by Lavigueur (1976) reflect the targeted child's improved behavior by an almost total elimination of negative verbalizations and noncompliance with the onset of the initial parental intervention. His positive affect (smiling, laughing, singing, dancing) and constructive, cooperative play—categories of behavior that had been observed but not directly treated—showed the most pronounced increase during those treatment phases where the parents and the sibling acted as therapists. Of particular interest, however, was the behavior of the sibling himself. During the first treatment phase where only the parents were managing the contingencies, the mother had attended to the targeted child far more frequently than to his brother, at which that boy had shown a marked decrease in positive verbalizations and affect. At the investigators' request, the parents then equalized their attention to the two children and the sibling now not only again became more positive in affect and verbalization but also more consistent as a change agent for his brother's behavior. What is more, when he started being involved as his brother's therapist, working on increasing his positive verbalizations and decreasing his negative statements, the content of the boy's own speech changed in that direction. Later on, when he also became involved in the treatment of noncompliance, his own noncompliance decreased and his positive affect showed an increase. Not only need siblings of children in treatment not develop untoward reactions, but by judiciously involving them in the treatment plan one may actually be able to turn this experience to a constructive end.

A GLIMPSE INTO THE FUTURE

As we have seen, children's problem behaviors can be changed in a positive direction by professional therapists, by parents who are trained to act as therapists for their own children, and even by interventions on the part of their siblings. A hint of where this development might lead comes from a laboratory study by Grusec and Kuczynski (1977) who showed that children's compliance with instructions can be increased if they are taught to impose negative consequences on themselves contingent on their own noncompliant behavior. Working with boys and girls between the ages of 7 and 11, these experimenters taught each child to play a miniature bowling game on which the scores could be surreptitiously controlled while the child was led to believe that the score was a function of skill. All children were presented with a response-cost contingency, being given a large supply of pennies at the onset of the game. From this supply coins were removed for obtaining a "low," losing score. With the pennies remaining at the end of the game the child was allowed to buy a prize from an array of toys and games that varied in value, the better ones costing more money.

In one experimental condition the response-cost punishment was administered by the experimenter who removed the pennies from the supply when the child had a low score. In a second condition, the experimenter merely suggested that the child take some pennies from the bowl for a low score, while in a third condition the child was directly instructed to do so. Following this training, the children were asked to continue playing the game by themselves while the experimenter either left the room or attended to some other activity. This test showed that children who had punished themselves during the training session, either on the basis of the experimenter's suggestion or instruction, continued to punish themselves for low scores significantly more severely (in terms of the number of pennies they took from themselves) than those whose punishment had been administered by the experimenter.

The question whether such self-punishment would affect behavior other than that involved in the game on which the children had been trained was investigated in a second experiment. Here different children were trained on the bowling game, using the procedure already described, and then tested for compliance with instructions. Following training on the bowling game each child was left alone with two toys, a very attractive one that the experimenter had instructed the child not to touch and an unattractive one to which no such prohibition had been attached. During a 9-minute period, while the children were alone in the room with these toys, they were observed through a one-way mirror and their compliance with the instruction not to play with the attractive toy was recorded. This revealed that 34 of the 72 children in this experiment complied with the instructions. Among those who deviated, the ones who had "voluntarily" punished themselves, that is those to whom self-punishment had merely been suggested by the experimenter, spent significantly less time playing with the forbidden toy than did those whose punishment had been either directed or administered by the experimenter.

Grusec and Kuczynski (1977) conclude from their work that training in self-punishment that minimizes the role of an outsider and actively involves the child in the role of punitive agent appears capable of promoting self-punishment and compliance. In the absence of a rewarded group and of a control group that had experienced neutral consequences during training it is, of course, impossible to tell whether the results obtained by these investigators are unique to self-punishment but the study suggests that we may some day be able to increase children's compliance by giving them experiences that involve self-administered, mild punishment. In combination with the self-monitoring, self-evaluation, and self-reinforcement which Spates and Kanfer (1977) studied in a different context, and the various modes of teaching children to manage their own behavior that O'Leary and Dubey (1974) and Rosenbaum and Drabman (1979) have reviewed, we may ultimately learn how to help children achieve the valuable social skill we call self-control.

Recapitulation

Whenever one person undertakes to intervene in the life of another, be it in the context of training, teaching, correction, or therapy, issues of ethics and values are involved because such intervention is an intrusion that may violate the other person's integrity as a human being. While no therapy is ever value-free and although therapists must always be sensitive to ethical issues, these matters are accentuated when the focus of intervention is a child's noncompliant behavior. We therefore preceded the material in this chapter with a discussion of ethics and values, and of the rights of children who are clients in therapy. It was stressed that a therapist must take care to avoid reducing a child's noncompliance when this occurs in the face of unreasonable or irrational parental expectations or demands. Since intervention with noncompliant children often involves teaching their parents effective methods for changing behavior, the therapist must recognize the ethical dilemma posed by the potential abuse to which knowledge of these methods might be put.

Various studies were reviewed that demonstrated the feasibility of increasing compliance with parental requests by the systematic manipulations of the contingencies of reinforcement. However, important as attention to the consequences of a child's behavior is, it seems at least as crucial to examine the antecedents, particularly those represented by the manner in which a parent issues requests and instructions. Parents who complain about the noncompliant behavior of their children often employ vague, nonspecific circumlocutions of what they want their child to do. When they are taught to issue requests in direct, unambiguous terms and to be consistent in the consequences with which they follow the child's response to a request, noncompliance can usually be reduced. Teaching these and similar child-management approaches to parents does not seem difficult and can be done either in individual or in group sessions. Once parents employ these approaches in the home, they affect not only the behavior of the child about whom help was originally sought, because positive changes have also been reported in that child's siblings and in the cohesion of the total family. The effective use of a child's sibling in helping reduce oppositional and other aversive behavior has also been demonstrated. This led us to ask whether ultimately children might not be helped to become agents of their own behavior change in which case they might then be said to be exerting self-control.

References

Adams, M. J., & Shepp, B. E. Selective attention and the breadth of learning: A developmental study. *Journal of Experimental Child Psychology*, 1975, *20*, 168–180.

Adelson, R., Liebert, R. M., Poulos, R. W., & Herskovitz, A. A modeling film to reduce children's fear of dental treatment. *International Association for Dental Research Abstracts*, March, 1972, p. 114.

Agras, W. S., Barlow, T. H., Chapin, H. N. Abel, G. G., & Leitenberg, H. Behavior modification of anorexia nervosa. *Archives of General Psychiatry*, 1974, *30*, 343–352.

Alexander, A. B. Systematic relaxation and flow rates in asthmatic children: Relationship to emotional precipitants and anxiety. *Journal of Psychosomatic Research*, 1972, *16*, 405–410.

Alexander, A. B., Chai, H., Creer, T. L., Miklich, D. R., Renne, C. M., & Cardoso, R. R. deA. The elimination of chronic cough by response suppression shaping. *Journal of Behavior Therapy and Experimental Psychiatry*, 1973, *4*, 75–80.

Alexander, A. B., Cropp, G. J. A., & Chai, H. Effects of relaxation training on pulmonary mechanics in children with asthma. *Journal of Applied Behavior Analysis*, 1979, *12*, 27–35.

Alexander, A. B., Miklich, D. R., & Hershkoff, H. The immediate effects of systematic relaxation training on peak expiratory flow rates in asthmatic children. *Psychosomatic Medicine*, 1972, *34*, 388–394.

Alexander, J. F., Barton, C., Schiavo, R. S., & Parsons, B. V. Systems-behavioral intervention with families of delinquents: Therapist characteristics, family behavior, and outcome. *Journal of Consulting and Clinical Psychology*, 1976, *44*. 656–664.

Alexander, J. F., & Parsons, B. V. Short-term behavioral intervention with delinquent families: Impact on family process and recidivism. *Journal of Abnormal Psychology*, 1973, *81*, 219–225.

Allen, K. E., & Harris, F. R. Elimination of a child's excessive scratching by training the mother in reinforcement procedures. *Behaviour Research and Therapy*, 1966, *4*, 79–84.

Allen, K. E., Hart, B. M., Buell, J. S., Harris, F. R., & Wolf, M. M. Effects of social reinforcement on isolate behavior of a nursery school child. *Child Development*, 1964, *35*, 511–518.

Altman, K., Haavik, S., & Cook, J. W. Punishment of self-injurious behavior in natural settings using contingent aromatic ammonia. *Behaviour Research and Therapy*, 1978, *16*, 85–96.

Anthony, W. Z. Brief intervention in a case of childhood trichotillomania by self-monitoring. *Journal of Behavior Therapy and Experimental Psychiatry*, 1978, *9*, 173–175.

Aragona, J., Cassady, J., & Drabman, R. S. Treating overweight children through parental training and contingency contracting. *Journal of Applied Behavior Analysis*, 1975, *8*, 269–278.

Arnold, J. E., Levine, A. G., & Patterson, G. R. Changes in sibling behavior following family intervention. *Journal of Consulting and Clinical Psychology*, 1975, *43*, 683–688.

Atkeson, B. M., & Forehand, R. Parent behavioral training for problem children: An examination of studies using multiple outcome measures. *Journal of Abnormal Child Psychology*, 1978, *6*, 449–460.

Ayllon, T., Garber, S., & Pisor, K. The elimination of discipline problems through a combined school–home motivational system. *Behavior Therapy*, 1975, *6*, 616–626.

Ayllon, T., Layman, D., & Kandel, H. J. A behavioral–educational alternative to drug control of hyperactive children. *Journal of Applied Behavior Analysis*, 1975, *8*, 137–146.

Ayllon, T., Simon, S. J., & Wildman, R. W., II. Instructions and reinforcement in the elimination of encopresis: A case study. *Journal of Behavior Therapy and Experimental Psychiatry*, 1975, *6*, 235–238.

Ayllon, T., Smith, D., & Rogers, M. Behavioral management of school phobia. *Journal of Behavior Therapy and Experimental Psychiatry*, 1970, *1*, 125–138.

Azrin, N. H., & Foxx, R. M. *Toilet Training In Less Than a Day*. New York: Simon & Schuster, 1974.

Azrin, N. H., Gottlieb, L., Hughart, L., Wesolowski, M. D., & Rahn, T. Eliminating self-injurious behavior by educative procedures. *Behaviour Research and Therapy*, 1975, *13*, 101–111.

Azrin, N. H., Hontos, P. T., & Besalel-Azrin, V. Elimination of enuresis without a conditioning apparatus: An extension by office instruction of the child and parents. *Behavior Therapy*, 1979, *10*, 14–19.

Azrin, N. H., & Nunn, R. G. Habit reversal: A method of eliminating nervous habits and tics. *Behaviour Research and Therapy*, 1973, *11*, 619–628.

Azrin, N. H., & Powers, M. A. Eliminating classroom disturbances of emotionally disturbed children by positive practice procedures. *Behavior Therapy*, 1975, *6*, 525–534.

Azrin, N. H., Sneed, T. J., & Foxx, R. M. Dry-bed training: Rapid elimination of childhood enuresis. *Behaviour Research and Therapy*, 1974, *12*, 147-156.

Azrin, N. H., & Thienes, P. M. Rapid elimination of enuresis by intensive learning without a conditioning apparatus. *Behavior Therapy*, 1978, *9*, 342-354.

Azrin, N. H., & Wesolowski, M. D. Theft reversal: An overcorrection procedure for eliminating stealing by retarded persons. *Journal of Applied Behavior Analysis*, 1974, *7*, 577-581.

Bach, R., & Moylan, J. J. Parents administered behavior therapy for inappropriate urination and encopresis: A case study. *Journal of Behavior Therapy and Experimental Psychiatry*, 1975, *6*, 239-241.

Bachman, J. A. Self-injurious behavior: A behavioral analysis. *Journal of Abnormal Psychology*, 1972, *80*, 211-224.

Baer, D. M., & Guess, D. Receptive training of adjectival inflections in mental retardates. *Journal of Applied Behavior Analysis*, 1971, *4*, 129-139.

Baer, D. M., & Sherman, J. Reinforcement control of generalized imitation in young children. *Journal of Experimental Child Psychology*, 1964, *1*, 37-49.

Bailey, J. S., Wolf, M. M., & Phillips, E. L. Home-based reinforcement and the modification of pre-delinquents' classroom behavior. *Journal of Applied Behavior Analysis*, 1970, *3*, 223-233.

Baker, B. L. Symptom treatment and symptom substitution in enuresis. *Journal of Abnormal Psychology*, 1969, *74*, 42-49.

Balaschak, B. A. Teacher-implemented behavior modification in a case of organically based epilepsy. *Journal of Consulting and Clinical Psychology*, 1976, *44*, 218-223.

Ball, T. S., & Irwin, A. E. A portable, automated device applied to training a hyperactive child. *Journal of Behavior Therapy and Experimental Psychiatry*, 1976, *7*, 185-187.

Bandura, A. Psychotherapy as a learning process. *Psychological Bulletin*, 1961, *58*, 143-159.

Bandura, A. *Principles of Behavior Modification*. New York: Holt, Rinehart & Winston, 1969.

Bandura, A. Vicarious and self-reinforcement processes. In R. Glaser (Ed.), *The Nature of Reinforcement*. New York: Academic Press, 1971. Pp. 228-278.

Bandura, A. *Aggression: A social learning analysis*. Englewood Cliffs, N.J.: Prentice-Hall, 1973.

Bandura, A. Self-efficacy: Toward a unifying theory of behavioral change. *Psychological Review*, 1977, *84*, 191-215. (a)

Bandura, A. *Social Learning Theory*. Englewood Cliffs, N.J.: Prentice-Hall, 1977. (b)

Bandura, A., Blanchard, E. B., & Ritter, B. Relative efficacy of desensitization and modeling approaches for inducing behavioral, affective, and attitudinal changes. *Journal of Personality and Social Psychology*, 1969, *13*, 173-199.

Bandura, A., Grusec, J. E., & Menlove, F. L. Vicarious extinction of avoidance behavior. *Journal of Personality and Social Psychology*, 1967, *5*, 16-23.

Bandura, A., & Menlove, F. L. Factors determining vicarious extinction of avoidance behavior through symbolic modeling. *Journal of Personality and Social Psychology*, 1968, *8*, 99-108.

Bandura, A., Ross, D., & Ross, S. A. Imitation of film-mediated aggressive models. *Journal of Abnormal and Social Psychology*, 1963, *66*, 3-11.

Barkley, R. A., Hasting, J. E., Tousel, R. E., & Tousel, S. E. Evaluation of a token system for juvenile delinquents in a residential setting. *Journal of Behavior Therapy and Experimental Psychiatry*, 1976, *7*, 227–230.

Bauermeister, J. J., & Jemail, J. A. Modification of "elective mutism" in the classroom setting: A case study. *Behavior Therapy*, 1975, *6*, 246–250.

Baum, M. Extinction of avoidance responding through response prevention (flooding). *Psychological Bulletin*, 1970, *74*, 276–284.

Begelman, D. A., & Hersen, M. Critique of Obler and Terwilliger's "Systematic desensitization with neurologically impaired children with phobic disorders." *Journal of Consulting and Clinical Psychology*, 1971, *37*, 10–13.

Bemis, K. M. Current approaches to the etiology and treatment of anorexia nervosa. *Psychological Bulletin*, 1978, *85*, 593–617.

Bernal, M. E., Duryee, J. S., Pruett, H. L., & Burns, B. J. Behavior modification and the Brat syndrome. *Journal of Consulting and Clinical Psychology*, 1968, *32*, 447–455.

Bernal, M. E., & North, J. A. A survey of parent training manuals. *Journal of Applied Behavior Analysis*, 1978, *11*, 533–544.

Bhanji, S., & Thompson, J. Operant conditioning in the treatment of anorexia nervosa: A review and retrospective study of 11 cases. *British Journal of Psychiatry*, 1974, *124*, 166–172.

Blanchard, E. B. The relative contribution of modeling, informational influences, and physical contact in the extinction of phobic behavior. *Journal of Abnormal Psychology*, 1970, *76*, 55–61.

Block, J., Block, J. H., & Harrington, D. M. Some misgivings about the Matching Familiar Figures Test as a measure of reflection-impulsivity. *Developmental Psychology*, 1974, *10*, 611–632.

Bollard, R. J., & Woodroffe, P. The effect of parent-administered dry-bed training on nocturnal enuresis in children. *Behaviour Research and Therapy*, 1977, *15*, 159–165.

Bolstad, O. D., & Johnson, S. M. Self-regulation in the modification of disruptive behavior. *Journal of Applied Behavior Analysis*, 1972, *5*, 443–454.

Bornstein, P. H., & Quevillon, R. P. The effects of a self-instructional package on overactive preschool boys. *Journal of Applied Behavior Analysis*, 1976, *9*, 179–188.

Borden, M., Hall, R. V., & Mitts, B. The effect of self-recording on the classroom behavior of two eighth-grade students. *Journal of Applied Behavior Analysis*, 1971, *4*, 191–199.

Brown, P., & Elliott, R. Control of aggression in a nursery school class. *Journal of Experimental Child Psychology*, 1965, *2*, 103–107.

Bucher, B., & Reaume, J. Generalization of reinforcement effects in a token program in the home. *Behavior Modification*, 1979, *3*, 63–72.

Buell, J., Stoddard, P., Harris, F., & Baer, D. M. Collateral social development accompanying reinforcement of outdoor play in a preschool child. *Journal of Applied Behavior Analysis*, 1968, *1*, 167–173.

Burchard, J., & Barrera, F. An analysis of time-out and response cost in a programmed environment. *Journal of Applied Behavior Analysis*, 1972, *5*, 271–282.

Burchard, J. D., & Harig, P. T. Behavior modification and juvenile delinquency. In H. Leitenberg (Ed.), *Handbook of Behavior Modification and Behavior Therapy*. Englewood Cliffs, N.J.: Prentice-Hall, 1976, Pp. 405–452.

Burchard, J., & Tyler, V., Jr. The modification of delinquent behavior through operant conditioning, *Behaviour Research and Therapy*, 1965, *2*, 245–250.

Butler, J. F. Treatment of encopresis by overcorrection. *Psychological Reports*, 1977, *40*, 639–646.

Carr, E. G. The motivation of self-injurious behavior: A review of some hypotheses. *Psychological Bulletin*, 1977, *84*, 800–816.

Carr, E. G., Newsom, C. D. & Binkoff, J. A. Stimulus control of self-destructive behavior in a psychotic child. *Journal of Abnormal Child Psychology*, 1976, *4*, 139–153.

Carr, E. G., Schreibman, L., & Lovaas, O. I. Control of echolalic speech in psychotic children. *Journal of Abnormal Child Psychology*, 1975, *3*, 331–351.

Chomsky, N. *Aspects of the Theory of Syntax*. Cambridge: M. I. T. Press, 1965.

Christopherson, E. R., Arnold, C. M., Hill, D. W., & Quilitich, H. R. The home point system: Token reinforcement procedures for application by parents of children with behavior problems. *Journal of Applied Behavior Analysis*, 1972, *5*, 485–497.

Christy, P. R. Does use of tangible rewards with individual children affect peer observers? *Journal of Applied Behavior Analysis*, 1975, *8*, 187–196.

Ciminero, A. R., Calhoun, K. S., & Adams, H. E. (Eds.), *Handbook of Behavioral Assessment*. New York: Wiley, 1977.

Clark, H. B., Rowbury, T., Baer, A. M., & Baer, D. M. Timeout as a punishing stimulus in continuous and intermittent schedules. *Journal of Applied Behavior Analysis*, 1973, *6*, 443–455.

Clement, P.W. Elimination of sleepwalking in a 7-year-old boy. *Journal of Consulting and Clinical Psychology*, 1970, *34*, 22–26.

Clifton C., & Bogartz, R. Selective attention during dichotic listening by pre-school children. *Journal of Experimental Child Psychology*, 1968, *6*, 483–491.

Cone, J. D. Assessing the effectiveness of programmed generalization. *Journal of Applied Behavior Analysis*, 1973, *6*, 713–718.

Cohen, H. L., & Filipczak, J. *A New Learning Environment: A case for learning*. San Francisco: Jossey Bass, 1971.

Collins, R. W. Importance of the bladder-cue buzzer contingency in the conditioning treatment for enuresis. *Journal of Abnormal Psychology*, 1973 *82*, 299–308.

Comptom, R. D. Changes in enuretics accompanying treatment by the conditioned response technique. *Dissertation Abstracts*, 1968, *28* (7-A), 2549.

Conners, C. K. A teacher rating scale for use in drug studies with children. *American Journal of Psychiatry*, 1969, *126*, 884–888.

Conroy, R. L., & Weener, P. The development of visual and auditory selective attention using the central-incidental paradigm. *Journal of Experimental Child Psychology*, 1976, *22*, 400–407.

Corte, H. E., Wolf, M. M., & Locke, B. J. A comparison of procedures for eliminating self-injurious behavior of retarded adolescents. *Journal of Applied Behavior Analysis*, 1971, *4*, 201–213.

Crane, N. L., & Ross, L. E. A developmental study of attention to cue redundancy introduced following discrimination learning. *Journal of Experimental Child Psychology*, 1967, *5*, 1–15.

Creer, T. L. The use of time-out from positive reinforcement procedure with asthmatic children. *Journal of Psychosomatic Research*, 1970, *14*, 117–120.

Croghan, L., & Musante, G. J. The elimination of a boy's high-building phobia by *in vivo* desensitization and game playing. *Journal of Behavior Therapy and Experimental Psychiatry*, 1975, *6*, 87–88.

Crowley, C. P., & Armstrong, P. M. Positive practice, overcorrection and behavior rehearsal in the treatment of three cases of encopresis. *Journal of Behavior Therapy and Experimental Psychiatry*, 1977, *8*, 411–416.

Dalton, A. J., Rubino, C. A., & Hislop, M. W. Some effects of token rewards on school achievement of children with Down's syndrome. *Journal of Applied Behavior Analysis*, 1973, *6*, 251–259.

Davidson, W. S., II, & Seidman, E. Studies of behavior modification and juvenile delinquency: A review, methodological critique, and social perspective. *Psychological Bulletin*, 1974, *81*, 998–1011.

Davis, M. H., Saunders, D. R., Creer, T. L., & Chai, H. Relaxation training facilitated by biofeedback apparatus as a supplemental treatment of bronchial asthma. *Journal of Psychosomatic Research*, 1973, *17*, 121–128.

Davison, G. C. Homosexuality: The ethical challenge. *Journal of Consulting and Clinical Psychology*, 1976, *44*, 157–162.

Davison, G. C., & Wilson, G. T. Processes of fear-reduction in systematic desensitization: Cognitive and social reinforcement factors in humans. *Behavior Therapy*, 1973, *4*, 1–21.

DeLeon, G., & Mandell, W. A comparison of conditioning and psychotherapy in the treatment of functional enuresis. *Journal of Clinical Psychology*, 1966, *22*, 326–330.

DeLeon, G., & Sacks, S. Conditioning functional enuresis: A four year follow-up. *Journal of Consulting and Clinical Psychology*, 1972, *39*, 299–300.

Devany, J., & Rincover, A. *Experimental analysis of ethical issues: 1. Using self-stimulation as a reinforcer in the treatment of developmentally delayed children.* Paper presented at the meeting of the Association for Advancement of Behavior Therapy, Chicago, November 1978.

De Villiers, J. G., & Naughton, J. M. Teaching a symbol language to autistic children. *Journal of Consulting and Clinical Psychology*, 1974, *42*, 111–117.

Dineen, J. P., Clark, H. B., & Risley, T. R. Peer tutoring among elementary students: Educational benefits to the tutor. *Journal of Applied Behavior Analysis*, 1977, *10*, 231–238.

Doke, L. A., & Epstein, L. H. Oral overcorrection: Side effects and extended applications. *Journal of Experimental Child Psychology*, 1975, *20*, 496–511.

Doleys, D. M. Behavioral treatments for nocturnal enuresis in children: A review of the recent literature. *Psychological Bulletin*, 1977, *84*, 30–54.

Doleys, D. M., Ciminero, A. R., Tollison, J. W., Williams, C. L., & Wells, K. C. Drybed training and retention control training: A comparison. *Behavior Therapy*, 1977, *8*, 541–548.

Douglas, V. I. Stop, look and listen: The problem of sustained attention and impulse control in hyperactive and normal children. *Canadian Journal of Behavioral Science*, 1972, *4*, 259–281.

Drabman, R. S., & Lahey, B. B. Feedback in classroom behavior modification: Effects on the target and her classmates. *Journal of Applied Behavior Analysis*, 1974, *7*, 591–598.

Drabman, R., & Spitalnik, R. Social isolation as a punishment procedure: A controlled study. *Journal of Experimental Child Psychology*, 1973, *16*, 236–249. (a)

Drabman, R., & Spitalnik, R. Training a retarded child as a behavioral teaching assistant. *Journal of Behavior Therapy and Experimental Psychiatry*, 1973, *4*, 269–272. (b)

Drabman, R. S., Spitalnik, R., & O'Leary, K. D. Teaching self-control to disruptive children. *Journal of Abnormal Psychology*, 1973, *82*, 10–16.

Drabman, R., Spitalnik, R., & Spitalnik, K. Sociometric and disruptive behavior as a function of four types of token reinforcement programs. *Journal of Applied Behavior Analysis*, 1974, *7*, 93–101.

Dublin, J., Elton, C., & Berzins, J. Some personality and aptitudinal correlates of the "A–B" therapist scale. *Journal of Consulting and Clinical Psychology*, 1969, *33*, 739–745.

Dusek, J. B. The effects of labeling and pointing on children's selective attention. *Developmental Psychology*, 1978, *14*, 115–116.

Edelman, R. I. Operant conditioning treatment of encopresis. *Journal of Behavior Therapy and Experimental Psychiatry*, 1971, *2*, 71–73.

Egeland, B. Training impulsive children in the use of more efficient scanning techniques. *Child Development*, 1974, *45*, 165–171.

Egeland, B. Effects of errorless training on teaching children to discriminate letters of the alphabet. *Journal of Applied Psychology*, 1975, *60*, 533–536.

Egeland, B., & Winer, K. Teaching children to discriminate letters of the alphabet through errorless discrimination training. *Journal of Reading Behavior*, 1974, *6*, 142–150.

Epstein, L. H., Doke, L. A., Sajwaj, T. E., Sorrell, S., & Rimmer, B. Generality and side effects of overcorrection. *Journal of Applied Behavior Analysis*, 1974, *7*, 385–390.

Epstein, R., & Goss, C. M. A self-control procedure for the maintenance of nondisruptive behavior in an elementary school child. *Behavior Therapy*, 1978, *9*, 109–117.

Evans, B. A. A case of trichotillomania in a child treated in a home token program. *Journal of Behavior Therapy and Experimental Psychiatry*, 1976, *7*, 197–198.

Eyberg, S. M., & Johnson, S. M. Multiple assessment of behavior modification with families: Effects of contingency contracting and order of treated problems. *Journal of Consulting and Clinical Psychology*, 1974, *42*, 594–606.

Eysenck, H. J. *The Dynamics of Anxiety and Hysteria.* New York: Praeger, 1957.

Favell, J. E., McGimsey, J. F., & Jones, M. L. The use of physical restraint in the treatment of self-injury and as positive reinforcement. *Journal of Applied Behavior Analysis*, 1978, *11*, 225–241.

Felixbrod, J. J., & O'Leary, K. D. Effects of reinforcement on children's academic behavior as a function of self-determined and externally imposed contingencies. *Journal of Applied Behavior Analysis*, 1973, *6*, 241–250.

Ferster, C. B. Arbitrary and natural reinforcement. *Psychological Record*, 1967, *17*, 341–347.

Ferster, C. B., & DeMyer, M. K. A method for the experimental analysis of behavior of autistic children. *American Journal of Orthopsychiatry*, 1962, *32*, 89–98.

Finley, W. W., Besserman, R. L., Bennett, L. F., Clapp, R. K., & Finley, P. M. The effect of continuous, intermittent, and "placebo" reinforcement on the effectiveness of the conditioning treatment for enuresis nocturna. *Behaviour Research and Therapy*, 1973, *11*, 289–297.

Finley, W. W., Wansley, R. A., & Blenkarn, M. M. Conditioning treatment of enuresis using a 70% intermittent reinforcement schedule. *Behaviour Research and Therapy*, 1977, *15*, 419–427.

Firestone, P. The effects and side effects of timeout on an aggressive nursery school child. *Journal of Behavior Therapy and Experimental Psychiatry*, 1976, *7*, 79–81.

Fixsen, D. L., Phillips, E. L., Phillips, E. A., & Wolf, M. M. *The teaching-family model of group home treatment*. Paper presented at the meeting of the American Psychological Association, Honolulu, Hawaii, September, 1972.

Fixsen, D. L., Phillips, E. L., & Wolf, M. M. Achievement Place: The reliability of self-reporting and peer-reporting and their effects on behavior. *Journal of Applied Behavior Analysis*, 1972, *5*, 19–30.

Fixsen, D. L., Phillips, E. L., & Wolf, M. M. Achievement Place: Experiments in self-government with pre-delinquents. *Journal of Applied Behavior Analysis*, 1973, *6*, 31-47.

Flanagan, S., Adams, H. E., & Forehand, R. A comparison of four instructional techniques for teaching parents to use time-out. *Behavior Therapy*, 1979, *10*, 94–102.

Forehand, R. Child noncompliance to parental commands: Behavioral analysis and treatment. In M. Hersen, R. M. Eisler, & P. M. Miller (Eds.), *Progress in Behavior Modification* (Vol. 5). New York: Academic Press, 1977. Pp. 111–147.

Forehand, R., & Atkeson, B. M. Generality of treatment effects with parents as therapists: A review of assessment and implementation procedures. *Behavior Therapy*, 1977, *8*, 575–593.

Forehand, R., & King, H. E. Preschool children's non-compliance: Effects of short-term behavior therapy. *Journal of Community Psychology*, 1974, *2*, 42–44.

Forehand, R., & King, H. E. Noncompliant children: Effects of parent training on behavior and attitude change. *Behavior Modification*, 1977, *1*, 93–109.

Forehand, R., Roberts, M. W., Doleys, D. M., Hobbs, S. A., & Resick, P. A. An examination of disciplinary procedures with children. *Journal of Experimental Child Psychology*, 1976, *21*, 109–120.

Forehand, R., Sturgis, E. T., McMahon, R. J., Aguar, D., Green, K., Wells, K. C., & Breiner, J. Parent behavioral training to modify child noncompliance. *Behavior Modification*, 1979, *3*, 3–25.

Forehand, R., Wells, K. C., & Sturgis, E. T. Predictors of child noncompliant behavior in the home. *Journal of Consulting and Clinical Psychology*, 1978, *46*, 179.

Foxx, R. M., & Azrin, N. H. Restitution: A method of eliminating aggressive-disruptive behaviors of retarded and brain damaged patients. *Behaviour Research and Therapy*, 1972, *10*, 15–27.

Foxx, R. M., & Azrin, N. H. Dry pants: A rapid method of toilet training children. *Behaviour Research and Therapy*, 1973, *11*, 435–442. (a)

Foxx, R. M., & Azrin, N. H. The elimination of autistic self-stimulatory behavior by overcorrection. *Journal of Applied Behavior Analysis*, 1973, *6*, 1–14. (b)

Friedling, C., & O'Leary, S. G. Effects of self-instructional training on second- and third-grade hyperactive children: A failure to replicate. *Journal of Applied Behavior Analysis*, 1979, *12*, 211–219.

Gardner, R. A., & Gardner, B. T. Teaching sign language to a chimpanzee. *Science*, 1969, *165*, 664–672.

Geffen, G., & Sexton, M. A. The development of auditory strategies of attention. *Developmental Psychology*, 1978, *14*, 11–17.

Gelber, H., & Meyer, V. Behavior therapy and encopresis: The complexities involved in treatment. *Behaviour Research and Therapy*, 1965, *2*, 227–231.

Gelfand, D. M. Social withdrawal and negative emotional states: Behavior therapy. In B. B. Wolman, J. Egan, & A. O. Ross (Eds.), *Handbook of Treatment of Mental Disorders in Childhood and Adolescence*, Englewood Cliffs, N.J.: Prentice-Hall, 1978, Pp. 330–353.

Gelfand, D. M., & Hartmann, D. P. Behavior therapy with children: A review and evaluation of research methodology. *Psychological Bulletin*, 1968, *69*, 204–215.

Gelfand, D. M., & Hartmann, D. P. *Child Behavior Analysis and Therapy*. New York: Pergamon, 1975.

Gesell, A. The conditioned reflex and the psychiatry of infancy. *American Journal of Orthopsychiatry*, 1938, *8*, 19–29.

Gibson, E. *Principles of Perceptual Learning and Development*. New York: Appleton-Century-Crofts, 1969.

Gibson, E. J. The ontogeny of reading. *American Psychologist*, 1970, *25*, 136–143.

Gibson, E. J. Trends in perceptual development: Implications for the reading process. In A. D. Pick (Ed.), *Minnesota Symposia on Child Psychology* (Vol. 8). Minneapolis, MN: University of Minnesota Press, 1975. Pp. 24–54.

Gibson, E. J., & Levin, H. *The Psychology of Reading*. Cambridge, MA: MIT Press, 1975.

Glogower, F., & Sloop, E. W. Two strategies of group training of parents as effective behavior modifiers. *Behavior Therapy*, 1976, *7*, 177–184.

Goldfried, M. R. Systematic desensitization as training in self-control. *Journal of Consulting and Clinical Psychology*, 1971, *37*, 228–234.

Goldfried, M. R., & Davison, G. C. *Clinical Behavior Therapy*. New York: Holt, Rinehart & Winston, 1976.

Goren, E. R., Romanczyk, R. G., & Harris, S. L. A functional analysis of echolalic speech. *Behavior Modification*, 1977, *1*, 481–498.

Gottman, J., Gonso, J., & Rasmussen, B. Social interaction, social competence and friendship in children. *Child Development*, 1975, *46*, 708–718.

Gottman, J., Gonso, J., & Schuler, P. Teaching social skills to isolated children. *Journal of Abnormal Child Psychology*, 1976, *4*, 179–197.

Gray, J. S. A biological view of behavior modification. *Journal of Educational Psychology*, 1932, *23*, 611–620.

Graziano, A. M. Behavior therapy. In B. B. Wolman, J. Egan, & A. O. Ross (Eds.), *Handbook of Treatment of Mental Disorders in Childhood and Adolescence*. Englewood-Cliffs, N.J.: Prentice-Hall, 1978. Pp. 28–46.

Graziano, A. M., Mooney, K. C., Huber, C., & Ignasiak, D. Self-control instruction for children's fear-reduction. *Journal of Behavior Therapy and Experimental Psychiatry*, 1979, *10*, 221–227.

Green, K. D., Forehand, R., & McMahon, R. J. Parental manipulation of compliance and non-compliance in normal and deviant children. *Behavior Modification*, 1979, *3*, 245–266.

Grusec, J. E., & Kuczynski, L. Teaching children to punish themselves and effects on subsequent compliance. *Child Development*, 1977, *48*, 1296–1300.

Hagen, J. W., & Hale, G. A. The development of attention in children. In A. D. Pick (Ed.), *Minnesota Symposia on Child Psychology*, vol. 7. Minneapolis: University of Minnesota Press, 1973, Pp. 117–140.

Hale, G. A., & Taweel, S. S. Age differences in children's performance on measures of component selection and incidental learning. *Journal of Experimental Child Psychology*, 1974, *18*, 107–116.

Hall, R. V., Axelrod, S., Tyler, L., Grief, E., Jones F. C., & Robertson, R. Modification of behavior problems in the home with a parent as observer and experimenter. *Journal of Applied Behavior Analysis*, 1972, *5*, 53–64.

Hallahan, D. P., & Kauffman, J. M. *Introduction to Learning Disabilities: A Psychobehavioral Approach.* Englewood Cliffs, N.J.: Prentice-Hall, 1976.

Hallahan, D. P., Kauffman, J. M., & Ball, D. W. Developmental trends in recall of central and incidental auditory material. *Journal of Experimental Child Psychology*, 1974, *17*, 409–421.

Hallsten, E. A., Jr. Adolescent anorexia nervosa treated by desensitization. *Behaviour Research and Therapy*, 1965, *3*, 87–91.

Halmi, K. A., Powers, P., & Cunningham, S. Treatment of anorexia nervosa with behavior modification. *Archives of General Psychiatry*, 1975, *32*, 93–95.

Hampe, E., Noble, H., Miller, L. C., & Barrett, C. L. Phobic children one and two years posttreatment. *Journal of Abnormal Psychology*, 1973, *82*, 446–453.

Harris, B. Whatever happened to Little Albert? *American Psychologist*, 1979, *34*, 151–160.

Harris, L. S., & Purohit, A. P. Bladder training and enuresis: A controlled trial. *Behaviour Research and Therapy*, 1977, *15*, 485–490.

Harris, S. L. Teaching language to nonverbal children—with emphasis on problems of generalization. *Psychological Bulletin*, 1975, *82*, 565–580.

Harris, S. L., & Ersner-Hershfield, R. Behavioral suppression of seriously disruptive behavior in psychotic and retarded patients: A review of punishment and its alternatives. *Psychological Bulletin*, 1978, *85*, 1352–1375.

Harris, S. L., & Romanczyk, R. G. Treating self-injurious behavior of a retarded child by overcorrection. *Behavior Therapy*, 1976, *7*, 235–239.

Harris, V. W., & Sherman, J. A. Effects of peer tutoring and consequences on the math performance of elementary classroom students. *Journal of Applied Behavior Analysis*, 1973, *6*, 587–597.

Hatzenbuehler, L. C., & Schroeder, H. E. Desensitization procedures in the treatment of childhood disorders. *Psychological Bulletin*, 1978, *85*, 831–844.

Hawkins, R. P., Peterson, R. F., Schweid, E., & Bijou, S. W. Behavior therapy in the home: Amelioration of problem parent–child relations with the parent in a therapeutic role. *Journal of Experimental Child Psychology*, 1966, *4*, 99–107.

Heiman, J. R., Fischer, M. J., & Ross, A. O. A supplementary behavioral program to improve deficient reading performance. *Journal of Abnormal Child Psychology*, 1973, *1*, 390–399.

Henek, T., & Miller, L. K. The effects of display conditions upon developmental trends in incidental learning. *Child Development*, 1976, *47*, 1214–1218.

Hersen, M. Behavior modification approach to a school-phobia case. *Journal of Clinical Psychology*, 1970, *20*, 395–402.

Hersen, M., & Barlow, D. H. *Single-case Experimental Designs: Strategies for Studying Behavior Change*. New York: Pergamon, 1976.

Herson, M., & Bellack, A. (Eds.), *Behavioral Assessment: A Practical Handbook*. Elmsford, N.Y.: Pergamon, 1976.

Hobbs, S. A., & Forehand, R. Important parameters in the use of timeout with children: A re-examination. *Journal of Behavior Therapy and Experimental Psychiatry*, 1977, *8*, 365–370.

Hobbs, S. A., Forehand, R., & Murray, R. G. Effects of various durations of timeout on the noncompliant behavior of children. *Behavior Therapy*, 1978, *9*, 652–656.

Hobbs, T. R., & Holt, M. M. The effect of token reinforcement on the behavior of delinquents in cottage settings. *Journal of Applied Behavior Analysis*, 1976, *9*, 189–198.

Holland, C. J. Elimination by the parents of fire-setting behaviour in a seven-year-old boy. *Behaviour Research and Therapy*, 1969, *7*, 135–137.

Horton, L. E. Generalization of aggressive behavior in adolescent delinquent boys. *Journal of Applied Behavior Analysis*, 1970, *3*, 205–211.

Humphrey, L. L., Karoly, P., & Kirschenbaum, D. S. Self-management in the classroom: Self-imposed response cost versus self-reward. *Behavior Therapy*, 1978, *9*, 592–601.

Humphreys, L., Forehand, R., McMahon, R., & Roberts, M. Parent behavioral training to modify child noncompliance: Effects on untreated siblings. *Journal of Behavior Therapy and Experimental Psychiatry*, 1978, *9*, 235–238.

Hung, D. W. Using self-stimulation as reinforcement for autistic children. *Journal of Autism and Childhood Schizophrenia*, 1978, *8*, 355–366.

Hutzell, R. R., Platzek, D., & Logue, P. E. Control of symptoms of Gilles de la Tourette's syndrome by self-monitoring. *Journal of Behavior Therapy and Experimental Psychiatry*, 1974, *5*, 71–76.

Ince, L. P. The use of relaxation training and a conditioned stimulus in the elimination of epileptic seizures in a child: A case study. *Journal of Behavior Therapy and Experimental Psychiatry*, 1976, *7*, 39–42.

Ingersoll, B., & Curry, F. Rapid treatment of persistent vomiting in a 14-year-old female by shaping and time-out. *Journal of Behavior Therapy and Experimental Psychiatry*, 1977, *8*, 305–307.

Jakibchuk, Z., & Smeriglio, V. L. The influence of symbolic modeling on the social behavior of preschool children with low levels of social responsiveness. *Child Development*, 1976, *47*, 838–841.

James, L. E., & Foreman, M. E. A–B status of behavior therapy technicians as related to success of Mowrer's conditioning treatment for enuresis. *Journal of Consulting and Clinical Psychology*, 1973, *41*, 224–229.

Jehu, D., Morgan, R. T. T., Turner, R. K., & Jones, A. A controlled trial of treatment of nocturnal enuresis in residential homes for children. *Behaviour Research and Therapy*, 1977, *15*, 1–16.

Jenkins, W. O., & Stanley, J. C., Jr., Partial reinforcement: A review and critique. *Psychological Bulletin*, 1950, *47*, 193–234.

Jesness, C. F., & DeRisi, W. J. Some variations in techniques of contingency management in a school for delinquents. In J. S. Stumphauzer (Ed.), *Behavior Therapy with Delinquents*. Springfield, IL: Thomas, 1973, Pp. 196–235.

Jesness, C. F., DeRisi, W. J., McCormick, P. M., & Wedge, R. F. *The Youth Center Research Project*. Sacramento, CA: American Justice Institute, 1972.

Johnson, M., & Bailey, J. S. Cross-age tutoring: Fifth graders as arithmetic tutors for kindergarten children. *Journal of Applied Behavior Analysis,* 1974, *7*, 223–232.

Johnston, J. M. Punishment of human behavior. *American Psychologist*, 1972, *27*, 1033–1054.

Jones, H. G. The behavioural treatment of enuresis nocturna. In H. J. Eysenck (Ed.), *Behaviour Therapy and the Neuroses*. London: Pergamon, 1960. Pp. 377–403.

Jones, M. C. A laboratory study of fear: The case of Peter. *Pedagogical Seminary,* 1924, *31*, 308–315. (a)

Jones, M. C. The elimination of children's fears. *Journal of Experimental Psychology*, 1924, *7*, 383–390. (b)

Kagan, J. Reflection-impulsivity: The generality of conceptual tempo. *Journal of Abnormal Psychology*, 1966, *71*, 17–24.

Kagan, J., Pearson, L., & Welch, L. The modification of an impulsive tempo. *Journal of Educational Psychology*, 1966. *57*, 359–365.

Kanfer, F. H., Karoly, P., & Newman, A. Reduction of children's fear of the dark by competence-related and situational threat-related verbal cues. *Journal of Consulting and Clinical Psychology*, 1975, *43*, 251–258.

Kanfer, F. H., & Phillips, J. S. *Learning Foundations of Behavior Therapy*. New York: Wiley, 1970.

Karoly, P., & Rosenthal, M. Training parents in behavior modification: Effects on perceptions of family interaction and deviant child behavior. *Behavior Therapy*, 1977, *8*, 406–410.

Kaufman, K. F., & O'Leary, K. D. Reward, cost, and self-evaluation procedures for disruptive adolescents in a psychiatric hospital school. *Journal of Applied Behavior Analysis,* 1972, *5*, 293–309.

Kazdin, A. E. *The Token Economy: A Review and Evaluation*. New York: Plenum, 1977.

Kazdin, A. E. *Research Design in Clinical Psychology*, New York: Harper & Row, 1980.

Kelly, J. A., & Drabman, R. S. Generalizing response suppression of self-injurious behavior through an overcorrection punishment procedure: A case study. *Behavior Therapy*, 1977, *8*, 468–472.

Kendall, P. C., & Finch, A. J., Jr. A cognitive-behavioral treatment for impulse control: A case study. *Journal of Consulting and Clinical Psychology*, 1976, *44*, 852–857.

Kendall, P. C., & Finch, A. J., Jr. A cognitive-behavioral treatment for impulsivity: A group comparison study. *Journal of Consulting and Clinical Psychology*, 1978, *46*, 110–118.

Kennedy, W. A. School phobia: Rapid treatment of fifty cases. *Journal of Abnormal Psychology*, 1965, *70*, 285–289.

Kent, R. N., & O'Leary, K. D. A controlled evaluation of behavior modification with conduct problem children. *Journal of Consulting and Clinical Psychology*, 1976, *44*, 586–596.

Kimmel, H. D., & Kimmel, E. An instrumental conditioning method for the treatment of enuresis. *Journal of Behavior Therapy and Experimental Psychiatry*, 1970, *1*, 121–122.

Kingsley, R. G., & Shapiro, J. A comparison of three behavioral programs for the control of obesity in children. *Behavior Therapy*, 1977, *8*, 30–36.

Kirigin, K. A., Braukmann, C. J., Fixsen, D. L., Phillips, E. L., & Wolf, M. M. Is community-based correction effective: An evaluation of Achievement Place. Paper presented at the meeting of the American Psychological Association, Chicago, 1975.

Klier, J. L., & Harris, S. L. Self-stimulation and learning in autistic children: Physical or functional incompatibility. *Journal of Applied Behavior Analysis*, 1977, *10*, 311.

Knapp, T. J. The Premack Principle in human experimental and applied settings. *Behaviour Research and Therapy*, 1976, *14*, 133–147.

Knapp, T. J., & Wells, L. A. Behavior therapy for asthma. A review. *Behaviour Research and Therapy*, 1978, *16*, 103–115.

Koegel, R. L. & Covert, A. The relationship of self-stimulation to learning in autistic children. *Journal of Applied Behavior Analysis*, 1972, *5*, 381–387.

Koegel, R. L., Firestone, P. B., Kramme, K. W., & Dunlap, G. Increasing spontaneous play by suppressing self-stimulation in autistic children. *Journal of Applied Behavior Analysis*, 1974, *7*, 521–528.

Koegel, R. L., & Rincover, A. Some detrimental effects of using extra stimuli to guide learning in normal and autistic children. *Journal of Abnormal Child Psychology*, 1976, *4*, 59–71.

Koegel, R. L., & Schreibman, L. Teaching autistic children to respond to simultaneous multiple cues. *Journal of Experimental Child Psychology*, 1977, *24*, 299–311.

Koegel, R. L., & Wilhelm, H. Selective responding to the components of multiple visual cues by autistic children. *Journal of Experimental Child Psychology*, 1973, *15*, 442–453.

Koenigsberg, R. S. An evaluation of visual versus sensorimotor methods for improving orientation discrimination for letter reversal by preschool children. *Child Development*, 1973, *44*, 764–769.

Kohlenberg, R. J. The punishment of persistent vomiting. *Journal of Applied Behavior Analysis*, 1970, *3*, 241–245.

Kohlenberg, R. J. Operant conditioning of human anal sphincter pressure. *Journal of Applied Behavior Analysis*, 1973, *6*, 201–208.

Koocher, G. P. (Ed.), *Children's Rights and the Mental Health Professions.* New York: Wiley, 1976.

Kornhaber, R. C., & Schroeder, H. E. Importance of model similarity on extinction of avoidance behavior in children. *Journal of Consulting and Clinical Psychology*, 1975, *43*, 601–607.

Krasner, L. The behavioral scientist and social responsibility: No place to hide. *Journal of Social Issues*, 1965, *21*, 9–30.

Krasner, L. Behavioral modification: Ethical issues and future trends. In H. Leitenberg (Ed.) *Handbook of Behavior Modification and Behavior Therapy*. Englewood Cliffs, N.J.: Prentice-Hall, 1976. Pp. 627–649.

Krumboltz, J. D., & Krumboltz, H. B. *Changing Children's Behavior.* Englewood Cliffs, N.J.: Prentice-Hall, 1972.

Lahey, B. B. & Drabman, R. S. Facilitation of the acquisition and retention of sight-word vocabulary through token reinforcement. *Journal of Applied Behavior Analysis*, 1974, *7*, 307–312.

Lahey, B. B., McNees, M. P., & Brown, C. C. Modification of deficits in reading for comprehension. *Journal of Applied Behavior Analysis*, 1973, *6*, 475–480.

Lahey, B. B., McNees, M. P., & McNees, M. C. Control of an obscene "verbal tic" through timeout in an elementary school classroom. *Journal of Applied Behavior Analysis*, 1973, *6*, 101–104.

Lahey, B. B., Stempniak, M., Robinson, E. J., & Tyroler, M. J. Hyperactivity and learning disabilities as independent dimensions of child behavior problems. *Journal of Abnormal Psychology*, 1978, *87*, 333–340.

Lang, P. J. The mechanics of desensitization and the laboratory study of fear. In C. M. Franks (Ed.), *Behavior Therapy: Appraisal and Status.* New York: McGraw-Hill, 1969. Pp. 160–191.

Lang, P. J., & Melamed, B. G. Avoidance conditioning therapy of an infant with chronic ruminative vomiting: Case report. *Journal of Abnormal Psychology*, 1969, *74*, 1–8.

Lavigueur, H. The use of siblings as an adjunct to the behavioral treatment of children in the home with parents as therapists. *Behavior Therapy*, 1976, *7*, 602–613.

Lazarus, A. A. The elimination of children's phobias by deconditioning. *Medical Proceedings of South Africa*, 1959, *5*, 261–265.

Lazarus, A. A., & Abramovitz, A. The use of "emotive imagery" in the treatment of children's phobias. In L. P. Ullmann & L. Krasner (Eds.), *Case Studies in Behavior Modification.* New York: Holt, 1965. Pp. 300–304.

Lazarus, A. A., Davison, G. C., & Polefka, D. A. Classical and operant factors in the treatment of a school phobia. *Journal of Abnormal Psychology*, 1965, *70*, 225–229.

Ledwidge, B. Cognitive behavior modification: A step in the wrong direction? *Psychological Bulletin*, 1978, *85*, 353–375.

Leitenberg, H. Is time-out from positive reinforcement an aversive event? *Psychological Bulletin*, 1965, *64*, 428–441.

Leitenberg, H. Behavioral approaches to treatment of neuroses. In H. Leitenberg (Ed.), *Handbook of Behavior Modification and Behavior Therapy.* Englewood Cliffs, N.J.: Prentice-Hall, 1976. Pp. 124–167.

Leitenberg, H., Agras, S., & Thomson, L. E. A sequential analysis of the effect of selective positive reinforcement in modifying anorexia nervosa. *Behaviour Research and Therapy*, 1968, *6*, 211–218.

Leitenberg, H., & Callahan, E. J. Reinforced practice and reduction of different kinds of fears in adults and children. *Behaviour Research and Therapy*, 1973, *11*, 19–30.

Levine, F. M., & Fasnacht, G. Token rewards may lead to token learning. *American Psychologist*, 1974, *29*, 816–820.

Lewis, S. A comparison of behavior therapy techniques in the reduction of fearful avoidance behavior. *Behavior Therapy*, 1974, *5*, 648–655.

Lichstein, K. L., & Schreibman, L. Employing electric shock with autistic children. *Journal of Autism and Childhood Schizophrenia*, 1976, *6*, 163–174.

Lovaas, O. I. *The Autistic Child: Language Development Through Behavior Modification*. New York: Irvington, 1977.

Lovaas, O. I., Freitag, G., Gold, V. J., & Kassorla, I. C. Experimental studies in childhood schizophrenia: Analysis of self-destructive behavior. *Journal of Experimental Child Psychology*, 1965, *2*, 67–84.

Lovaas, O. I., Freitag, G., Kinder, M. I., Rubenstein, B. D., Schaeffer, B., & Simmons, J. Q. Establishment of social reinforcers in two schizophrenic children on the basis of food. *Journal of Experimental Child Psychology*, 1966, *4*, 109–125.

Lovaas, O. I., Koegel, R., Simmons, J. Q., & Long, J. S. Some generalization and follow-up measures on autistic children in behavior therapy. *Journal of Applied Behavior Analysis*, 1973, *6*, 131–166.

Lovaas, O. I., Litrownik, A., & Mann, R. Response latencies to auditory stimuli in autistic children engaged in self-stimulatory behavior. *Behaviour Research and Therapy*, 1971, *9*, 39–49.

Lovaas, O. I., & Newsom, C. D. Behavior modification with psychotic children. In H. Leitenberg (Ed.), *Handbook of Behavior Modification and Behavior Therapy*. Englewood Cliffs, N.J.: Prentice-Hall, 1976. Pp. 303–360.

Lovaas, O. I., Schaeffer, B., & Simmons, J. Q. Building social behavior in autistic children by use of electric shock. *Journal of Experimental Research in Personality*, 1965, *1*, 99–109.

Lovaas, O. I., & Schreibman, L. Stimulus overselectivity of autistic children in a two stimulus situation. *Behaviour Research and Therapy*, 1971, *9*, 305–310.

Lovaas, O. I., Schreibman, L., Koegel, R., & Rehm, R. Selective responding by autistic children to multiple sensory input. *Journal of Abnormal Psychology*, 1971, *77*, 211–222.

Lovaas, O. I., & Simmons, J. Q. Manipulation of self-destruction in three retarded children. *Journal of Applied Behavior Analysis*, 1969, *2*, 143–157.

Lovaas, O. I., Young, D. B., & Newsom, C. D. Childhood psychosis: Behavioral treatment. In B. B. Wolman, J. Egan, & A. O. Ross (Eds.), *Handbook of Treatment of Mental Disorders in Childhood and Adolescence*. Englewood Cliffs, N.J.: Prentice-Hall, 1978. Pp. 385–420.

Lovibond, S. H. *Conditioning and Enuresis*. Oxford: Pergamon, 1964.

Lovibond, S. H. Critique of Turner, Young and Rachman's conditioning treatment of enuresis. *Behaviour Research and Therapy*, 1972, *10*, 287–289.

Lovitt, T. C., & Curtiss, K. A. Academic response rate as a function of teacher- and self-imposed contingencies. *Journal of Applied Behavior Analysis*, 1969, *2*, 49-53.

Lowitz, G. H., & Suib, M. R. Generalized control of persistent thumbsucking by differential reinforcement of other behavior. *Journal of Behavior Therapy and Experimental Psychiatry*, 1978, *9*, 343–346.

MacDonald, M. L. Multiple impact behavior therapy in a child's dog phobia. *Journal of Behavior Therapy and Experimental Psychiatry*, 1975, *6*, 317–322.

MacDonough, T. S., & Forehand, R. Response-contingent time out: Important parameters in behavior modification with children. *Journal of Behavior Therapy and Experimental Psychiatry*, 1973, *4*, 231–236.

McLaughlin, J. G., & Nay, W. R. Treatment of trichotillomania using positive coverants and response cost: A case study. *Behavior Therapy*, 1975, *6*, 87–91.

Madsen, C. H., Becker, W. C., & Thomas, D. R. Rules, praise, and ignoring: Elements of elementary classroom control. *Journal of Applied Behavior Analysis*, 1968, *1*, 139–150.

Marlowe, R. H., Madsen, C. H., Jr., Bowen, C. E., Reardon, R. C., & Logue, P. E. Severe classroom behavior problems: Teachers or counsellors. *Journal of Applied Behavior Analysis*, 1978, *11*, 53–66.

Mash, E. J., & Terdal, L. G. (Eds.), *Behavior-therapy Assessment: Diagnosis, Design, and Evaluation*. New York: Springer, 1976.

Meichenbaum, D. *Cognitive-behavior Modification: An Integrative Approach*. New York: Plenum, 1977.

Meichenbaum, D., & Asarnow, J. Cognitive-behavior modification and metacognitive development: Implications for the classroom. In P. Kendall & S. Hollon (Eds.), *Cognitive-behavioral Interventions: Theory, Research, and Procedures*. New York: Academic Press, 1979.

Meichenbaum, D., & Goodman, J. Training impulsive children to talk to themselves: A means of developing self-control. *Journal of Abnormal Psychology*, 1971, *77*, 115–126.

Melamed, B. G., & Siegel, L. J. Reduction of anxiety in children facing hospitalization and surgery by use of filmed modeling. *Journal of Consulting and Clinical Psychology*, 1975, *43*, 511–521.

Miller, L. C., Barrett, C. L., Hampe, E., & Noble, H. Comparison of reciprocal inhibition, psychotherapy, and waiting list control for phobic children. *Journal of Abnormal Psychology*, 1972, *79*, 269–279

Miller, N. E., & Dollard, J. *Social Learning and Imitation*. New Haven: Yale University Press, 1941.

Morgan, J., & O'Brien, J. S. The counterconditioning of a vomiting habit by sips of gingerale. *Journal of Behavior Therapy and Experimental Psychiatry*, 1972, *3*, 135–137.

Morgan, R. T. T. Relapse and therapeutic response in the conditioning treatment of enuresis: A review of recent findings on intermittent reinforcement, overlearning and stimulus intensity. *Behaviour Research and Therapy*, 1978, *16*, 273–279.

Morgan, R. T. T., & Young, G. C. Parental attitudes and the conditioning treatment of childhood enuresis. *Behaviour Research and Therapy*, 1975, *13*, 197–199.

Morris, R. J. *Behavior Modification with Children: A Systematic Guide*. Cambridge, MA: Winthrop, 1976.

Mowrer, O. H., & Mowrer, W. M. Enuresis—A method for its study and treatment. *American Journal of Orthopsychiatry*, 1938, *8*, 436–459.

Muellner, S. R. Development of urinary control in children: A new concept in cause, prevention, and treatment of primary enuresis. *Journal of Urology*, 1960, *84*, 714–716.

Mulick, J. A., Hoyt, P., Rojahn, J., & Schroeder, S. R. Reduction of a "nervous habit" in a profoundly retarded youth by increasing toy play. *Journal of Behavior Therapy and Experimental Psychiatry*, 1978, *9*, 381–385.

Neisworth, J. T., & Moore, F. Operant treatment of asthmatic responding with the parent as therapist. *Behavior Therapy*, 1972, *3*, 95–99.

Nordquist, V. M. The modification of a child's enuresis: Some response–response relationships. *Journal of Applied Behavior Analysis*, 1971, *4*, 241–247.

Nordyke, N. S., Baer, D. M., Etzel, B. C., & LeBlanc, J. M. Implications of the stereotyping and modification of sex role. *Journal of Applied Behavior Analysis*, 1977, *10*, 553-557.

Novick, J. Symptomatic treatment of acquired and persistent enuresis. *Journal of Abnormal Psychology*, 1966, *71*, 363-368.

Obler, M., & Terwilliger, R. F. Pilot study of the effectiveness of systematic desensitization with neurologically impaired children with phobic disorders. *Journal of Consulting and Clinical Psychology*, 1970, *34*, 314-318.

O'Brien, F., Bugle, C., & Azrin, N. H. Training and maintaining a retarded child's proper eating. *Journal of Applied Behavior Analysis*, 1972, *5*, 67-72.

O'Connor, R. D. Modification of social withdrawal through symbolic modeling. *Journal of Applied Behavior Analysis*, 1969, *2*, 15-22.

O'Connor, R. D. Relative efficacy of modeling, shaping, and the combined procedures for modification of social withdrawal. *Journal of Abnormal Psychology*, 1972, *79*, 327-334.

O'Leary, K. D., Becker, W. C., Evans, M. B., & Saudargas, R. A. A token reinforcement program in a public school: A replication and systematic analysis. *Journal of Applied Behavior Analysis*, 1969, *2*, 3-13.

O'Leary, K. D., Kaufman, K. F., Kass, R. E., & Drabman, R. The effects of loud and soft reprimands on the behavior of disruptive children. *Exceptional Children*, 1970, *37*, 145-155.

O'Leary, K. D., & O'Leary, S. G. *Classroom Management: The Successful Use of Behavior Modification*. 2nd edition. Elmsford, N.Y.: Pergamon, 1977.

O'Leary, K. D., Pelham, W. E., Rosenbaum, A., & Price, G. H. Behavioral treatment of hyperkinetic children: An experimental evaluation of its usefulness. *Clinical Pediatrics,* 1976, *15*, 510-515.

O'Leary, K. D., & Turkewitz, H. Methodological errors in marital and child treatment research. *Journal of Consulting and Clinical Psychology*, 1978, *46*, 747-758.

O'Leary, K. D., Turkewitz, H., & Taffel, S. J. Parent and therapist evaluation of behavior therapy in a child psychological clinic. *Journal of Consulting and Clinical Psychology*, 1973, *41*, 279-283.

O'Leary, K. D., & Wilson, G. T. *Behavior Therapy: Application and Outcome*. Englewood Cliffs, N.J.: Prentice-Hall, 1975.

O'Leary, S. G., & Dubey, D. R. Applications of self-control procedures by children: A review. *Journal of Applied Behavior Analysis*, 1979, *12*, 449-465.

O'Leary, S. G., & O'Leary, K. D. Behavior modification in the school. In H. Leitenberg (Ed.), *Handbook of Behavior Modification and Behavior Therapy*. Englewood Cliffs, N.J.: Prentice-Hall, 1976. Pp. 475-515.

Ollendick, T. H., & Matson, J. L. Overcorrection: An overview. *Behavior Therapy*, 1978, *9*, 830-842.

Palkes, H., Stewart, M. A., & Freedman, J. Improvement in maze performance of hyperactive boys as a function of verbal-training procedures. *Journal of Special Education*, 1971, *5*, 337-342.

Palkes, H., Stewart, M., & Kahana, B. Porteus maze performance of hyperactive boys after training in self-directed verbal commands. *Child Development*, 1968, *39*, 817-829.

Parke, R. D. Rules, roles, and resistance to deviation: Recent advances in punishment, discipline, and self-control. In A. D. Pick (Ed.), *Minnesota Symposia on Child Psychology* (Vol. 8). Minneapolis, MN: University of Minnesota Press, 1975. Pp. 111–143.

Paschalis, A. Ph., Kimmel, H. D., & Kimmel, E. Further study of diurnal instrumental conditioning in the treatment of enuresis nocturna. *Journal of Behavior Therapy and Experimental Psychiatry*, 1972, *3*, 253–256.

Patterson, G. R. *Families: Applications of Social Learning to Family Life*. Champaign, IL: Research Press, 1971.

Patterson, G. R. Interventions for boys with conduct problems: Multiple settings, treatments, and criteria. *Journal of Consulting and Clinical Psychology*, 1974, *42*, 471–481.

Patterson, G. R., Cobb, J. A., & Ray, R. S. Direct intervention in the classroom: A set of procedures for the aggressive child. In F. Clark, D. Evans, & L. Hamerlynck (Eds.), *Implementing Behavioral Programs for Schools and Clinics*. Champaign, IL: Research Press, 1972.

Patterson, G. R., Cobb, J. A., & Ray, R. S. A social engineering technology for re-training the families of aggressive boys. In H. E. Adams & I. P. Unikel (Eds.), *Issues and Trends in Behavior Therapy*. Springfield, IL: Thomas, 1973. Pp. 139-210.

Patterson, G. R., & Fleischman, M. J. Maintenance of treatment effects: Some considerations concerning family systems and follow-up data. *Behavior Therapy*, 1979, *10*, 168–185.

Patterson, G. R., & Gullion, M. E. *Living with Children: New Methods for Parents and Teachers*. Champaign, IL. Research Press, 1968.

Patterson, G. R., Jones, R., Whittier, J., & Wright, M. A. A behavior modification technique for the hyperactive child. *Behaviour Research and Therapy*, 1965, *2*, 217–226.

Patterson, G. R., Littman, R. A., & Bricker, W. Assertive behavior in children: A step toward a theory of aggression. *Monographs of the Society for Research in Child Development*, 1967, *32*, 5, (Whole #113).

Patterson, G. R., & Reid, J. B. Reciprocity and coercion: Two facets of social systems. In C. Neuringer & J. L. Michael (Eds.), *Behavior Modification in Clinical Psychology*. New York: Appleton-Century-Crofts, 1970. Pp. 133–177.

Patterson, G. R., & Reid, J. B. Intervention for families of aggressive boys: A replication study. *Behaviour Research and Therapy*, 1973, *11*, 383–394.

Paul, G. L. Behavior modification research: Design and tactics. In C. M. Franks (Ed.), *Behavior Therapy: Appraisal and Status*. New York: McGraw-Hill, 1969, Pp. 29–62.

Peed, S., Roberts, M., & Forehand, R. Evaluation of the effectiveness of a standardized parent training program in altering the interaction of mothers and their non-compliant children. *Behavior Modification*, 1977, *1*, 323–350.

Pelham, W. E. Behavioral treatment of hyperkinesis. *American Journal of Diseases of Children*, 1976, *130*, 565.

Pelham, W. E., & Ross, A. O. Selective attention in children with reading problems: A developmental study of incidental learning. *Journal of Abnormal Child Psychology*, 1977, *5*, 1–8.

Pendergrass, V. Timeout from positive reinforcement following persistent, high-rate behavior in retardates. *Journal of Applied Behavior Analysis*, 1972, *5*, 85–91.

Phillips, E. L. Achievement Place: Token reinforcement procedures in a home-style rehabilitation setting for "pre-delinquent" boys. *Journal of Applied Behavior Analysis*, 1968, *1*, 213–223.

Phillips, E. L., Phillips, E. A., Fixsen, D. L., & Wolf, M. M. Achievement Place: Modification of the behaviors of pre-delinquent boys within a token economy. *Journal of Applied Behavior Analysis*, 1971, *4*, 45–59.

Pick, A. D., Frankel, D. G., & Hess, V. L. *Children's Attention: The Development of Selectivity*. Chicago: University of Chicago Press, 1975.

Pinkston, E. M., Reese, N. M., LeBlanc, J. M., & Baer, D. M. Independent control of a preschool child's aggression and peer interaction by contingent teacher attention. *Journal of Applied Behavior Analysis*, 1973, *6*, 115–124.

Plachetta, K. E. Encopresis: A case study utilizing contracting, scheduling, and self-charting. *Journal of Behavior Therapy and Experimental Psychiatry*, 1976, *7*, 195–196.

Plummer, S., Baer, D. M., & LeBlanc, J. M. Functional considerations in the use of procedural timeout and an effective alternative. *Journal of Applied Behavior Analysis*, 1977, *10*, 689–705.

Pomerantz, P. B., Peterson, N. T., Marholin II, D., & Stern, S. Bath time for Ben: The *in vivo* elimination of a childhood phobia by a paraprofessional at home. *Journal of Behavior Therapy and Experimental Psychiatry*, 1977, *8*, 417–421.

Porteus, S. E. *Qualitative Performance in the Maze Test*. Vineland, N.J.: Smith, 1942.

Premack, D. A. Toward empirical behavior laws: I. Positive reinforcement. *Psychological Review*, 1959, *66*, 219–233.

Premack, D. A. A functional analysis of language. *Journal of the Experimental Analysis of Behavior*, 1970, *14*, 107–125.

Pressey, S. L. A third and fourth contribution to the coming "industrial revolution" in education. *School and Society*, 1932, *36*.

Purcell, K., Brady, K., Chai, H., Muser, J., Molk, L., Gordon, N., & Means, J. The effect on asthma in children of experimental separation from the family. *Psychosomatic Medicine*, 1969, *31*, 144–164.

Rachlin, H. *Introduction to Modern Behaviorism*. San Francisco: Freeman, 1970.

Ramp, E., Ulrich, R., Dulaney, S. Delayed timeout as a procedure for reducing disruptive classroom behavior: A case study. *Journal of Applied Behavior Analysis*, 1971, *4*, 235–239.

Reid, J. B., & Hendriks, A. F. Preliminary analysis of the effectiveness of direct home intervention for the treatment of predelinquent boys who steal. In L. A. Hamerlynck, L. C. Handy, & E. J. Mash (Eds.), *Behavior Change: Methodology, Concepts, and Practice*. Champaign, IL: Research Press, 1973. Pp. 209–220.

Rekers, G. A. Stimulus control over sex-typed play in cross-gender identified boys. *Journal of Experimental Child Psychology*, 1975, *20*, 136–148.

Rekers, G. A. A typical gender development and psychosocial adjustment. *Journal of Applied Behavior Analysis*, 1977, *10*, 559–571.

Rekers, G. A., & Lovaas, O. I. Behavioral treatment of deviant sex-role behaviors in a male child. *Journal of Applied Behavior Analysis*, 1974, *7*, 173–190.

Rekers, G. A., Lovaas, O. I., & Low, B. The behavioral treatment of a "transsexual" preadolescent boy. *Journal of Abnormal Child Psychology*, 1974, *2*, 99–116.

Rekers, G. A., & Varni, J. W. Self-monitoring and self-reinforcement processes in a pre-transsexual boy. *Behaviour Research and Therapy*, 1977, *15*, 177–180. (a)

Rekers, G. A., & Varni, J. W. Self-regulation of gender-role behaviors: A case study. *Journal of Behavior Therapy and Experimental Psychiatry*, 1977, *8*, 427–432. (b)

Repp, A. C., & Deitz, S. M. Reducing aggressive and self-injurious behavior of institutionalized retarded children through reinforcement of other behaviors. *Journal of Applied Behavior Analysis*, 1974, *7*, 313–325.

Reppucci, N. D., & Clingempeel, W. G. Methodological issues in research with correctional populations. *Journal of Consulting and Clinical Psychology*, 1978, *46*, 727–746.

Reppucci, N. D., & Saunders, J. T. Social psychology of behavior modification: Problems of implementation in natural settings. *American Psychologist*, 1974, *29*, 649–660.

Resick, P. A., Forehand, R., & McWhorter, A. Q. The effect of parental treatment with one child on an untreated sibling. *Behavior Therapy*, 1976, *7*, 544–548.

Reynolds, B. S., Newsom, C. D., & Lovaas, O. I. Auditory overselectivity in autistic children. *Journal of Abnormal Child Psychology*, 1974, *2*, 253–263.

Rincover, A. Sensory extinction: A procedure for eliminating self-stimulatory behavior in autistic children. *Journal of Abnormal Child Psychology*, 1978, *6*, 299–310.

Rincover, A., Cook, R., Peoples, A., & Packard, D. Sensory extinction and sensory reinforcement principles for programming multiple adaptive behavior change. *Journal of Applied Behavior Analysis*, 1979, *12*, 221–233.

Rincover, A., & Koegel, R. L. Research on the education of autistic children: Recent advances and future directions. In B. Lahey & A. Kazdin (Eds.), *Advances in Child Clinical Psychology* (Vol. 1). New York: Plenum, 1977. Pp. 329–359.

Rinn, R. C., Vernon, J. C., & Wise, M. J. Training parents of behaviorally-disturbed children in groups: A three years' program evaluation. *Behavior Therapy*, 1975, *6*, 378–387.

Risley, T. R. The effects and side effects of punishing the autistic behaviors of a deviant child. *Journal of Applied Behavior Analysis*, 1968, *1*, 21–34.

Risley, T., & Wolf, M. Establishing functional speech in echolalic children. *Behaviour Research and Therapy*, 1967, *5*, 73–88.

Ritter, B. The group desensitization of children's snake phobias using vicarious and contact desensitization procedures. *Behaviour Research and Therapy*, 1968, *6*, 1–6.

Roberts, M. W., McMahon, R. J., Forehand, R., & Humphreys, L. The effect of parental instruction-giving on child compliance. *Behavior Therapy*, 1978, *9*, 793–798.

Romanczyk, R. G., Diament, C., Goren, E. R., Trunell, G., & Harris, S. L. Increasing isolate and social play in severely disturbed children: Intervention and postintervention effectiveness. *Journal of Autism and Childhood Schizophrenia*, 1975, *5*, 57–70.

Romanczyk, R. G., & Goren, E. Severe self-injurious behavior: The problem of clinical control. *Journal of Consulting and Clinical Psychology*, 1975, *43*, 730–739.

Rosen, A. C., Rekers, G. A., & Bentler, P. M. Ethical issues in the treatment of children. *Journal of Social Issues*, 1978, *34*, 122–136.

Rosenbaum, A., O'Leary, K. D., & Jacob, R. G. Behavior intervention with hyperactive children: Group consequences as a supplement to individual contingencies. *Behavior Therapy*, 1975, *6*, 315–323.

Rosenbaum, M. S., & Drabman, R. S. Self-control training in the classroom: A review and critique. *Journal of Applied Behavior Analysis*, 1979, *12*, 467–485.

Rosenthal, T. L., & Bandura, A. Psychological modeling: Theory and practice. In S. L. Garfield and A. E. Bergin (Eds.), *Handbook of Psychotherapy and Behavior Change* (2nd ed.). New York: Wiley, 1978. Pp. 621–658.

Ross, A. O. *The Practice of Clinical Child Psychology*. New York: Grune & Stratton, 1959.

Ross, A. O. Learning theory and therapy with children. *Psychotherapy: Theory, Research and Practice*, 1964, *1*, 102–108.

Ross, A. O. The rights of children as psychotherapy patients. In G. P. Koocher (Chair). *Children's Rights and the Psychologist's Role*. Symposium presented at the meeting of the American Psychological Association, New Orleans, Louisiana, 1974.

Ross, A. O. *Psychological Aspects of Learning Disabilities and Reading Disorders*. New York: McGraw-Hill, 1976.

Ross, A. O. *Psychological Disorders of Children: A Behavioral Approach to Theory, Research, and Therapy* (2nd ed.). New York: McGraw-Hill, 1980.

Ryback, D., & Staats, A. W. Parents as behavior therapy-technicians in treating reading deficits (dyslexia). *Journal of Behavior Therapy and Experimental Psychiatry*, 1970, *1*, 109–119.

Sajwaj, T., Libet, J., & Agras, S. Lemon-juice therapy: The control of life-threatening rumination in a six-month-old infant. *Journal of Applied Behavior Analysis*, 1974, *7*, 557–563.

Salter, A. *Conditioned Reflex Therapy*. New York: Farrar, Straus, & Giroux, 1949.

Sanders, M. R., & Glynn, T. Functional analysis of a program for training high and low preference peers to modify disruptive classroom behavior. *Journal of Applied Behavior Analysis*, 1977, *10*, 503.

Sanok, R. L., & Ascione, F. R. Behavioral interventions for childhood elective mutism: An evaluative review. *Child Behavior Therapy*, 1979, *1*, 49–68.

Saposnek, D. T., & Watson, L. S., Jr. The elimination of the self-destructive behavior of a psychotic child: A case study. *Behavior Therapy*, 1974, *5*, 79–89.

Scarboro, M. E., & Forehand, R. Effects of two types of response-contingent time-out on compliance and oppositional behavior of children. *Journal of Experimental Child Psychology*, 1975, *19*, 252–264.

Schover, L. R., & Newsom, C. D. Overselectivity, developmental level, and overtraining in autistic and normal children. *Journal of Abnormal Child Psychology*, 1976, *4*, 289–298.

Schreibman, L. Effects of within-stimulus and extra-stimulus prompting on discrimination learning in autistic children. *Journal of Applied Behavior Analysis*, 1975, *8*, 91–112.

Schreibman, L., & Carr, E. G. Elimination of echolalic responding to questions through the training of generalized verbal response. *Journal of Applied Behavior Analysis*, 1978, *11*, 453–463.

Schreibman, L., Koegel, R. L., & Craig, M. S. Reducing stimulus overselectivity in autistic children. *Journal of Abnormal Child Psychology*. 1977, *5*, 425–436.

Schreibman, L., & Lovaas, O. I. Overselective response to social stimuli by autistic children. *Journal of Abnormal Child Psychology*, 1973, *1*, 152–168.

Schumaker, J., & Sherman, J. A. Training generative verb usage by imitation and reinforcement procedures. *Journal of Applied Behavior Analysis*, 1970, *3*, 273–287.

Schwartz, G. J. College students as contingency managers for adolescents in a program to develop reading skills. *Journal of Applied Behavior Analysis*, 1977, *10*, 645–655.

Shafto, F., & Sulzbacher, S. Comparing treatment tactics with a hyperactive preschool child: Stimulant medication and programmed teacher intervention. *Journal of Applied Behavior Analysis*, 1977, *10*, 13–20.

Shapiro, D., & Surwit, R. S. Learned control of physiological function and disease. In H. Leitenberg (Ed.), *Handbook of Behavior Modification and Behavior Therapy*. Englewood Cliffs, N.J.: Prentice-Hall, 1976. Pp. 74–123.

Shepp, B. E., & Swartz, K. B. Selective attention and the processing of integral and nonintegral dimensions: A developmental study. *Journal of Experimental Child Psychology*, 1976, *22*, 73–85.

Sibley, S. A. Reading rate and accuracy of retarded readers as a function of fixed-ratio schedules of conditioned reinforcement. *Dissertation Abstracts*, 1967, *27*, 4114–4115.

Siegel, A. W. Variables affecting incidental learning in children. *Child Development*, 1968, *39*, 957–968.

Skinner, B. F. *The Behavior of Organisms: An Experimental Analysis*, New York: Appleton-Century-Crofts, 1938.

Skinner, B. F. *Science and Human Behavior*. New York: Macmillan, 1953.

Skinner, B. F. *Verbal Behavior*. New York: Appleton-Century-Crofts, 1957.

Slaby, R. G., & Crowley, C. G. Modification of cooperation and aggression through teacher attention to children's speech. *Journal of Experimental Child Psychology*, 1977, *23*, 442–458.

Sleator, E. K., & von Neumann, A. W. Methylphenidate in the treatment of hyperkinetic children. *Clinical Pediatrics*, 1974, *13*, 19–24.

Smith, L. B., Kemler, D. G., & Aronfreed, J. Developmental trends in voluntary selective attention: Differential effects of source distinctness. *Journal of Experimental Child Psychology*, 1975, *20*, 352–362.

Smith, R. E., & Sharpe, T. M. Treatment of a school phobia with implosive therapy. *Journal of Consulting and Clinical Psychology*, 1970, *35*, 239–243.

Snyder, J. J. Reinforcement analysis of interaction in problem and nonproblem families. *Journal of Abnormal Psychology*, 1977, *86*, 528–535.

Solnick, J. V., Rincover, A., & Peterson, C. R. Some determinants of the reinforcing and punishing effects of time-out. *Journal of Applied Behavior Analysis*, 1977, *10*, 415–424.

Solomon, R. L., & Brush, E. S. Experimentally derived conceptions of anxiety and aversion. In M. R. Jones (Ed.), *Nebraska Symposium on Motivation*. Lincoln NE: University of Nebraska Press, 1956. Pp. 212–305.

Solomon, R. W., & Wahler, R. G. Peer reinforcement control of classroom problem behavior. *Journal of Applied Behavior Analysis*, 1973, *6*, 49–56.

Spates, C. R., & Kanfer, F. H. Self-monitoring, self-evaluation and self-reinforcement in children's learning: A test of a multi-stage self-regulation model. *Behavior Therapy*, 1977, *8*, 9–16.

Sprague, R. L., & Sleator, E. K. Methylphenidate in hyperkinetic children: Differences in dose effects on learning and social behavior. *Science*, 1977, *198*, 1274–1276.

Staats, A. W., & Butterfield, W. H. Treatment of nonreading in a culturally deprived juvenile delinquent: An application of reinforcement principles. *Child Development*, 1965, *36*, 925–942.

Staats, A. W., Minke, K. A., Finley, J. R., Wolf, M. M., & Brooks, L. O. A. Reinforcer system and experimental procedure for the laboratory study of reading acquisition. *Child Development*, 1964, *35*, 209–231.

Staats, A. W., Minke, K. A., Goodwin, W., & Landeen, J. Cognitive behavior modification: "Motivated learning" reading treatment with sub-professional therapy-technicians. *Behaviour Research and Therapy*, 1967, *5*, 283–299.

Stabler, B., & Warren, A. B. Behavioral contracting in treating trichotillomania: Case note. *Psychological Reports*, 1974, *34*, 401–402.

Stampfl, G., & Levis, D. J. Essentials of implosive therapy: A learning-theory-based psychodynamic behavioral therapy. *Journal of Abnormal Psychology*, 1967, *72*, 496–503.

Starfield, B., & Mellits, E. D. Increase in functional bladder capacity and improvement in enuresis. *Journal of Pediatrics*, 1968, *72*, 483–487.

Stawar, T. L. Fable mod: Operantly structured fantasies as an adjunct in the modification of fire-setting behavior. *Journal of Behavior Therapy and Experimental Psychiatry*, 1976, *7*, 285–287.

Stevens-Long, J., & Rasmussen, M. The acquisition of simple and compound sentence structure in an autistic child. *Journal of Applied Behavior Analysis*, 1974, *7*, 473–479.

Stevens-Long, J., Schwarz, J. L., & Bliss, D. The acquisition and generalization of compound sentence structure in an autistic child. *Behavior Therapy*, 1976, *7*, 397–404.

Stokes, T. F., & Baer, D. M. An implicit technology of generalization. *Journal of Applied Behavior Analysis*, 1977, *10*, 349–367.

Stokes, T. F., Baer, D. M., & Jackson, R. L. Programming the generalization of a greeting response in four retarded children. *Journal of Applied Behavior Analysis*, 1974, *7*, 599–610.

Stolz, S. B., & Associates. *Ethical Issues in Behavior Modification.* Report of the American Psychological Association Commission. San Francisco: Jossey-Bass, 1978.

Strain, P. S. An experimental analysis of peer social initiations on the behavior of withdrawn preschool children: Some training and generalization effects. *Journal of Abnormal Child Psychology*, 1977, *5*, 445–455.

Strain, P. S., Shores, R. E., & Timm, M. A. Effects of peer social initiation on the behavior of withdrawn preschool children. *Journal of Applied Behavior Analysis*, 1977, *10*, 289–298.

Strain, P. S., & Timm, M. A. An experimental analysis of social interaction between a behaviorally disordered preschool child and her classroom peers. *Journal of Applied Behavior Analysis*, 1974, *7*, 583–590.

Stuart, R. B. Behavioral contracting with the families of delinquents. *Journal of Behavior Therapy and Experimental Psychiatry*, 1971, *2*, 1–11.

Stuart, R. B., & Davis, B. *Slim Chance in a Fat World: Behavioral Control of Obesity.* Champaign, IL: Research Press, 1972.

Stuart, R. B., Jayaratne, S., & Tripodi, T. Changing adolescent deviant behavior through reprogramming the behaviour of parents and teachers: An experimental evaluation. *Canadian Journal of Behavioural Science,* 1976, *8,* 132–144.

Stuart, R. B., & Lott, L. A., Jr. Behavioral contracting with delinquents: A cautionary note. *Journal of Behavior Therapy and Experimental Psychiatry,* 1972, *3,* 161–169.

Stuart, R. B., Tripodi, T., Jayaratne, S., & Camburn, D. An experiment in social engineering in serving the families of predelinquents. *Journal of Abnormal Child Psychology,* 1976, *4,* 243–261.

Stunkard, A. J., & Mahoney, M. J. Behavioral treatment of eating disorders. In H. Leitenberg (Ed.), *Handbook of Behavior Modification and Behavior Therapy.* Englewood Cliffs, N.J.: Prentice-Hall, 1976. Pp. 45–73.

Switzer, E. B., Deal, T. E., & Bailey, J. S. The reduction of stealing in second graders using a group contingency. *Journal of Applied Behavior Analysis,* 1977, *10,* 267–272.

Tarver, S. G., Hallahan, D. P., Kauffman, J. M., & Ball, D. W. Verbal rehearsal and selective attention in children with learning disabilities: A developmental lag. *Journal of Experimental Child Psychology,* 1976, *22,* 375–385.

Tasto, D. L. Systematic desensitization, muscle relaxation and visual imagery in the counterconditioning of a four-year-old phobic child. *Behaviour Research and Therapy,* 1969, *7,* 409–411.

Tate, B. G., & Baroff, G. S. Aversive control of self-injurious behavior in a psychotic boy. *Behaviour Research and Therapy,* 1966, *4,* 281–287.

Taylor, P. D., & Turner, R. K. A clinical trial of continuous, intermittent and overlearning "bell and pad" treatments for nocturnal enuresis. *Behaviour Research and Therapy,* 1975, *13,* 281–293.

Terrace, H. Discrimination learning with and without "errors." *Journal of the Experimental Analysis of Behavior,* 1963, *6,* 1–27.

Terwilliger, R. F., & Obler, M. Comment on research in behavior therapy. *Journal of Consulting and Clinical Psychology,* 1971, *37,* 14–15.

Tharp, R. G., & Wetzel, R. J. *Behavior Modification in the Natural Environment.* New York: Academic Press, 1969.

Thoresen, C. E., & Mahoney, M. J. *Behavioral Self-control.* New York: Holt, Rinehart, & Winston, 1974.

Tomlinson, A. The treatment of bowel retention by operant procedures: A case study. *Journal of Behavior Therapy and Experimental Psychiatry,* 1970, *1,* 83–85.

Torgesen, J., & Goldman, T. Verbal rehearsal and short-term memory in reading-disabled children. *Child Development,* 1977, *48,* 56–60.

Tucker, G. H., O'Dell, S. L., & Suib, M. R. Control of selective echolalia via the instatement of a general alternative response. *Behaviour Research and Therapy,* 1978, *16,* 302–306.

Turkewitz, H., O'Leary, K. D., & Ironsmith, M. Generalization and maintenance of appropriate behavior through self-control. *Journal of Consulting and Clinical Psychology,* 1975, *43,* 577–583.

Turner, R. K. Conditioning treatment of nocturnal enuresis. In I. Kolvin, R. C. Mac-

Keith, & S. R. Meadow (Eds.), *Bladder Control and Enuresis.* Philadelphia: Lippincott, 1973. Pp. 24–35.

Turner, R. K., Rachman, S., & Young, G. Conditioning treatment of enuresis: A rejoinder to Lovibond. *Behaviour Research and Therapy,* 1972, *10,* 291–292.

Turner, R. K., Young, G. C., & Rachman, S. Treatment of nocturnal enuresis by conditioning techniques. *Behaviour Research and Therapy,* 1970, *8,* 367–381.

Tyler, V. O., Jr., & Brown, G. D. The use of swift, brief isolation as a group control device for institutionalized delinquents. *Behaviour Research and Therapy,* 1967, *5,* 1–9.

Tyler, V. O., Jr., & Brown, G. D. Token reinforcement of academic performance with institutionalized delinquent boys. *Journal of Educational Psychology,* 1968, *59,* 164–168.

Van Hoose, W. H., & Kottler, J. A. *Ethical and Legal Issues in Counseling and Psychotherapy.* San Francisco: Jossey-Bass, 1977.

Varni, J. W., & Henker, B. A self-regulation approach to the treatment of three hyperactive boys. *Child Behavior Therapy,* 1979, *1.* 171–192.

Wahler, R. G. Oppositional children: A quest for parental reinforcement control. *Journal of Applied Behavior Analysis,* 1969, *2,* 159–170. (a)

Wahler, R. G. Setting generality: Some specific and general effects of child behavior therapy. *Journal of Applied Behavior Analysis,* 1969, *2,* 239–246. (b)

Wahler, R. G. Some structural aspects of deviant child behavior. *Journal of Applied Behavior Analysis,* 1975, *8,* 27–42.

Wahler, R. G., Berland, R. M., & Coe, T. D. Generalization processes in child behavior change. In B. B. Lahey & A. E. Kazdin (Eds.), *Advances in Clinical Child Psychology* (Vol. 2). New York: Plenum, 1979. Pp. 35–69.

Wahler, R. G., Leske, G., & Rogers, E. S. The insular family: A deviance support system for oppositional children. In L. A. Hamerlynck (Ed.), *Behavioral Systems for the Developmentally Disabled: I. School and Family Environments.* New York: Bruner/Mazel, 1979. Pp. 102–127.

Walker, H. M., & Buckley, N. K. Programming generalization and maintenance of treatment effects across time and across settings. *Journal of Applied Behavior Analysis,* 1972, *5,* 209–224.

Walter, H., & Gilmore, S. K. Placebo versus social learning effects in parent training procedures designed to alter the behaviours of aggressive boys. *Behaviour Research and Therapy,* 1973, *4,* 361–377.

Watson, J. B., & Rayner, R. Conditioned emotional reactions. *Journal of Experimental Psychology,* 1920, *3,* 1–14.

Wechsler, D. *Wechsler Intelligence Scale for Children.* New York: The Psychological Corp., 1949.

Weiher, R. G., & Harman, R. E. The use of omission training to reduce self-injurious behavior in a retarded child. *Behavior Therapy,* 1975, *6,* 261–268.

Weil, G., & Goldfried, M. R. Treatment of insomnia in an eleven-year-old child through self-relaxation. *Behavior Therapy,* 1973, *4,* 282–284.

Weinrott, M. R., Corson, J. A., & Wilchesky, M. Teacher-mediated treatment of social withdrawal. *Behavior Therapy,* 1979, *10,* 281–294.

Weiss, A. R. A behavioral approach to the treatment of adolescent obesity. *Behavior Therapy*, 1977, *8*, 720–726.

Wells, K. C., Forehand, R., Hickey, K., & Green, K. D. Effects of a procedure derived from the overcorrection principle on manipulated and nonmanipulated behaviors. *Journal of Applied Behavior Analysis*, 1977, *10*, 679–687.

Werry, J. S., Weiss, G., & Douglas, V. Studies on the hyperactive child: I. Some preliminary findings. *Canadian Psychiatric Association Journal*, 1964, *9*, 120–130.

Wetzel, R. Use of behavioral techniques in a case of compulsive stealing. *Journal of Consulting Psychology*, 1966, *30*, 367–374.

Wheeler, A. J., & Sulzer, B. Operant training and generalization of a verbal response form in a speech deficient child. *Journal of Applied Behavior Analysis*, 1970, *3*, 139–147.

Wheeler, M. E., & Hess, K. W. Treatment of juvenile obesity by successive approximation control of eating. *Journal of Behavior Therapy and Experimental Psychiatry*, 1976, *7*, 235–241.

White, G. D., Nielsen, G., & Johnson, S. M. Timeout duration and the suppression of deviant behavior in children. *Journal of Applied Behavior Analysis*, 1972, *5*, 111–120.

White, W. C., Jr., & Davis, M. T. Vicarious extinction of phobic behavior in early childhood. *Journal of Abnormal Child Psychology*, 1974, *2*, 25–32.

Wilhelm, H., & Lovaas, O. I. Stimulus overselectivity: A common feature in autism and mental retardation. *American Journal of Mental Deficiency*, 1976, *81*, 26–31.

Williams, C. L., Doleys, D. M., & Ciminero, A. R. A two-year follow-up of enuretic children treated with dry bed training. *Journal of Behavior Therapy and Experimental Psychiatry*, 1978, *9*, 285–286.

Winett, R. A., & Winkler, R. C. Current behavior modification in the classroom: Be still, be quiet, be docile. *Journal of Applied Behavior Analysis*, 1972, *5*, 499–504.

Winkler, R. C. What types of sex-role behavior should behavior modifiers promote? *Journal of Applied Behavior Analysis*, 1977, *10*, 549–552.

Wish, P. A., Hasazi, J. E., & Jurgela, A. R. Automated direct deconditioning of a childhood phobia. *Journal of Behavior Therapy and Experimental Psychiatry*, 1973, *4*, 279–283.

Witmer, L. Clinical psychology. *The Psychological Clinic*, 1907, *1*, 1–9.

Wolpe, J. *Psychotherapy by Reciprocal Inhibition.* Stanford, CA: Stanford University Press, 1958.

Wolpe, J. *The Practice of Behavior Therapy.* New York: Pergamon, 1969.

Wright, L., & Walker, C. E. A simple behavioral treatment program for psychogenic encopresis. *Behaviour Research and Therapy*, 1978, *16*, 209–212.

Wulbert, M., & Dries, R. The relative efficacy of methylphenidate (Ritalin) and behavior-modification techniques in the treatment of a hyperactive child. *Journal of Applied Behavior Analysis*, 1977, *10*, 21–31.

Wulbert, M., Nyman, B. A., Snow, D., & Owen, Y. The efficacy of stimulus fading and contingency management in the treatment of elective mutism: A case study. *Journal of Applied Behavior Analysis*, 1973, *6*, 435–441.

Young, G. C. The treatment of childhood encopresis by conditioned gastro-ileal reflex training. *Behaviour Research and Therapy*, 1973, *11*, 499–503.

Young, G. C., & Morgan, R. T. T. Overlearning in the conditioning treatment of enuresis. *Behaviour Research and Therapy*, 1972, *10*, 147–151.

Yule, W., Sacks, B., & Hersov, L. Successful flooding treatment of a noise phobia in an eleven-year-old. *Journal of Behavior Therapy and Experimental Psychiatry*, 1974, *5*, 209–211.

Zaslow, R. W., & Breger, L. A theory and treatment of autism. In L. Breger (Ed.), *Clinical-Cognitive Psychology: Models and Integrations.* Englewood Cliffs, N.J.: Prentice-Hall, 1969. Pp. 246–291.

Zeilberger, J., Sampen, S. E., & Sloane, H. N., Jr. Modification of a child's problem behaviors in the home with the mother as therapist. *Journal of Applied Behavior Analysis*, 1968, *1*, 47–53.

Zelniker, T., & Oppenheimer, L. Effect of different training methods on perceptual learning in impulsive children. *Child Development*, 1976, *47*, 492–497.

Zigler, E., & Balla, D. Developmental course of responsiveness to social reinforcement in normal children and institutionalized retardates. *Developmental Psychology*, 1972, *6*, 66–73.

Zlutnick, S., Mayville, W. J., & Moffat, S. Modification of seizure disorders: The interruption of behavioral chains. *Journal of Applied Behavior Analysis*, 1975, *8*, 1–12.

Name Index

Subject Index

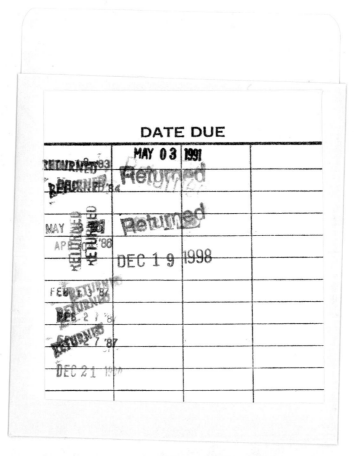